Interstitial Lung Disease and Autoimmune Lung Diseases

Editors

KEVIN K. BROWN
ARYEH FISCHER
JEFFREY J. SWIGRIS

IMMUNOLOGY AND ALLERGY CLINICS OF NORTH AMERICA

www.immunology.theclinics.com

Consulting Editor
RAFEUL ALAM

November 2012 • Volume 32 • Number 4

ELSEVIER

1600 John F. Kennedy Blvd., ● Suite 1800 ● Philadelphia, PA 19103-2899.
http://www.theclinics.com

IMMUNOLOGY AND ALLERGY CLINICS OF NORTH AMERICA Volume 32, Number 4
November 2012 ISSN 0889-8561, ISBN-13: 978-1-4557-4846-4

Editor: Pamela Hetherington

Immunology and Allergy Clinics of North America (ISSN 0889-8561) is published quarterly by Elsevier Inc., 360 Park Avenue South, New York, NY 10010-1710. Months of issue are February, May, August, and November. Periodicals postage paid at New York, NY and additional mailing offices. Subscription prices are $294.00 per year for US individuals, $417.00 per year for US institutions, $139.00 per year for US students and residents, $361.00 per year for Canadian individuals, $202.00 per year for Canadian students, $518.00 per year for Canadian institutions, $409.00 per year for international individuals, $518.00 per year for international institutions, $202.00 per year for international students. To receive student/resident rate, orders must be accompanied by name of affiliated institution, date of term, and the *signature* of program/residency coordinator on institution letterhead. Orders will be billed at individual rate until proof of status is received. Foreign air speed delivery is included in all *Clinics* subscription prices. All prices are subject to change without notice. **POSTMASTER:** Send address changes to *Immunology and Allergy Clinics of North America,* Elsevier Health Sciences Division, Subscription Customer Service, 3251 Riverport Lane, Maryland Heights, MO 63043. **Customer Service: 1-800-654-2452 (U.S. and Canada); 314-447-8871 (outside U.S. and Canada). Fax: 314-447-8029. E-mail: journalscustomerservice-usa@elsevier.com (for print support); journalsonlinesupport-usa@elsevier.com (for online support).**

Reprints. For copies of 100 or more, of articles in this publication, please contact the Commercial Reprints Department, Elsevier Inc., 360 Park Avenue South, New York, New York 10010-1710. Tel. (212) 633-3812, Fax: (212) 462-1935, E-mail: reprints@elsevier.com.

Immunology and Allergy Clinics of North America is covered in MEDLINE/PubMed (Index Medicus), Current Contents/Life Sciences, Science Citation Index, ISI/BIOMED, Chemical Abstracts, and EMBASE/Excerpta Medica.

Printed and bound by CPI Group (UK) Ltd, Croydon, CR0 4YY

Transferred to digital print 2012

Contributors

CONSULTING EDITOR

RAFEUL ALAM, MD, PhD
Professor and Chief, Division of Allergy and Immunology, National Jewish Health, and Professor, University of Colorado Denver, Denver, Colorado

GUEST EDITORS

KEVIN K. BROWN, MD
Associate Professor of Medicine, Autoimmune and Interstitial Lung Disease Program, National Jewish Health, Denver, Colorado

ARYEH FISCHER, MD
Autoimmune and Interstitial Lung Disease Program; Associate Professor of Medicine, Division of Rheumatology, National Jewish Health, Denver, Colorado

JEFFREY J. SWIGRIS, DO, MS
Associate Professor of Medicine, National Jewish Health, Denver, Colorado

AUTHORS

JENNIFER BIERACH, MD
Section of Allergy, Pulmonary and Critical Care Medicine, Department of Medicine, University of Wisconsin School of Medicine and Public Health, Madison, Wisconsin

FRANCESCO BONELLA, MD
Department of Pneumology/Allergy, Ruhrlandklinik, University Hospital, Essen, Germany

KEVIN K. BROWN, MD
Associate Professor of Medicine, Autoimmune and Interstitial Lung Disease Program, National Jewish Health, Denver, Colorado

RODRIGO CARTIN-CEBA, MD
Assistant Professor, Division of Pulmonary and Critical Care, Department of Internal Medicine, Mayo Clinic, Rochester, Minnesota

JEAN-FRANÇOIS CORDIER, MD
Service de pneumologie, Hospices Civils de Lyon, Centre de référence national des maladies pulmonaires rares, Hôpital Louis Pradel, Lyon Cedex, France; Université de Lyon, Université Lyon I, INRA, UMR754 INRA-Vetagrosup EPHE IFR 128, Lyon, France

ULRICH COSTABEL, MD, PhD
Professor of Medicine, Department of Pneumology/Allergy, Ruhrlandklinik, University Hospital, Essen, Germany

VINCENT COTTIN, MD, PhD
Service de pneumologie, Hospices Civils de Lyon, Centre de référence national des maladies pulmonaires rares, Hôpital Louis Pradel, Lyon Cedex, France; Université de Lyon, Université Lyon I, INRA, UMR754 INRA-Vetagrosup EPHE IFR 128, Lyon, France

DANIEL A. CULVER, DO
Respiratory Institute, Cleveland Clinic, Cleveland, Ohio

SONYE K. DANOFF, MD, PhD
Associate Professor, Division of Pulmonary and Critical Care Medicine, Co-Director, Johns Hopkins Interstitial Lung Disease Clinic, Johns Hopkins University School of Medicine, Baltimore, Maryland

JOAO A. DE ANDRADE, MD
Associate Professor of Medicine, Interstitial Lung Disease Program, Division of Pulmonary, Allergy, and Critical Care Medicine, University of Alabama at Birmingham and Birmingham VA Medical Center, Birmingham, Alabama

EVANS R. FERNÁNDEZ PÉREZ, MD, MS
Assistant Professor of Medicine, Autoimmune Lung Center and Interstitial Lung Disease Program, Division of Pulmonary and Critical Care Medicine, National Jewish Health, Denver, Colorado

ARYEH FISCHER, MD
Autoimmune and Interstitial Lung Disease Program; Associate Professor of Medicine, Division of Rheumatology, National Jewish Health, Denver, Colorado

BRIAN T. GARIBALDI, MD
Instructor, Division of Pulmonary and Critical Care Medicine, Johns Hopkins University School of Medicine, Baltimore, Maryland

JOSUNE GUZMAN, MD, PhD
Professor of General and Experimental Pathology, General and Experimental Pathology, Ruhr-University, Bochum, Germany

PETER ILLEI, MD
Assistant Professor, Department of Pathology, Johns Hopkins University School of Medicine, Baltimore, Maryland

MEGAN L. KRAUSE, MD
Chief Medical Resident, Department of Internal Medicine, Mayo Clinic, Rochester, Minnesota

TOBY M. MAHER, MB, MSc, PhD, MRCP
Consultant Physician and Honorary Senior Lecturer, Interstitial Lung Disease Unit, Royal Brompton Hospital; National Heart and Lung Institute, Imperial College; Centre for Respiratory Research, University College London, London, United Kingdom

KEITH C. MEYER, MD, MS, FACP, FCCP
UW Lung Transplant & Advanced Pulmonary Disease Program; Interstitial Lung Disease Program, Interstitial Lung Disease Clinic; Adult Cystic Fibrosis Program, Adult Cystic Fibrosis Clinic; Section of Allergy, Pulmonary and Critical Care Medicine, Department of Medicine, University of Wisconsin School of Medicine and Public Health, Madison, Wisconsin

SHINICHIRO OHSHIMO, MD, PhD
Department of Molecular and Internal Medicine, Graduate School of Biomedical Sciences, Hiroshima University, Japan

AMY L. OLSON, MD
Assistant Professor of Medicine, Autoimmune and Interstitial Lung Disease Program, National Jewish Health, Denver, Colorado

TOBIAS PEIKERT, MD
Assistant Professor, Division of Pulmonary and Critical Care, Departments of Internal Medicine and Immunology, Mayo Clinic, Rochester, Minnesota

ULRICH SPECKS, MD
Professor, Division of Pulmonary and Critical Care, Department of Internal Medicine, Mayo Clinic, Rochester, Minnesota

JASON S. ZOLAK, MD
Chief Fellow, Division of Pulmonary, Allergy, and Critical Care Medicine, University of Alabama at Birmingham, Birmingham, Alabama

Contents

> The diffuse parenchymal lung diseases (DPLDs) are a group of more than 200 diverse conditions; therefore achieving an exact diagnosis is frequently challenging. However, with the advent of novel, disease-specific therapies, an accurate diagnosis in DPLD is of growing importance. The recognition that many of the DPLDs have distinctive high-resolution computed tomography appearances has greatly reduced the need for biopsy, although in cases of uncertainty, histologic assessment remains an important tool. Ultimately, the diagnostic assessment of DPLD is best undertaken through an interstitial lung disease multidisciplinary team meeting that brings together physicians, thoracic radiologists, and pathologists.

> Idiopathic pulmonary fibrosis (IPF) is a chronic lung disease of unknown cause characterized by progressive scarring of the lung parenchyma and relentless loss of lung function. The diagnosis depends on close collaboration between clinicians, radiologists, and pathologists. No therapies approved by the Food and Drug Administration are available for IPF, and an analysis of completed clinical trials has demonstrated that the clinical course of IPF is largely unpredictable. Until therapies that improve survival become available, measures to preserve function and quality of life should be considered, and gastroesophageal reflux should be treated aggressively.

> Sarcoidosis is a multisystem granulomatous syndrome with a vast range of clinical manifestations. Since the first description of sarcoidosis in 1869, it has simultaneously intrigued and perplexed generations of physicians. Because sarcoidosis can occur variably in any organ and does not always adhere to classic descriptions, both diagnosis of sarcoidosis and attribution of symptoms can be extremely challenging. The management of sarcoidosis requires consideration of the expected course. Medication is considered when there is risk of irreversible vital organ damage, substantial progression, or symptoms that are affecting quality of life. Recently, a range of steroid-sparing therapies have been adopted for sarcoidosis.

Interstitial Lung Disease and Autoimmune Lung Diseases

IMMUNOLOGY AND ALLERGY CLINICS OF NORTH AMERICA

FORTHCOMING ISSUES

February 2013
Conditions Mimicking Asthma
Eugene Choo, *Guest Editor*

May 2013
Aspirin and NSAID-Induced Respiratory Diseases
Donald Stevenson, MD,
and Marek Kowalski, MD, *Guest Editors*

RELATED INTEREST

Clinics in Chest Medicine June 2012 (Volume 33, 2)
Bronchiectasis
Mark L. Metersky, MD, and Anne E. O'Donnell, MD, *Guest Editors*

DOWNLOAD Free App!

Review Articles
THE CLINICS

NOW AVAILABLE FOR YOUR iPhone and iPad

Preface

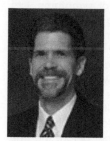
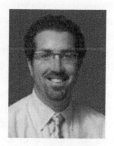
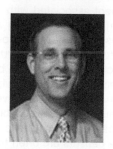

Kevin K. Brown, MD   Aryeh Fischer, MD   Jeffrey J. Swigris, DO, MS
Guest Editors

The interstitial, or diffuse parenchymal, lung diseases are a large group of outwardly similar disorders, sharing many clinical, physiologic, and chest imaging features. However, outward appearances are deceiving; on closer inspection, marked differences exist in clinical context, radiographic pattern, pathologic features, therapeutic responsiveness, and prognosis. So, the differential for the patient with exertional dyspnea and bilateral lung opacities include dozens of these unique respiratory diseases. In this issue of *Immunology and Allergy Clinics of North America*, we review our current understanding of the common and a few of the uncommon members of this group.

For the clinician, the evaluation of the patient with persistent cough, dyspnea, or wheeze and diffusely abnormal chest imaging is always a challenge. Each piece of information; the clinical context, the findings from tests of pulmonary physiology and gas exchange, the pattern seen on high-resolution computerized tomographic scanning, and the pathologic pattern seen in transbronchial or surgical lung biopsy specimens is important in our search for the diagnosis. Dr Maher provides us with a map for this clinical maze, highlighting the importance of each piece of information and where it fits. Idiopathic pulmonary fibrosis (IPF) is the most common of the idiopathic interstitial pneumonias and the prototypical chronic progressive fibrosing interstitial lung disease (ILD). Distilling the explosion of clinical research on IPF over the past decade, Drs Zolak and de Andrade review our current understanding of this increasingly common problem and our search for a beneficial therapy. Dr Culver provides us with a state-of-the-art review of the most common ILD, sarcoidosis. Every clinician who deals with respiratory complaints has seen this disease. Enigmatic in its origins, the clinical manifestations of this systemic granulomatous disease range from self-limited asymptomatic chest imaging findings to progressive fibrosis. When evaluating the patient with ILD, one cannot overemphasize the importance of the history. It is here where the clinical context is defined and potentially relevant environmental, occupation, and avocational exposures are identified. Drs Ohshimo, Bonella, Guzman, and Costabel provide us with an exhaustive review of the exposure-related diffuse lung disease hypersensitivity pneumonitis. Often confused with IPF, the identification of hypersensitivity pneumonitis can be life-saving.

Immunol Allergy Clin N Am 32 (2012) xi–xii
http://dx.doi.org/10.1016/j.iac.2012.09.001
0889-8561/12/$ – see front matter
immunology.theclinics.com

The subsequent articles review less common, but equally compelling, forms of ILD. Eosinophilic infiltration can occur in any of the anatomic compartments of the lung, with each compartment associated with a different constellation of symptoms. Drs Cottin and Cordier make this confusing area of eosinophilic lung disorders understandable. Drs Krause, Cartin-Ceba, Specks, and Peikert summarize our current understanding of diffuse alveolar hemorrhage and the pulmonary vasculitides. This potentially deadly group of diseases are both inflammatory and destructive but may have a benign presentation. The otherwise healthy patient who wheezes is almost always assumed to have asthma; however, hidden in the asthma epidemic are the patients with small airways disease or bronchiolitis. Drs Garibaldi, Illei, and Danoff provide us with clinical insight into these unique disorders. Pathologically inflammatory or fibrotic, these patients are often treated for months or longer before the true diagnosis is appreciated. Dr Fernandez-Perez reminds us that respiratory disease in the immunodeficient host is not solely due to infection and highlights that the noninfectious complications of the primary immunodeficiencies are poorly understood and uncommonly recognized. Drs. Olson, Brown, and Fischer discuss the complex intersection of lung disease with the systemic connective tissue diseases. Finally, Dr Meyer orients us to the therapeutic options and strategies when using immunosuppressive therapy in the autoimmune lung diseases.

In summarizing our current clinical knowledge, we recognize the outstanding combined efforts of these authors and know that you will gain an appreciation for and greater insight into the diverse world of ILD.

Kevin K. Brown, MD
Professor of Medicine
National Jewish Health
1400 Jackson Street
Denver, CO 80206, USA

Aryeh Fischer, MD
Associate Professor of Medicine
National Jewish Health
1400 Jackson Street
Denver, CO 80206, USA

Jeffrey J. Swigris, DO, MS
Associate Professor of Medicine
National Jewish Health
1400 Jackson Street
Denver, CO 80206, USA

E-mail addresses:
BrownK@NJHealth.org (K.K. Brown)
FischerA@NJHealth.org (A. Fischer)
SwigrisJ@NJHealth.org (J.J. Swigris)

Foreword
Interstitial Lung Diseases

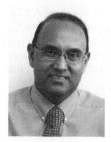

Rafeul Alam, MD, PhD
Consulting Editor

Interstitial lung diseases represent a diverse group of diseases that encompass inflammatory to fibrotic processes. Inflammatory processes frequently occur in response to exogenous instigators, such drugs, microbial and parasitic organisms, chemicals, and environmental and occupational agents. While the purpose of lung inflammation occurring in response to inhaled agents (microbial and nonmicrobial) is understood, the same is not true for drug-induced hypersensitivity pneumonitis. Why the immune response against a noninhaled medication takes place in the lung is not immediately clear. Possible mechanisms include a relative increase in lung bioavailability, altered lung antigenicity, and/or increased tissue accessibility due to lung vasculature damage. Lung is one of the most heavily vascularized tissues, so a systemic inflammatory response manifesting heavily in the lung would not be a surprise.

Interstitial lung diseases also occur as a consequence of systemic autoimmune diseases. Again the pathological process may vary from inflammatory to fibrotic processes. The inflammatory response may range from select leukocytic (eosinophilic, neutrophilic, lymphocytic, and mixed) to granulomatous. What determines the type of lung response is not totally clear. Perhaps the type of the T-helper immune response (Th1/Th2/Th17) contributes to the quality of the response. Advances have been made in noninvasive imaging procedures, which help decide the next step of diagnostic procedure. Newer immunosuppressive agents as well as biologics are allowing better disease control with less toxicity.[1] It has been reported that the vasculitis-dominant form of Wegener's granulomatosis (renamed granulomatosis with polyangiitis) responds better to anti-B-cell therapy than the granulomatous form of the disease.[2] The multisystem nature of clinical manifestation in autoimmune diseases has always made the diagnostic process difficult. The application of mathematical modeling, such as the artificial neural network, has been shown to improve the accuracy of the diagnosis.[3,4] These advances are likely to make a significant impact on our knowledge

Supported by NIH grants RO1 AI091614, PPG HL 36577, and N01 HHSN272200700048C.

Immunol Allergy Clin N Am 32 (2012) xiii–xiv
http://dx.doi.org/10.1016/j.iac.2012.08.009
0889-8561/12/$ – see front matter

and clinical practice. To update us on the advances in diagnosis and management of this diverse group of diseases, I have invited three guest editors—Drs Kevin Brown, Jeff Swigris, and Aryeh Fischer, who bring outstanding expertise in pulmonary and autoimmune lung diseases.

Rafeul Alam, MD, PhD
Division of Allergy and Immunology
National Jewish Health and University of Colorado Denver
1400 Jackson Street
Denver, CO 80206, USA

E-mail address:
alamr@njhealth.org

REFERENCES

1. Gadola SD, Gross WL. Vasculitis in 2011: the renaissance of granulomatous inflammation in AAV. Nat Rev Rheumatol 2012;8:74-6.
2. Holle JU, Dubrau C, Herlyn K, et al. Rituximab for refractory granulomatosis with polyangiitis (Wegener's granulomatosis): comparison of efficacy in granulomatous versus vasculitic manifestations. Ann Rheum Dis 2012;71:327-33.
3. Schmitt WH, Linder R, Reinhold-Keller E, et al. Improved differentiation between Churg-Strauss syndrome and Wegener's granulomatosis by an artificial neural network. Arthritis Rheum 2001;44:1887-96.
4. Linder R, Orth I, Hagen EC, et al. Differentiation between Wegener's granulomatosis and microscopic polyangiitis by an artificial neural network and by traditional methods. J Rheumatol 2011;38:1039-47.

A Clinical Approach to Diffuse Parenchymal Lung Disease

Toby M. Maher, MB, MSc, PhD, MRCP[a,b,c]

KEYWORDS

- Diffuse parenchymal lung diseases • Interstitial lung disease • Multidisciplinary team
- Alveolar parenchym

KEY POINTS

- Although individual DPLDs tend to be rare or orphan conditions, as a group they contribute up to 15% of the case load in the average general respiratory clinic.
- Diagnosis relies on the careful integration of history, clinical examination and key investigation findings. In the majority of cases HRCT is diagnostic but in a significant minority histological assessment is required.
- The interstitial lung disease multi-disciplinary team meeting is central to the diagnosis of DPLD and brings together clinicians, thoracic radiologists and thoracic pathologists.
- Development of disease specific therapies (e.g. pirfenidone for idiopathic pulmonary fibrosis and rapamycin for lymphangioleiomyomatosis) has increased the importance of early, accurate diagnosis in individuals with suspected DPLD.

INTRODUCTION

Diffuse parenchymal lung disease (DPLD) is an umbrella term covering more than 200 separate disorders, all of which are characterized by either inflammation or fibrosis of the alveolar parenchyma (the space bounded on one side by the alveolar epithelium and on the other by the capillary endothelium) or by a small number of diseases that result in alveolar filling. Individually, most of the DPLDs are very rare, but collectively it has been estimated that they contribute up to 15% of the cases in general respiratory clinics.[1] The most common of the DPLDs, idiopathic pulmonary fibrosis (IPF) and sarcoidosis, have an incidence of 7.4 to 15 per 100,000 population, whereas at the other extreme, conditions like alveolar proteinosis or alveolar microlithiasis have

Disclosures: I am in receipt of an unrestricted academic industry grant from GSK. In the last 3 years, I have received advisory board or consultancy fees from Actelion, Boehringer Ingelheim, GSK, Respironics, and Sanofi-Aventis.
a Interstitial Lung Disease Unit, Royal Brompton Hospital, Sydney Street, London, SW3 6NP, UK; b National Heart and Lung Institute, Imperial College, Emmanuel Kaye Building, 1B Manresa Rd, London SW3 6LP, UK; c Centre for Respiratory Research, University College London, 5 University Street, London WC1E 6FF, UK
E-mail address: t.maher@rbht.nhs.uk

Immunol Allergy Clin N Am 32 (2012) 453–472
http://dx.doi.org/10.1016/j.iac.2012.08.004
0889-8561/12/$ – see front matter © 2012 Elsevier Inc. All rights reserved.

immunology.theclinics.com

an estimated incidence of less than 1 per 1 million population.[2–5] The causes of the different DPLDs vary considerably, ranging from inhalational exposure (eg, the pneumoconioses), autoimmune disease (eg, rheumatoid-associated lung disease), granulomatous conditions, and a large number of diseases of unknown causes (eg, IPF). **Fig. 1** provides a schematic for broadly categorizing the different DPLDs.

In addition to differing incidences and causes, the DPLDs have a distinct range of disease behaviors, carry widely varying prognoses, and respond differently to therapy. At one extreme, acute interstitial pneumonia (AIP) develops rapidly, inevitably progresses to respiratory failure, is poorly responsive to treatment, and carries a mortality rate in excess of 50%. Sarcoidosis, by contrast, may develop entirely asymptomatically, and even in symptomatic cases, it may regress fully without the need for treatment.

Despite these differences in causes, progression, and treatment response, the presentation of many of the DPLDs is broadly similar. Most present with progressive breathlessness and cough, Clinical examination in DPLD frequently discloses fine, bibasal end-inspiratory crepitations. The similarity of presentation but differences in treatment response and outcomes make the precise diagnosis of individual DPLDs challenging. Advances in medical diagnostics and in pharmacotherapy have enhanced both the importance and possibility of early, precise diagnosis. Even so, the diagnosis of DPLD relies on the traditional medical approach of careful integration of the medical history with examination findings and the results of key investigations. In many cases, this integration is best performed in the context of a multidisciplinary team (MDT) meeting consisting of the physician, thoracic radiologist, and pathologist. This article provides an overview of the key aspects of diagnosis in DPLD and covers in greater detail the typical presentation and diagnosis of specific DPLDs.

HISTORY

The usual starting point for considering a diagnosis of DPLD is when a patient presents with dyspnea and either fine crepitations on chest auscultation or a plain chest radiograph demonstrating diffuse interstitial shadowing. In either context, before embarking on a full diagnostic DPLD work-up, it is important to exclude conditions that may mimic DPLD. These conditions include infection (especially in immunocompromised subjects), malignancy (including pulmonary lymphoma, alveolar cell carcinoma, and lymphangitis carcinomatosis), and pulmonary edema. In an individual with suspected DPLD, the clinical history provides important clues as to potential diagnoses, should guide further investigations, and provides information on disease severity and potentially prognosis.

PRESENTING HISTORY

As noted, almost all patients with a DPLD present with dyspnea. The speed of onset of breathlessness can be important in distinguishing several of the DPLDs. Rapid-onset breathlessness (ie, during a period of ≤4 weeks) is a characteristic of a few DPLDs, including AIP and cryptogenic organizing pneumonia. In both conditions, patients can go from asymptomatic to being in respiratory failure during only a few weeks. In most DPLDs, the onset of dyspnea is much more insidious and progresses slowly during a period of several months to years. In conditions such as IPF, inexorable progression of dyspnea is the rule; however, in diseases like sarcoidosis, symptoms may wax and wane, whereas in acute or subacute hypersensitivity pneumonitis, breathlessness typically has a temporal relationship to a relevant exposure. A common ancillary symptom is that of cough. Frequently, this tends to be dry, although

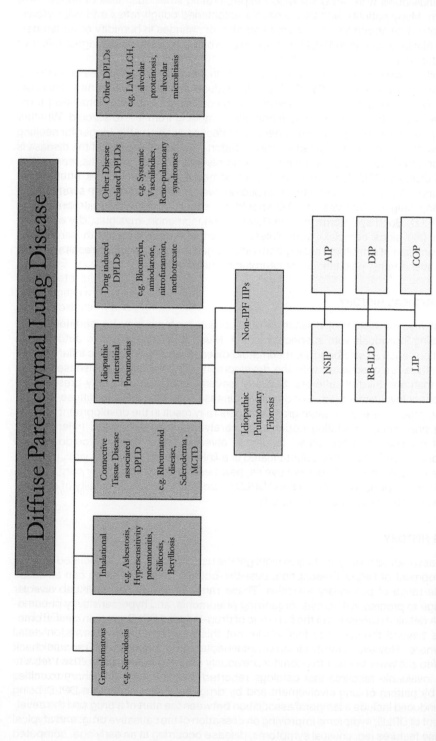

Fig. 1. A schematic for the general classification of the DPLDs. *Abbreviations:* COP, cryptogenic organizing pneumonia; LIP, lymphocytic interstitial pneumonia; MCTD, mixed connective tissue disease.

many individuals with DPLD will report expectorating small quantities of nonpurulent sputum. Many patients with DPLD have a heightened cough reflex and will typically be troubled by strong smells, cigarette smoke, or changes in humidity or air temperature. Similarly, cough in DPLD may be exacerbated by gastroesophageal reflux or postnasal drip.[6]

Ancillary symptoms occur commonly and in many cases indicates a systemic condition giving rise to the DPLD. Often, individuals presenting with a new diagnosis of DPLD will report an initial prodromal illness consisting of constitutional symptoms and general malaise. This is seen in conditions ranging from IPF to sarcoid. Whether this represents a coexistent viral or bacterial infection acting as the trigger for seeking medical assistance or is a systemic manifestation heralding the onset of the disease is unclear. Individuals presenting with systemic disease such as vasculitis, connective tissue disease (CTD) (eg, polymyositis), or some cases of sarcoidosis often report profound constitutional symptoms including weight loss, drenching sweats, and disabling fatigue. Features of CTD should be sought in all individuals presenting with DPLD. Such symptoms include Raynaud phenomenon, myalgias, dry eyes and mouth (the sicca complex), arthralgias, and arthritis. Individuals with sarcoidosis may complain of symptoms arising from other organ systems including rashes, uveitis, lymphadenopathy, palpitations, or neurologic phenomena.

PAST MEDICAL HISTORY

A past medical history of disease in other organ systems may be pertinent when assessing individuals with suspected DPLD. Most obviously, systemic autoimmune conditions such as scleroderma, rheumatoid disease, and the idiopathic inflammatory myopathies are associated with the development of interstitial lung disease (ILD) in more than one-third of sufferers. Similarly, several renal disorders may present with pulmonary involvement (eg, Goodpasture disease may present with diffuse alveolar hemorrhage, whereas Wegener granulomaosis may result in the development of organizing pneumonia, cavitating nodules, or, rarely, pulmonary fibrosis). Inflammatory bowel disease has been linked to diffuse alveolar hemorrhage, sarcoidosis, and pulmonary fibrois. Less well substantiated is a link between hepatitis C virus infection and pulmonary fibrosis. Recurrent uveitis, new neurologic symptoms, or cardiomyopathy in an individual with unexplained DPLD all point toward the possibility of sarcoidosis, vasculitis, or an undiagnosed CTD.

DRUG HISTORY

The past medical history might also highlight the use of medications associated with the development of DPLD. Prescription, over-the-counter, and illicit drugs can all cause a wide range of pulmonary toxicities. These range in severity from diffuse alveolar damage to progressive fibrosis, organizing pneumonia, and hypersensitivity pneumonitis. A detailed discussion of the full range of drug-induced DPLDs seen in clinical practice is beyond the scope of this article, but this topic has been reviewed in detail elsewhere.[7] However, any physician who suspects a drug-induced DPLD should check the Web site www.pneumotox.com for previously reported associations. This Web site is an invaluable resource that catalogs reported drug-induced pulmonary toxicities both by pattern of lung involvement and by drug. Important clues to a DPLD being drug induced include a temporal association between the start of a drug and the development of DPLD, symptoms improving on cessation of the causative drug, and atypical disease features (eg, unusual symptoms, disease occurring at an early age, computed tomography [CT] appearances not fitting the pattern of any recognized DPLD, or a biopsy specimen showing unusual features or marked eosinophilic infiltration).

Several commonly used drugs may cause DPLD, and patients with such cases will be encountered several times a year in a typical respiratory service.[8] The antibiotic nitrofurantoin, when used long term (usually for recurrent urinary tract infection), can cause a widespread peripherally based organizing pneumonia with marked architectural distortion (**Fig. 2**), which typically resolves on stopping the drug. Many chemotherapeutic agents used in oncology therapy can cause DPLD that may range from rapid-onset diffuse alveolar damage to chronic fibrosis. Bleomycin is probably the best-recognized chemotherapy capable of causing DPLD. The antiarrhythmic amiodarone is another well-recognized cause of DPLD. Unlike the fibrosis induced by bleomycin, which tends to relate to cumulative dose, the interstitial disease triggered by amiodarone is idiosyncratic in onset and may occur shortly after initiation of treatment or in individuals who have been receiving stable treatment for many years. People with rheumatoid disease seem to be uniquely susceptible to drug-induced lung disease. The folate inhibitor methotrexate can cause a range of pulmonary abnormalities including progressive fibrosis and hypersensitivity pneumonitis. Most cases of methotrexate-induced DPLD occur in individuals with rheumatoid. Similarly, other antirheumatic drugs, including gold, sulfasalazine, penicillamine, and infliximab may cause DPLD; again, this seems to occur most frequently in individuals being treated for rheumatoid. Although relatively few drugs account for most cases of drug-induced lung disease, it is important to consider that any drug may have the potential to cause DPLD. This is especially the case for novel agents that may not yet have been reported in the literature as causing pulmonary side effects.

FAMILY HISTORY

Although most DPLDs occur sporadically, several have an underlying genetic basis. IPF, the most frequent DPLD, occurs in individuals with an affected first-degree relative in 2% to 5% of cases.[9] Several genetic abnormalities have been implicated in such familial cases including single nucleotide polymorphisms (SNPs) in the genes encoding for surfactant protein C, telomerase, and MUC5B.[10–13] The rare congenital syndromes of Hermansky-Pudlak syndrome and dyskeratosis congenita are associated with a range of abnormalities that includes the development of fibrosis indistinguishable from IPF.[11,14] In both conditions, this affects individuals in their third or

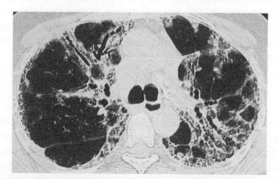

Fig. 2. CT scan of a 58-year-old woman receiving long-term nitrofurantoin for treatment of recurrent urinary tract infection. Scan demonstrates bilateral bands of consolidation with reticular change and architectural distortion. These appearances are typical of those seen in nitrofurantoin-induced lung disease.

fourth decade. Sarcoidosis occurs more commonly in certain racial groups, suggesting a genetic component, and SNPs in several human leukocyte antigen loci have been implicated in the development of sarcoid.[15] Although familial disease is much less common in sarcoid than in IPF, it remains the case that individuals with an affected first-degree relative have a higher odds ratio for developing the condition than do individuals with no family history. The CTDs shows a similar weak genetic association. Lymphangioleiomyomatosis (LAM), a rare DPLD causing cystic lung destruction in women with an incidence of approximately 1 per 1 million population, either occurs sporadically or, in 50% of cases, is associated with the autosomal dominant neurocutaneous condition tuberous sclerosis.[16] Unique among the DPLDs, there is a genetic test for tuberous sclerosis, and this should be undertaken in all individuals with LAM in whom there is a suspicion of tuberous sclerosis.

EXPOSURE HISTORY

A wide range of environmental, domestic, and industrial exposures have been implicated in the development of many of the DPLDs. Cigarette smoking, in addition to causing emphysema, may induce a range of DPLDs.[17] Pulmonary Langerhans cell histiocytosis (LCH) is a rare DPLD characterized by parenchymal nodules and cystic lung destruction that occurs only in smokers.[18] Desquamative interstitial pneumonia (DIP), a condition characterized by marked macrophage proliferation and associated interstitial fibrosis, almost always occurs in smokers (with the small remainder of cases being autoimmune related). Respiratory bronchiolitis ILD (RBILD) is another smoking-driven DPLD, and it seems likely that a proportion of cases of nonspecific interstitial pneumonitis are also smoking related. IPF, while not being directly smoking related, tends to occur most commonly in individuals with a substantial smoking history. Almost 80% of people with the condition are current smokers or ex-smokers.[19]

Health and safety legislation has resulted in a decrease in work-related DPLDs. Pneumoconioses, particularly coal miner's lung, used to be frequent occurrences in mining towns. Asbestosis is becoming a rare disease in the developed world now that the pneumotoxic effects of asbestos have been recognized.[20] Work-related exposure to molds remains an important cause of hypersensitivity pneumonitis.[21] Epidemiologic studies point to work-based exposure to wood and metal dust as being important risk factors for the development of IPF. Beryllium, used principally in the aerospace and nuclear industries, can cause berylliosis, a multisystem granulomatous disease that is indistinguishable from sarcoidosis. Within the domestic environment, birds (usually parrots, budgerigars, or pigeons) may trigger the development of hypersensitivity pneumonitis. Similarly, chronic mold exposure, such as occurs in "hot-tub lung," may cause hypersensitivity pneumonitis.

EXAMINATION

Clinical examination in DPLD frequently provides important findings that allow the list of potential differential diagnoses to be narrowed further and provides clues about the development of disease-related complications. Hypertrophic pulmonary osteoarthropathy (finger clubbing) occurs in several DPLDs. It is most common in IPF and DIP, affecting approximately 50% to 60% of individuals with these conditions. By contrast, in sarcoidosis clubbing is very unusual and tends to occur only in association with severe progressive pulmonary disease with a usual interstitial pneumonia (UIP) pattern of fibrosis.[22]

RESPIRATORY EXAMINATION

On respiratory examination, the typical auscultatory finding in DPLD is that of fine, usually basal, end-inspiratory crepitations. The finding of "squawks", short, high-pitched musical sounds most frequently heard toward the end of inspiration, suggests coexistent bronchiolitis and, in the context of DPLD, strongly suggests a diagnosis of hypersensitivity pneumonitis. Interestingly, in sarcoidosis, even in individuals with extensive radiographic abnormalities, respiratory examination is often unremarkable. In one study, less than 20% of individuals with chronic fibrotic sarcoid had any auscultatory abnormalities.[23] Individuals with pulmonary alveolar proteinosis may have surprisingly few findings on clinical examination despite extensive disease. Other signs of note on respiratory examination include tachypnea, hypoxia, and cyanosis in individuals with advanced DPLD. Pneumothorax may be a presenting feature in DPLDs with a cystic component such as pulmonary LCH and LAM. Pleural effusions may be seen in LAM and CTDs with a pleural component (eg, rheumatoid disease or systemic lupus erythematosus [SLE]). Pleural effusions may also occur as a rare presenting feature of sarcoidosis and asbestos-related disease but, when seen in other DPLDs such as IPF or chronic hypersensitivity pneumonitis (HP), suggest the development of a second pathologic condition.

CARDIAC EXAMINATION

Cardiovascular examination in DPLD is, in general, targeted at detecting signs of pulmonary hypertension including a loud second pulmonary heart sound, a murmur of tricuspid regurgitation, and peripheral edema. In some systemic conditions giving rise to DPLD, there may be signs of cardiac involvement (eg, conduction abnormalities and dysrhythmias in sarcoidosis, dilated cardiomyopathy in sarcoidosis, myocarditis in Churg-Strauss syndrome, or pericardial effusions or constrictive pericarditis in Churg-Strauss syndrome, SLE, or rheumatoid disease).

OTHER ORGAN SYSTEMS

The development of DPLD may be the first manifestation of a systemic CTD. In such cases, affected individuals may have other systemic signs that point to a unifying diagnosis. These include evidence of arthritis or arthropathy, changes associated with Raynaud phenomenon, skin involvement (which may be seen in sarcoidosis, SLE, and dermatomyositis), neurologic findings (SLE, Churg-Strauss syndrome, and sarcoidosis), or hepatosplenomegaly (eg, sarcoidosis).

INVESTIGATIONS

In many cases of DPLD, the history and clinical examination provide an important indication as to the likely diagnosis. In such cases, performed investigations will simply be confirmatory and should also be directed at providing an indication of baseline disease severity that can then be used to gauge treatment response and longitudinal disease behavior. In a significant minority of patients with DPLD, however, the diagnosis will remain unclear, and carefully targeted investigations should help refine diagnosis. In individuals with advanced disease or with multisystem conditions, additional screening investigations may be necessary to define other organ involvement and to exclude the development of disease related complications. A general algorithm for the investigation of DPLD is provided in **Fig. 3.**

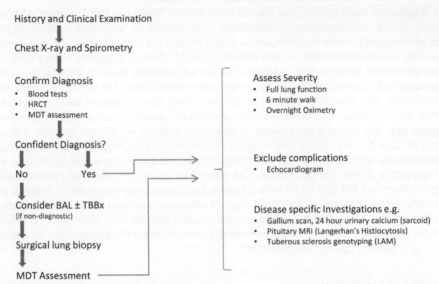

Investigation of Suspected DPLD

History and Clinical Examination

Chest X-ray and Spirometry

Confirm Diagnosis
- Blood tests
- HRCT
- MDT assessment

Confident Diagnosis?

No   Yes

Consider BAL ± TBBx
(if non-diagnostic)

Surgical lung biopsy

MDT Assessment

Assess Severity
- Full lung function
- 6 minute walk
- Overnight Oximetry

Exclude complications
- Echocardiogram

Disease specific Investigations e.g.
- Gallium scan, 24 hour urinary calcium (sarcoid)
- Pituitary MRI (Langerhan's Histiocytosis)
- Tuberous sclerosis genotyping (LAM)

Fig. 3. A schematic outlining a broad approach to the diagnostic assessment of suspected DPLD. Initial assessment is targeted at confirming a diagnosis whilst subsequent investigations aim to quantify disease severity and to exclude disease specific complications or other organ involvement. Interstitial lung disease multi-disciplinary team meeting is a key component of the diagnostic pathway in suspected DPLD. *Abbreviations*; HRCT – high resolution computed tomography; MDT – multi-disciplinary team; BAL – bronchoalveolar lavage; TBBx – trans bronchial biopsy; LAM – lymphangioleiomyomatosis.

BLOOD TESTS

Blood tests may occasionally be helpful in diagnosing the cause of DPLD. An eosinophilia may be seen on full blood count in Churg-Strauss syndrome and in eosinophilic pneumonia. Lymphopenia is common in active sarcoidosis. Serum calcium levels will be increased in 5% to 15% of cases of sarcoid. Serum angiotensin-converting enzyme levels, although lacking sensitivity, are, when increased, useful for monitoring disease activity in sarcoidosis. Antineutrophil cytoplasmic antibody levels are increased in a cytoplasmic pattern in Wegener's granulomatosis and in a perinuclear pattern in half of individuals with Churg-Strauss syndrome. Rheumatoid factor and an autoimmune profile should be checked for all patients with DPLD of unknown cause, because ILD is occasionally the initial manifestation of CTD. Creatine kinase is elevated in individuals with idiopathic inflammatory myositis as the underlying cause of their DPLD. Serum precipitins, although lacking in sensitivity and specificity, are occasionally useful in confirming a diagnosis of HP. Inflammatory markers are frequently raised in patients with DPLD and can provide a useful marker of treatment response. Increased serum brain natriuretic peptide levels point toward the development of secondary pulmonary hypertension and a worse prognosis in DPLD.[24] Genotyping can be helpful in suspected cases of tuberous sclerosis–associated LAM and in some cases of familial IPF.

RADIOLOGY

Almost all individuals with DPLD will have abnormalities on a plain chest radiograph. Although plain radiography provides a useful initial screening test for determining the presence of DPLD, it has been superseded in importance by high-resolution CT (HRCT). For many conditions, the HRCT appearance is sufficiently pathognomonic to allow a diagnosis to be made on the grounds of imaging alone, thus obviating surgical lung biopsy. The characteristic HRCT appearances of some of the individual DPLDs are described in **Table 1**.

BRONCHOSCOPY AND BRONCHOALVEOLAR LAVAGE

Bronchoscopy with bronchoalveolar lavage (BAL) provides an important adjunct to CT imaging in the diagnosis of DPLD. The American Thoracic Society (ATS) and European Respiratory Society (ERS) published detailed guidelines on the role of BAL in the diagnosis of DPLD.[25] BAL involves the instillation and aspiration, in 60-mL aliquots, of 240 mL of warmed saline, usually into the right middle lobe. The procedure enables

Table 1
Typical HRCT appearances of the more frequently occurring DPLDs

Disease	Typical HRCT Appearance
IPF	Bilateral, predominantly basal and subpleural reticulation associated with traction bronchiectasis and basal honeycombing with minimal ground glass attenuation.
NSIP	Bilateral, basal and symmetric, subpleural ground glass attenuation. May be associated reticulation and only rarely honeycomb change.
AIP	Patchy consolidation predominantly affecting dependent areas. Associated patchy ground glass attenuation with bronchial dilatation and architectural distortion.
Cryptogenic organizing pneumonia	Airspace consolidation: often multifocal and associated with ground glass attenuation.
Desquamative interstitial pneumonia	Widespread, patchy ground glass attenuation with a basal and peripheral predominance. Frequently associated with reticular change.
RBILD	Centrilobular nodules associated with patchy ground glass attenuation and thickening of the peripheral and central airway walls. Patients frequently also have evidence of centrilobular emphysema.
HP (acute)	Diffuse ground glass attenuation that may be associated with ill-defined centrilobular nodules and evidence of mosaic attenuation.
HP (chronic)	Evidence of fibrosis with reticular change, traction bronchiectasis, and occasional honeycombing. Fibrotic change does not tend to show any zonal predominance. In most cases, the fibrotic change is associated with mosaic attenuation and centrilobular nodules.
Pulmonary LCH	Multiple irregular cysts with variable wall thickness predominantly located in the upper and mid zones. In early disease, cysts are associated with interstitial nodules.
LAM	Multiple thin-walled regular cysts of variable size distributed evenly throughout both lung fields.

sampling of the alveolar compartment and permits identification of changes in the inflammatory cell component of the alveolar space. BAL is particularly helpful in identifying conditions characterized by either lymphocytic (eg, cryptogenic organizing pneumonia, HP, sarcoidosis, and lymphocytic interstitial pneumonitis) or eosinophilic (eg, eosinophilic lung disease or drug-induced lung disease) inflammation. In cases of IPF- or CTD-related nonspecific interstitial pneumonia (NSIP), BAL does not add to the diagnostic information provided by HRCT but does at least permit the exclusion of differential diagnoses such as chronic HP or sarcoid. In addition to the proportions of inflammatory cells, other features of the BAL can be helpful in diagnosing specific DPLDs. In HP, DIP, and drug-induced lung disease, the macrophages tend to have a foamy appearance. In the pneumoconioses, inclusion particles can sometime be seen within macrophages. Conditions characterized by diffuse alveolar hemorrhage (eg, the vasculitides or idiopathic pulmonary hemosiderosis) may show blood-stained return on BAL during periods of active hemorrhage or hemosiderin-laden macrophages during periods of disease quiescence. Individuals with PAP tend to return milky proteinacious BAL fluid, which on microscopic examination yields amorphous, periodic acid–Schiff–positive lipoproteinaceous material.

HISTOLOGIC EXAMINATION

For individuals in whom the combination of serologic testing, BAL, and HRCT is not diagnostic, it is generally necessary to obtain a tissue diagnosis. In individuals with a defined CTD, biopsy is very rarely necessary because the histologic findings, in most cases, do not subsequently affect the choice of therapy.

Once a decision has been made that tissue is required to facilitate diagnosis, then the type of biopsy that is necessary is, in part, dictated by the suspected diagnosis. For individuals with possible sarcoidosis, endobronchial, transbronchial, or even endobronchial ultrasound-guided biopsy of mediastinal lymph nodes may be sufficient to demonstrate the typical noncaseating granulomatous inflammation necessary to make a diagnosis. In cryptogenic organizing pneumonia, transbronchial biopsy may provide an adequate tissue sample for diagnosis. In some multisystem diseases (eg, sarcoidosis or the vasculitides), biopsy of extrapulmonary sites may provide an alternative route for confirming a diagnosis. However, for most cases of DPLD requiring histologic confirmation of diagnosis, it is necessary to undertake surgical lung biopsy. This can usually be obtained with video-assisted thoracoscopic surgery (VATS), which greatly reduces the invasiveness of the procedure. It is important to highlight the value of MDT communication with the thoracic surgeon before biopsy. Selection of biopsy sites based on the distribution of CT abnormality greatly improves the chances of obtaining diagnostic biopsy specimens at surgery. Furthermore, given the patchy nature of many of the DPLDs, biopsy specimens should be taken from at least 2 sites because this improves the sensitivity and specificity of biopsy in confirming the correct diagnosis. A description of the different histologic features of the various DPLDs is beyond the scope of this article but has been reviewed in detail elsewhere.[26,27]

PULMONARY PHYSIOLOGY

Pulmonary physiology testing, including measures of lung function, maximal pulmonary exercise testing, and 6-minute walk testing, does not tend to play a role in confirming a specific DPLD diagnosis but is important in defining disease severity and prognosis. These tests also provide important measures by which to subsequently assess response to therapy. In DPLD, spirometry tends to show a restrictive defect, although several conditions can also give rise to airflow obstruction. Sarcoidosis, in individuals with endobronchial disease or in those with perihilar fibrosis, is associated with airflow obstruction in up to a third of cases. Acute and subacute HP is also associated with obstructive spirometry, as are pulmonary LCH and LAM. Most patients with DPLD will also show impairment of gas transfer as demonstrated by a reduction in total lung diffusion of carbon monoxide. In IPF and fibrotic NSIP, longitudinal changes in FVC and total lung diffusion of carbon monoxide are important predictors of prognosis.[28,29]

Maximal pulmonary exercise testing can be helpful in identifying individuals with very early disease in whom HRCT abnormalities might not yet be apparent. Six-minute walk testing provides prognostic information in individuals with IPF. Those who desaturate to less than 88% or who walk less than 207 m have been shown to have a much worse prognosis.[30–32] The 6-minute walk may also be useful in discriminating those individuals with DPLD who might benefit from ambulatory oxygen therapy.[33] Both the 6-minute walk and maximal exercise tests may play a role in established disease in identifying individuals with DPLD who have developed secondary pulmonary hypertension (PH).[34–36]

CARDIAC INVESTIGATION

In most cases of DPLDs the role of cardiac investigation is to exclude the development of secondary PH. In PH, electrocardiogram may, in severe cases, show evidence of right-sided heart strain with right-axis deviation and a dominant R wave in the anterior chest leads. Echocardiogram provides a useful noninvasive screening test for PH with important measures being the gradient across the tricuspid valve (in those with measurable regurgitation), pulmonary acceleration time, right ventricular size, and visual estimation of right-sided heart function.[37,38] Right-sided heart catheterization, however, remains the gold standard for diagnosing PH and, in most cases, is necessary before therapy can be started. As noted earlier, a few multisystem conditions may present with cardiac involvement in addition to DPLD. In these cases, cardiac magnetic resonance (MR) imaging is quickly becoming the gold standard for defining the presence of cardiac disease.[39] In individuals with cardiac sarcoid who have received implantable defibrillators or pacemakers, positron emission tomography (PET) scanning can provide a useful method for assessing ongoing cardiac disease activity.[40]

THE MDT MEETING

During the past decade, there has been an increasing appreciation that the diagnosis of many of the DPLDs is best served by a combined clinical-radiological-pathologic MDT meeting.[41,42] There are few cases of DPLD in which a single clinical or investigation finding is diagnostic of a specific disease. It is also the case that in the diagnosis of the idiopathic interstitial pneumonias (IIPs), in particular, histologic examination lacks the sensitivity, specificity, and interobserver reproducibility to be considered a stand-alone gold standard.[43] Furthermore, the same histologic lesion can be associated with diseases of widely varying causes (eg, UIP is the histologic lesion of IPF and is seen in CTD-associated ILD, asbestosis, chronic HP, and, occasionally, sarcoidosis).[44] Therefore, integration of the clinical history and examination findings with the radiologic and, where appropriate, histologic findings in an MDT meeting greatly improves the reliability of the diagnostic process and in turn better identifies individuals with specific diagnoses and differing prognoses.[41,45] Although it remains an evolving field, there is literature emerging that supports the notion that specialist centers running ILD MDTs are able to improve outcomes for individuals presenting with DPLD of unknown cause; presumably through better case identification and therefore the administration of better-targeted therapy.[46]

DIAGNOSING SPECIFIC DPLDs

As a group of conditions, the IIPs are the most frequently occurring DPLDs, with IPF being the most common IIP. In 2001, an ATS/ERS consensus document defined the key characteristics of these conditions, and in so doing changed the categorization and nomenclature associated with this group of conditions (previously the different IIPs had been lumped together under the diagnostic umbrella of cryptogenic fibrosing alveolitis in the United Kingdom and Europe and of IPF in the United States).[26] Although the ATS/ERS document is currently being updated, it seems unlikely that there will be any fundamental changes to the classification of the IIPs in the near future. The reclassification of the IIPs was driven by the observation that the individual IIPs have widely differing prognoses and distinct radiologic and pathologic patterns (**Table 2**). As the most common IIP, IPF is covered in more detail below, and a description of the diagnostic features of the other IIPs is overviewed elsewhere.[1,26]

IDIOPATHIC PULMONARY FIBROSIS

IPF is a devastating and progressive disease with a median survival from diagnosis of 2.8 to 3.5 years.[44] Five-year survival is akin to that seen in many cancers. The condition has an incidence of 7.4 to 27.1 per 100,000 population and has during the past 30 years become more common.[2,3] The diagnosis and treatment of IPF have recently been addressed in an ATS/ERS/Japanese Respiratory Society/Latin American Thoracic Association consensus guideline.[19] As suggested by its name, the cause of IPF remains unknown but the condition is believed to develop as a consequence of aberrant activation of pathways involved in normal wound healing.[44,47]

IPF typically presents with progressive dyspnea, often with an associated dry cough. Two thirds of suffers are male and more than 80% are current or past smokers. More than half of affected individuals have finger clubbing, and almost all have bibasal fine end-inspiratory crepitations. Toward the final stages of the disease, most develop respiratory failure and more than half will have significant secondary pulmonary hypertension. In approximately two thirds, the HRCT findings (**Fig. 4**A; see **Table 1**) in the context of an appropriate clinical history are sufficient to confirm a diagnosis of IPF. In most requiring biopsy, the histologic lesion of IPF is that of UIP. The clinical course of IPF is, in approximately 8% of patients each year, punctuated by acute exacerbations.[48,49] These acute-onset episodes of rapid deterioration present with rapidly progressing dyspnea over days to a few weeks. Radiologically acute exacerbations are characterized by the development of diffuse ground glass attenuation on a background of the typical changes of IPF (see **Fig. 4**B). Histologically, acute exacerbations are characterized by the finding of diffuse alveolar damage; this is the same lesion seen in acute respiratory distress syndrome and AIP.

CTD-ASSOCIATED ILD

DPLD complicates CTD in as many as a third of cases.[50] Most commonly, the development of DPLD occurs following the manifestation of systemic symptoms and signs of CTD and usually within the first 6 to 12 months of disease onset. In a small minority, however, DPLD represents the first presentation of CTD, and so clinicians should be alert to this possibility when assessing any individual with apparently idiopathic DPLD.[51,52] Different CTDs manifest varying forms of ILD. Individuals with scleroderma

Table 2
Classification of the IIPs proposed by the ATS/ERS 2001 Consensus Committee

	IPF	NSIP	RBILD	DIP	Lymphocytic Interstitial Pneumonia	Cryptogenic Organizing Pneumonia	AIP
					Clinical Classification		
Histologic lesion	UIP	NSIP	RBILD	DIP	Lymphocytic interstitial pneumonia	Organizing pneumonia	Diffuse alveolar damage
Mean age of onset, y	65	50–55	40–50	40–50	40–50	55	50
Rate of onset	Insidious	Insidious	Insidious	Insidious	Insidious	Subacute	Acute
Prognosis	Poor	Intermediate	Good	Good	Intermediate	Good	Very poor

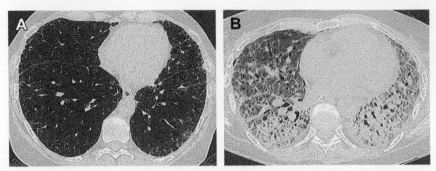

Fig. 4. A 64-year-old woman with IPF. The presenting CT (*A*) shows subpleural reticular change with traction bronchiectasis and limited ground glass attenuation. Two months later (*B*), the same patient presented with a 2-week history of rapidly deteriorating breathlessness. A repeat CT shows dramatic deterioration with new consolidation and diffuse ground glass attenuation. A biopsy confirmed diffuse alveolar damage on a background of UIP.

and mixed CTD most commonly develop the histologic lesion of NSIP (**Fig. 5**).[53,54] Those with idiopathic inflammatory myositis typically have combined organizing pneumonia that progresses to NSIP (**Fig. 6**).[54] By contrast to these conditions, individuals with rheumatoid disease frequently have fibrosis with the histologic pattern of UIP (which behaves clinically much like IPF, with inexorable progression of disease despite treatment).[55–57] Sjogren syndrome often gives rise to lymphocytic interstitial pneumonitis. Drug-induced lung disease should always be considered in those with CTD, especially rheumatoid disease, as many of the disease-modifying agents used to manage the CTDs are well documented as causes of DPLD.

The diagnosis of DPLD in known CTD can usually be confirmed on CT alone. Bronchoscopy and BAL can occasionally be useful in defining disease activity, particularly in DPLDs characterized by lymphocytic inflammation. In confirmed cases of CTD, surgical lung biopsy is rarely necessary and only then in cases where clinical or HRCT features are very atypical.[58] In patients without a known CTD, clues that the DPLD may be the first manifestation of a systemic disorder include extrathoracic symptoms such as arthropathy, arthritis, or those associated with Raynaud

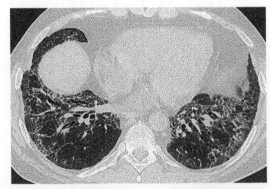

Fig. 5. An HRCT obtained in a 53-year-old woman with diffuse cutaneous systemic sclerosis. The CT shows basal reticular change and ground glass attenuation but a lack of honeycombing. The appearances are characteristic of those seen in scleroderma-associated NSIP.

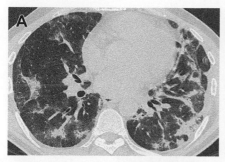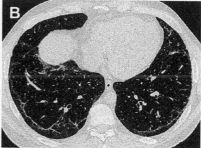

Fig. 6. An HRCT from a 34-year-old man presenting with Raynaud phenomenon and myalgia (A) shows appearances consistent with organizing pneumonia. A repeat scan 12 months later (B) demonstrates improvement in the previously noted consolidation but residual fibrosis in a pattern consistent with NSIP. This sequence of changes is typical of fibrosing organizing pneumonia in the context of antisynthetase syndrome.

phenomenon.[51,59] Similarly, clinical examination may disclose signs typical of CTD such as mechanic's hands in polymyositis. On serial CT, the finding of diffuse multifocal and peripheral organizing pneumonia progressing to an NSIP pattern of fibrosis is highly suggestive of antisynthetase syndrome. Blood autoimmune profiling may also provide important clues, particularly in individuals with autoantibodies suggestive of specific conditions (eg, anti-Scl70 antibody suggesting scleroderma in an individual with NSIP). On lung biopsy, an excess of inflammation and multiple lymphoid follicles on a background of either UIP or NSIP hints at the possibility of a forme fruste CTD-associated ILD.

HYPERSENSITIVITY PNEUMONITIS

HP (also known as extrinsic allergic alveolitis) is a syndrome caused by repeated exposure to respirable allergens. It may be acute, subacute, or chronic in presentation. The most common antigens causing HP are from birds (pigeons, parakeets, and budgerigars) and molds (ie, *Thermoactinomyces vulgaris*–the cause of farmer's lung). The overall incidence of HP is unknown; however, it may affect as many as 10% of individuals exposed to high levels of causative antigens.[60]

The diagnosis of acute HP relies on the temporal association between exposure and onset of symptoms, typically a period of 4 to 12 hours. Patients develop breathlessness and cough associated with flulike symptoms (chills, fevers, and myalgia). If examined during the acute phase, crepitations are frequently heard. Chest radiographs show diffuse ground glass attenuation. Without treatment, symptoms typically resolve during a few days (unless there is repeated or continuous antigen exposure). The diagnosis of subacute and chronic HP is harder because of the frequent lack of a temporal association between exposure and symptoms. Typically, in these forms of the condition, the exposure tends to be chronic and low grade. Affected individuals may present with symptoms and signs indistinguishable from those associated with IPF.[61] The finding of squawks on examination tends to occur in active disease and is an important clinical pointer toward a diagnosis of HP. On CT imaging, the classic findings of HP are those of centrilobular soft nodules, diffuse ground glass with evidence of gas trapping (mosaicism), and upper lobe predominance. In subacute and chronic disease, some or, less frequently, all of these features may be present combined with fibrosis in the form of reticular change, traction bronchiectasis, and occasionally honeycombing (**Fig. 7**). In an individual with CT features suggestive of

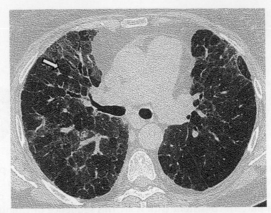

Fig. 7. An HRCT scan of a 34-year-old woman with chronic fibrotic hypersensitivity pneumonitis. The scan shows marked fibrotic change with subpleural reticulation and traction bronchiectasis. The striking gas trapping (mosaic attenuation - a region of which is indicated by the arrow) in this context is highly suggestive of a diagnosis of chronic HP.

NSIP or UIP, the finding of a BAL lymphocytosis greater than 20% raises the possibility of hypersensitivity pneumonitis as the underlying cause of fibrosis. Serum precipitins may highlight a hitherto unsuspected exposure. On biopsy, chronic HP may also be associated with a pattern indistinguishable from that of UIP or NSIP.[61,62] Clues that the underlying cause might be one of chronic HP are bronchocentricity of the fibrotic lesion, prominent lymphocytic inflammation, or airway-centered granulomas.

SARCOIDOSIS

Sarcoidosis, an idiopathic multisystem granulomatous disorder of unknown cause and protean manifestations, affects both genders equally and has a peak incidence in those between 20 and 39 years of age. The disease frequently presents with respiratory symptoms including dyspnea and cough and with ocular and skin lesions. Any organ of the body can be affected, but the lung, which is involved in more than 95% of cases, is the most common site for disease. Diagnosis can be challenging, both because sarcoidosis frequently "mimics" the presentation of other commoner conditions and because other known causes of granulomatous inflammation must be excluded. The diagnosis typically relies on histologic demonstration of noncaseating granulomatous inflammation in the context of a compatible clinical presentation and supportive ancillary investigations. Given the multiorgan nature of the condition, baseline screening investigations (eg, electrocardiogram, 24-hour urinary calcium estimation, and slit lamp examination of the eyes) should be performed according to symptoms. The guidelines produced by the ATS, ERS, and World Association for Sarcoidosis and Other Granulomatous Disorders provide a useful algorithm for approaching the diagnosis of suspected sarcoidosis.[63]

SUMMARY

The DPLDs are a group of conditions with widely varying causes and prognoses but overlapping clinical presentations. The development of disease-specific therapies (eg, pirfenidone for IPF, rituximab for CTD-associated ILD, sirolimus for LAM)[64–66] has greatly increased the importance of achieving a precise and early diagnosis as a means to guiding appropriate therapeutic interventions. In many cases, the individual DPLDs lack a single, specific diagnostic test, and as such, diagnosis relies on combining careful clinical assessment with the results of guided investigations. This integration of clinical and investigation findings is most effectively undertaken in the setting of an ILD MDT. There is a growing awareness of the important role played by the MDT in the diagnosis of DPLD. Improved access for patients to specialist ILD MDT services should lead to greater diagnostic precision at an earlier stage in disease for individual DPLDs, which in turn should permit prompt and more appropriately targeted therapy.

REFERENCES

1. Maher TM. Diffuse parenchymal lung disease. Medicine 2012;40:314–21.
2. Raghu G, Weycker D, Edelsberg J, et al. Incidence and prevalence of idiopathic pulmonary fibrosis. Am J Respir Crit Care Med 2006;174:810–6.
3. Navaratnam V, Fleming KM, West J, et al. The rising incidence of idiopathic pulmonary fibrosis in the U.K. Thorax 2011;66:462–7.
4. Borie R, Danel C, Debray MP, et al. Pulmonary alveolar proteinosis. Eur Respir Rev 2011;20:98–107.
5. Tachibana T, Hagiwara K, Johkoh T. Pulmonary alveolar microlithiasis: review and management. Curr Opin Pulm Med 2009;15:486–90.
6. Lee JS, Collard HR, Raghu G, et al. Does chronic microaspiration cause idiopathic pulmonary fibrosis? Am J Med 2010;123:304–11.
7. Camus P, Fanton A, Bonniaud P, et al. Interstitial lung disease induced by drugs and radiation. Respiration 2004;71:301–26.
8. Amar RK, Jick SS, Rosenberg D, et al. Drug-/radiation-induced interstitial lung disease in the United Kingdom general population: incidence, all-cause mortality, and characteristics at diagnosis. Respirology 2012;17(5):861–8.
9. Marshall RP, Puddicombe A, Cookson WO, et al. Adult familial cryptogenic fibrosing alveolitis in the United Kingdom. Thorax 2000;55:143–6.
10. Seibold MA, Wise AL, Speer MC, et al. A common MUC5B promoter polymorphism and pulmonary fibrosis. N Engl J Med 2011;364:1503–12.
11. Aubert G, Lansdorp PM. Telomeres and aging. Physiol Rev 2008;88:557–79.
12. Tredano M, Griese M, Brasch F, et al. Mutation of SFTPC in infantile pulmonary alveolar proteinosis with or without fibrosing lung disease. Am J Med Genet A 2004;126A:18–26.
13. Armanios MY, Chen JJ, Cogan JD, et al. Telomerase mutations in families with idiopathic pulmonary fibrosis. N Engl J Med 2007;356:1317–26.
14. Mahavadi P, Korfei M, Henneke I, et al. Epithelial stress and apoptosis underlie Hermansky-Pudlak syndrome-associated interstitial pneumonia. Am J Respir Crit Care Med 2010;182:207–19.
15. Sato H, Woodhead FA, Ahmad T, et al. Sarcoidosis HLA class II genotyping distinguishes differences of clinical phenotype across ethnic groups. Hum Mol Genet 2010;19:4100–11.
16. Johnson SR, Cordier JF, Lazor R, et al. European Respiratory Society guidelines for the diagnosis and management of lymphangioleiomyomatosis. Eur Respir J 2010;35:14–26.
17. Wells AU, Nicholson AG, Hansell DM. Challenges in pulmonary fibrosis {middle dot} 4: smoking-induced diffuse interstitial lung diseases. Thorax 2007;62:904–10.

18. Tazi A. Adult pulmonary Langerhans' cell histiocytosis. Eur Respir J 2006;27: 1272–85.
19. Raghu G, Collard HR, Egan JJ, et al. An official ATS/ERS/JRS/ALAT statement: idiopathic pulmonary fibrosis: evidence-based guidelines for diagnosis and management. Am J Respir Crit Care Med 2011;183:788–824.
20. Amar RK, Jick SS, Rosenberg D, et al. Incidence of the pneumoconioses in the United Kingdom general population between 1997 and 2008. Respiration 2012;84:200–6.
21. Zacharisen MC, Fink JN. Hypersensitivity pneumonitis and related conditions in the work environment. Immunol Allergy Clin North Am 2011;31:769–86, vii.
22. Adamali HI, Keir GJ, Nicholson A, et al. Evolution of pulmonary sarcoidosis to the clinical entity of idiopathic pulmonary fibrosis. Am J Respir Crit Care Med 2012; 185:A3005.
23. Baughman RP, Shipley RT, Loudon RG, et al. Crackles in interstitial lung disease. Comparison of sarcoidosis and fibrosing alveolitis. Chest 1991;100:96–101.
24. Corte TJ, Wort SJ, Gatzoulis MA, et al. Elevated brain natriuretic peptide predicts mortality in interstitial lung disease. Eur Respir J 2010;36:819–25.
25. Meyer KC, Raghu G, Baughman RP, et al. An official American Thoracic Society clinical practice guideline: the clinical utility of bronchoalveolar lavage cellular analysis in interstitial lung disease. Am J Respir Crit Care Med 2012;185: 1004–14.
26. American Thoracic Society/European Respiratory Society International Multidisciplinary Consensus Classification of the Idiopathic Interstitial Pneumonias. Am J Respir Crit Care Med 2002;165:277–304.
27. Myers JL, Katzenstein AL. Beyond a consensus classification for idiopathic interstitial pneumonias: progress and controversies. Histopathology 2009;54:90–103.
28. Zappala CJ, Latsi PI, Nicholson AG, et al. Marginal decline in forced vital capacity is associated with a poor outcome in idiopathic pulmonary fibrosis. Eur Respir J 2010;35:830–6.
29. du Bois RM, Weycker D, Albera C, et al. Ascertainment of individual risk of mortality for patients with idiopathic pulmonary fibrosis. Am J Respir Crit Care Med 2011;184(4):459–66.
30. Flaherty KR, Andrei AC, Murray S, et al. Idiopathic pulmonary fibrosis: prognostic value of changes in physiology and six-minute-walk test. Am J Respir Crit Care Med 2006;174:803–9.
31. Raghu G, Collard HR, Anstrom KJ, et al. Idiopathic pulmonary fibrosis: clinically meaningful primary endpoints in phase 3 clinical trials. Am J Respir Crit Care Med 2012;185:1044–8.
32. Swigris JJ, Wamboldt FS, Behr J, et al. The 6 minute walk in idiopathic pulmonary fibrosis: longitudinal changes and minimum important difference. Thorax 2010; 65:173–7.
33. Visca D, Montgomery A, de Lauretis A, et al. Ambulatory oxygen in interstitial lung disease. Eur Respir J 2011;38:987–90.
34. Fell CD, Liu LX, Motika C, et al. The prognostic value of cardiopulmonary exercise testing in idiopathic pulmonary fibrosis. Am J Respir Crit Care Med 2009;179(5): 402–7.
35. Boutou AK, Pitsiou GG, Trigonis I, et al. Exercise capacity in idiopathic pulmonary fibrosis: the effect of pulmonary hypertension. Respirology 2011;16:451–8.
36. Swigris JJ, Olson AL, Shlobin OA, et al. Heart rate recovery after six-minute walk test predicts pulmonary hypertension in patients with idiopathic pulmonary fibrosis. Respirology 2011;16:439–45.

37. Lau EM, Corte TJ. Pulmonary hypertension in 2012: contemporary issues in diagnosis and management. Panminerva Med 2012;54:11–28.
38. Corte TJ, Wort SJ, Macdonald PS, et al. Pulmonary function vascular index predicts prognosis in idiopathic interstitial pneumonia. Respirology 2012;17(4): 674–80.
39. Steckman DA, Schneider PM, Schuller JL, et al. Utility of cardiac magnetic resonance imaging to differentiate cardiac sarcoidosis from arrhythmogenic right ventricular cardiomyopathy. Am J Cardiol 2012;110:575–9.
40. Matthews R, Bench T, Meng H, et al. Diagnosis and monitoring of cardiac sarcoidosis with delayed-enhanced MRI and (18)F-FDG PET-CT. J Nucl Cardiol 2012;19:807–10.
41. Flaherty KR, King TE Jr, Raghu G, et al. Idiopathic interstitial pneumonia: what is the effect of a multidisciplinary approach to diagnosis? Am J Respir Crit Care Med 2004;170:904–10.
42. Bradley B, Branley HM, Egan JJ, et al. Interstitial lung disease guideline: the British Thoracic Society in collaboration with the Thoracic Society of Australia and New Zealand and the Irish Thoracic Society. Thorax 2008;63(Suppl 5):v1–58.
43. Nicholson AG, Addis BJ, Bharucha H, et al. Inter-observer variation between pathologists in diffuse parenchymal lung disease. Thorax 2004;59:500–5.
44. Maher TM, Wells AU, Laurent GJ. Idiopathic pulmonary fibrosis: multiple causes and multiple mechanisms? Eur Respir J 2007;30:835–9.
45. Flaherty KR, Andrei AC, King TE Jr, et al. Idiopathic interstitial pneumonia: do community and academic physicians agree on diagnosis? Am J Respir Crit Care Med 2007;175:1054–60.
46. Lamas DJ, Kawut SM, Bagiella E, et al. Delayed access and survival in idiopathic pulmonary fibrosis: a cohort study. Am J Respir Crit Care Med 2011;184:842–7.
47. King TE Jr, Pardo A, Selman M. Idiopathic pulmonary fibrosis. Lancet 2011;378: 1949–61.
48. Collard HR, Moore BB, Flaherty KR, et al. Acute exacerbations of idiopathic pulmonary fibrosis. Am J Respir Crit Care Med 2007;176:636–43.
49. Martinez FJ, Safrin S, Weycker D, et al. The clinical course of patients with idiopathic pulmonary fibrosis. Ann Intern Med 2005;142:963–7.
50. Fischer A, West SG, Swigris JJ, et al. Connective tissue disease-associated interstitial lung disease: a call for clarification. Chest 2010;138:251–6.
51. Corte TJ, Copley SJ, Desai SR, et al. Significance of connective tissue disease features in idiopathic interstitial pneumonia. Eur Respir J 2012;39:661–8.
52. Tzelepis GE, Toya SP, Moutsopoulos HM. Occult connective tissue diseases mimicking idiopathic interstitial pneumonias. Eur Respir J 2008;31:11–20.
53. Goh NS, Desai SR, Veeraraghavan S, et al. Interstitial lung disease in systemic sclerosis: a simple staging system. Am J Respir Crit Care Med 2008;177:1248–54.
54. Ingegnoli F, Lubatti C, Ingegnoli A, et al. Interstitial lung disease outcomes by high-resolution computed tomography (HRCT) in anti-Jo1 antibody-positive polymyositis patients: a single centre study and review of the literature. Autoimmun Rev 2012;11:335–40.
55. Olson AL, Swigris JJ, Sprunger DB, et al. Rheumatoid arthritis-interstitial lung disease-associated mortality. Am J Respir Crit Care Med 2011;183:372–8.
56. Kim EJ, Elicker BM, Maldonado F, et al. Usual interstitial pneumonia in rheumatoid arthritis-associated interstitial lung disease. Eur Respir J 2010;35:1322–8.
57. Kim EJ, Collard HR, King TE Jr. Rheumatoid arthritis-associated interstitial lung disease: the relevance of histopathologic and radiographic pattern. Chest 2009;136:1397–405.

58. Cottin V. Pragmatic prognostic approach of rheumatoid arthritis-associated interstitial lung disease. Eur Respir J 2010;35:1206–8.

59. Kinder BW, Collard HR, Koth L, et al. Idiopathic nonspecific interstitial pneumonia: lung manifestation of undifferentiated connective tissue disease? Am J Respir Crit Care Med 2007;176:691–7.

60. Chan AL, Juarez MM, Leslie KO, et al. Bird fancier's lung: a state-of-the-art review. Clin Rev Allergy Immunol 2012;43:69–83.

61. Myers JL. Hypersensitivity pneumonia: the role of lung biopsy in diagnosis and management. Mod Pathol 2012;25(Suppl 1):S58–67.

62. Herbst JB, Myers JL. Hypersensitivity pneumonia: role of surgical lung biopsy. Arch Pathol Lab Med 2012;136:889–95.

63. Hunninghake GW, Costabel U, Ando M, et al. ATS/ERS/WASOG statement on sarcoidosis. American Thoracic Society/European Respiratory Society/World Association of Sarcoidosis and other Granulomatous Disorders. Sarcoidosis Vasc Diffuse Lung Dis 1999;16:149–73.

64. Keir GJ, Maher TM, Hansell DM, et al. Severe interstitial lung disease in connective tissue disease: rituximab as rescue therapy. Eur Respir J 2012;40:641–8.

65. Maher TM. Pirfenidone in idiopathic pulmonary fibrosis. Drugs Today (Barc) 2010; 46:473–82.

66. McCormack FX, Inoue Y, Moss J, et al. Efficacy and safety of sirolimus in lymphangioleiomyomatosis. N Engl J Med 2011;364:1595–606.

Idiopathic Pulmonary Fibrosis

Jason S. Zolak, MD[a], Joao A. de Andrade, MD[a,b,c],*

KEYWORDS

- Idiopathic pulmonary fibrosis • Pathogenesis • Diagnosis • Management

KEY POINTS

- Progressive scarring of the lung parenchyma, and relentless loss of lung function leading to disabling dyspnea characterize idiopathic pulmonary fibrosis (IPF).
- The pathogenesis may be related to an aberrant wound healing process that starts in a genetically susceptible epithelium.
- The clinical course of IPF is unpredictable.
- No Food and Drug Administration approved therapies are available for IPF.
- Lung transplantation may be a viable option for a selected group of patients, and referral for evaluation should be considered at the time of diagnosis.

INTRODUCTION

Idiopathic pulmonary fibrosis (IPF) is a chronic lung disease of unknown cause characterized by progressive scarring of the lung parenchyma with a histologic pattern of usual interstitial pneumonia (UIP).[1] Clinically, it is manifested by progressive loss of lung function that leads to breathlessness and relentless functional limitation. It is a fatal disease with a median survival of only 3 years after the diagnosis,[2] and the incidence is estimated to be from 6.8 to 16.3 cases per 100 000 people.[3] IPF is more prevalent among older Caucasian men, with most cases being diagnosed in individuals older than 60 years.[3,4] To this date, no Food and Drug Administration–approved therapies are available for IPF.

The mortality rate associated with IPF has been increasing during the last few years, and a recent report estimates that it was approximately 50.8 deaths per million people between the years of 1992 and 2003.[5] If those numbers are correct, 40 000 people die

Funding sources: Dr Zolak: nil; Dr de Andrade: NIH/NHLBI (IPFnet), Intermune, Actelion, Fibrogen, Centocor, Immuneworks, Gilead, Boehringer-Ingelheim, and Celgene.
Conflict of interest: Nil.
^a Division of Pulmonary, Allergy, and Critical Care Medicine, University of Alabama at Birmingham, 1900 University Boulevard, THT 422, Birmingham, AL 35294-0006, USA; ^b Interstitial Lung Disease Program, Division of Pulmonary, Allergy, and Critical Care Medicine, University of Alabama at Birmingham, 1900 University Boulevard, THT 422, Birmingham, AL 35294-0006, USA; ^c Medical Intensive Care Unit, Birmingham VA Medical Center, Birmingham, AL, USA
* Corresponding author.
E-mail address: joao@uab.edu

Immunol Allergy Clin N Am 32 (2012) 473–485
http://dx.doi.org/10.1016/j.iac.2012.08.006
0889-8561/12/$ – see front matter Published by Elsevier Inc.

immunology.theclinics.com

of IPF every year in the United States alone, which is comparable with the mortality rates attributed to breast cancer.

In this review article, the authors discuss evolving concepts regarding the pathogenesis of IPF, describe the most current diagnostic and management strategies, and discuss some of the recent clinical trials that explored novel therapies for IPF.

PATHOGENESIS

The factors that determine the onset and progression of IPF are not completely understood. The last few years have seen a shift in the paradigms regarding the pathogenesis of IPF from chronic inflammation leading to progressive fibrosis to an abnormal wound healing process in which multiple factors interplay.[6] Supporting that concept, studies of gene expression profile patterns have demonstrated that, when compared with lungs with chronic hypersensitivity pneumonitis, which is characterized by a significant inflammatory component, IPF lungs have a shift toward extracellular matrix turnover and epithelium development, growth, and differentiation.[7] Moreover, older reports exploring antiinflammatory agents have largely failed to demonstrate a treatment benefit in IPF.[8–10]

Alveolar epithelial cells and the myofibroblast are thought to be the key target cells in the pathogenesis of IPF; there is growing evidence that genetic susceptibility, cellular senescence, endoplasmic reticulum stress and oxidative stress, as well as epigenetic factors associated with micro-RNAs are critical factors for the injury continuum that ultimately leads to the extensive fibrotic changes and loss of lung function seen in IPF. The authors focus the discussion on those emerging concepts.

A genetic component for the development of IPF is suggested because up to 20% of cases are reported to occur in families.[11,12] Mutations both in the surfactant protein C and an isoform of the surfactant protein A genes have been reported.[13–16] Both mutations are linked to abnormal processing and protein misfolding in alveolar epithelial cells with subsequent endoplasmic reticulum alveolar stress that leads to an increased predisposition to fibrosis in response to injury.[16]

IPF is rarely diagnosed in individuals younger than 50 years,[3] suggesting that it may be, at least in part, a disease related to the aging process. Corroborating this hypothesis, studies of both familial and so-called sporadic cases of IPF demonstrated the presence of telomere shortening, which has been associated with cellular senescence and a reduced capacity for epithelial repair.[17–19]

Oxidative stress is defined as an imbalance between excessive generation of reactive oxygen species and diminished ability to scavenge them. Oxidative stress plays a role in the development of fibrosis in several different organ systems and it is a feature of IPF.[20,21] Transforming growth factor (TGF)-β1, which is considered to be the premier profibrotic cytokine, can stimulate the production of Reactive Oxygen Species and myofibroblast differentiation in human lung fibroblasts.[22] It has been demonstrated that the bronchoalveolar lavage fluid of patients with IPF has increased levels of reactive oxygen species as well as diminished levels of glutathione compared with controls.[23] Furthermore, there have been reports of evidence of oxidative stress and damage in the lung tissue of patients with IPF.[21,24] It has been demonstrated that oxidative stress can induce cellular senescence and apoptosis[25,26]; when fibroblasts become senescent, they acquire an apoptosis-resistant phenotype and secrete higher levels of reactive oxygen species.[27] Lung myofibroblasts do undergo similar changes[28] and are likely implicated in the formation of the positive feedback loop that helps perpetuate a proinjury and profibrotic microenvironment in the IPF lung.

The endoplasmic reticulum (ER) is an intracellular organelle that is responsible for proper folding, processing and trafficking of secreted proteins. Additionally, it is involved in the production of steroids, synthesis of lipids and calcium homeostasis.[29] Several factors, such as reduced energy stores, accumulation of improperly folded mutant proteins, and oxidative stress, may induce ER stress in the form of an adaptive process called unfolded protein response (UPR).[30] UPR is meant to facilitate ER protein folding and degradation; but if the triggering factor is persistent, it can lead to cell death through apoptosis. ER stress has been proposed as an important component of the pathogenesis of IPF because evidence of it has been found in lung tissue from patients with both familial and sporadic IPF.[22,31] Similar findings have been reported in epithelial cells in IPF.[31] Recent reports propose that ER stress is involved in the differentiation of lung fibroblasts into myofibroblasts, a process that is critical for the persistent collagen and matrix deposition that ultimately leads to remodeling of the IPF lung.[22] Furthermore, several stressors that have been implicated in the pathogenesis of IPF, such as viral infections, cigarette smoking, surfactant protein mutations, and oxidative stress, are also potential triggers of ER stress.[32]

MicroRNAs (miRs) are noncoding small RNAs that bind to the untranslated regions of target genes in response to several cellular stimuli and, in doing so, repress the translation of target genes or induce degradation of a given target gene mRNA. Abnormal expression of miRs have been linked to the pathogenesis of several common entities, such as diabetes, cancer, and cardiovascular disease,[33–35] and specifically to fibrosing processes in different organs, including IPF lungs.[35–38] It has been suggested that the role of miRs in the pathogenesis of fibrotic processes may be caused by its effect in the biology of TGF-β1.[37] A recent study presented evidence that 3 members of the miR-200 family (miR-200a, miR-200b, miR-200c) were downregulated in the lungs of mice with bleomycin-induced fibrosis. Levels of miR-200a and mi-RNA-200c were also decreased in the lungs of patients with IPF. Importantly, members of the miR-200 family inhibited epithelial-mesenchymal transformation of alveolar epithelial cells induced by TGF-β1 and actually reversed the fibrogenic activity of fibroblasts from both mice with bleomycin-induced fibrosis and patients with IPF.[39]

Taken together, these recent reports suggest that a dysfunctional alveolar epithelium, generated by genetic and perhaps epigenetic susceptibility, aging, and/or external noxious stimuli, may lead to abnormal epithelium-mesenchymal interactions that create a sustained and self-perpetuating loop of injury through oxidative stress and perhaps ER stress, thereby preventing normal epithelial repair with progressive fibrosis and ultimate loss of lung function.

CLINICAL PRESENTATION AND DIAGNOSIS

Patients with IPF typically present with the gradual onset of dyspnea on exertion and persistent nonproductive cough. Systemic symptoms, such as weight loss, fevers, arthralgias, and myalgias, are rare and suggest another process, such as collagen vascular disease. The median duration of illness before diagnosis is 24 months.[40] Physical examination usually reveals late, fine inspiratory crackles (Velcrolike [Velcro USA, Inc, Manchester, New Hampshire]) on auscultation, and digital clubbing is present in approximately half of patients. Cardiac examination often remains normal in the absence of pulmonary hypertension.

Pulmonary function tests (PFTs) demonstrate a normal forced expiratory volume in the first second of expiration/forced vital capacity (FVC) ratio with a restrictive ventilatory defect caused by poorly compliant parenchyma with reduced diffusion capacity for carbon monoxide ($D_L CO$) and abnormal gas exchange. The main mechanism for hypoxemia at rest and with exercise in patients with IPF is ventilation-perfusion mismatch and not impaired diffusion as previously thought. Cardiopulmonary exercise testing may be more sensitive than resting PFTs in the detection of gas exchange abnormalities, and low maximum oxygen consumption on exercise testing correlates with an increased risk of death.[41]

In the appropriate clinical setting, a confident diagnosis of IPF can be made if a chest high-resolution CAT scan (HRCT) demonstrates bilateral and predominantly basal and subpleural reticulation, traction bronchiectasis, and honeycomb change (**Fig. 1**). Features that are inconsistent with IPF/UIP include upper/midlung predominance, peribronchovascular predominance, extensive ground-glass abnormality, profuse micronodules, discrete cysts, diffuse mosaic attenuation/air trapping, and consolidation in bronchopulmonary segments/lobes.[42] Unfortunately, a significant number of patients present with an HRCT that is atypical and require a surgical lung biopsy for a definitive diagnosis.[43,44]

The gross appearance of the lungs in IPF is characterized by a nodular pleural surface and the histopathology pattern is consistent with UIP. The histopathologic pattern of UIP includes the presence of temporal heterogeneity with areas of mature relatively acellular collagen bundles and areas of new fibrosis consisting of aggregates of fibroblasts in myxoid connective tissue called fibroblastic foci, honeycomb change, pleural involvement, and areas of normal lung (**Fig. 2**).

As one attempts to diagnose IPF and other types of interstitial lung disease, it is often helpful to think algorithmically. The evaluation begins with a careful and detailed history, physical examination, chest radiographs, pulmonary function testing, and serologic studies. This process should screen for systemic conditions associated with interstitial lung disease as well as environmental exposures and drug-related interstitial lung disease. The next step is obtaining an HRCT, and a confident diagnosis of UIP can be made if the typical features of UIP/IPF are present, abrogating the need for a surgical biopsy. If either the clinical presentation or the HRCT are atypical for IPF, then a surgical lung biopsy should be considered. Transbronchial biopsies are not thought to yield enough tissue and, therefore, are not usually indicated if IPF is suspected. A multidisciplinary discussion of the clinical information, radiographs, and histologic findings among experienced pulmonologists, radiologists, and pathologists

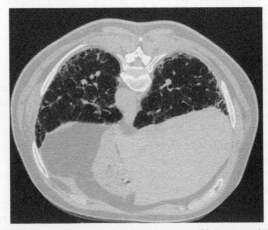

Fig. 1. Typical HRCT findings of IPF: pleural-based areas of honeycombing, coarse reticular opacities, and traction bronchiectasis.

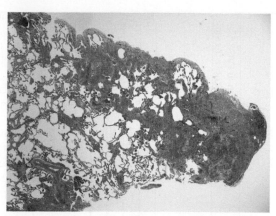

Fig. 2. Typical findings of usual interstitial pneumonia: temporal heterogeneity with areas of dense fibrosis (*right corner*), new fibrosis with fibroblast foci (*upper center, around airways*), bronchiolectasis, and early honeycombing (*upper center*), and areas of preserved alveolar architecture (*lower center*).

will increase diagnostic accuracy and is recommended as the method of choice for the diagnosis of IPF.[42,45]

CLINICAL TRIALS IN IPF

No approved therapies are available for IPF, and the process of drug discovery and drug development has been mired by several fundamental problems. Animal models of IPF using bleomycin-induced lung injury do not fully reproduce human disease, thereby making the interpretation of preclinical efficacy studies difficult. The scientific community continues to debate which outcome measures are clinically meaningful. Although all-cause mortality is clearly a meaningful end point for a clinical trial, those studies require larger numbers of patients, longer periods for enrollment and follow-up, and carry significant cost. Other measures, such as change in lung function over time, have been suggested as adequate surrogates for mortality but are yet to be rigorously validated.[46]

During the last 20 years, more than 3000 patients have been enrolled in clinical trials exploring novel therapies for IPF and most used different measures of change in lung physiology as the primary end point (**Table 1**). A few studies met their primary end point but none thus far have demonstrated a survival advantage or a clinically meaningful benefit in IPF. Another factor to consider as one interprets the results of the past IPF clinical trials is that most allowed the use of corticosteroids in the placebo arm.

To this date, only 3 phase III clinical trials in IPF have met their primary end point. The Study of the Effects of High-Dose N-Acetylcysteine (NAC) in Idiopathic Pulmonary Fibrosis (IFIGENIA) compared the effectiveness of 1-year combined antiinflammatory therapy of azathioprine and prednisone with or without the antioxidant NAC.[47] At the end of 1 year, patients randomized to the triple therapy arm had a statistically significant lower rate of decline in FVC and D_LCO compared with patients who took only prednisone and azathioprine. Although this study has been widely criticized for the lack of a placebo-only group and the significant rate of dropouts, it was used to inform a 3-arm (prednisone, azathioprine, NAC vs NAC alone vs placebo alone) randomized trial sponsored by the National Heart, Lung, and Blood Institute IPF Clinical Research Network (IPFnet), the Prednisone, Azathioprine, and N-Acetylcysteine (PANTHER)-IPF trial.

Table 1
Recent randomized clinical trials in IPF

Study	Drug	Entry Criteria	Primary End Point	n	Corticosteroids (CS) Allowed	Results
Raghu[77]	Interferon γ 1b	FVC >50, D_LCO >25	Progression-free survival	330	Yes	Negative
Azuma[52]	Pirfenidone	Age, oxygen saturation measured using pulse oximetry (SpO_2)	ΔSpO_2 six-minute walked test(6MWT)	109	Yes	Negative
Demedts[47]	Prednisone(Pred)/ azathioprine(AZA) ± NAC	FVC ≤80, D_LCO <80	Absolute (Abs) ΔFVC, D_LCO	182	Yes	Less deterioration in FVC and D_LCO with triple therapy
Kubo[50]	CS ± Anticoagulant	Decline with CS	Survival/time to death	56	Yes	Better survival in the anticoagulant group
King[78]	Bosentan	FVC ≥50, D_LCO ≥30	six-minute walk distance (6MWD)	158	Yes	Negative
Raghu[79]	Etanercept	FVC ≥45, D_LCO ≥25	Δ%FVC, D_LCO, A-a	88	No	Negative
King[80]	Interferon γ 1b	FVC ≥55, D_LCO ≥35	Survival	826	Yes	Negative
Daniels[81]	Imatinib	FVC ≥55, D_LCO ≥35	Disease progression/death	119	No	Negative
Noble[54]	Pirfenidone	FVC ≥50, D_LCO ≥35	Δ%FVC	435	Yes	Lower decline in FVC
Noble[54]	Pirfenidone	FVC ≥50, D_LCO ≥35	Δ%FVC	344	Yes	Negative
Taniguchi[53]	Pirfenidone	SpO_2 on 6MWT	ΔFVC	275	Yes	Lower decline in FVC for the group randomized to the higher dose of pirfenidone
Zisman[82]	Sildenafil	D_LCO <35	6MWD	180	Yes	Negative
Noth[51]	Warfarin	Progressive disease	Death/hospitalization/ decline in %FVC ≥10	145	Yes	Harmful
Raghu[48]	Pred/Aza/NAC	FVC ≥50, D_LCO ≥30	Δ%FVC	155	Yes	Harmful
Richeldi[83]	BIBF-1120	FVC ≥50, D_LCO 30–79	Rate of decline in FVC	432	Yes	Negative

Abbreviations: Abs, absolute; AZA, azathioprine; CS, corticosteroids; 6MWD, six-minute walked distance; 6MWT, six-minute walk test; NAC, N-acetylcysteine; SpO_2, oxygen saturation measured using pulse oximetry.

PANTHER-IPF is a randomized, double-blind, placebo-controlled trial that enrolled patients with mild to moderate IPF in a 1:1:1 ratio. An interim analysis conducted when approximately 50% of the data had been collected demonstrated a statistically significant increased risk of death and hospitalizations for patients randomized to the triple-therapy arm compared with those randomized to placebo. This finding prompted the data safety monitoring board to stop enrollment in the triple-therapy arm.[48] The study continued to recruit patients to both NAC and placebo arms and is expected to complete the follow-up in the fall of 2013. The results of PANTHER-IPF provide strong evidence against the use of antiinflammatory therapy for patients with IPF.

Many animal and human studies have supported the importance of the coagulation cascade in the pathogenesis of IPF.[49] Kubo and colleagues[50] conducted a prospective, randomized, open-label study of 64 patients with IPF with mild physiologic impairment recruited at the time of hospitalization. All patients had evidence of prior clinic deterioration and were taking corticosteroids at the time of enrollment. Patients were randomized to receive either corticosteroids alone (n = 33) or corticosteroids plus anticoagulation (n = 31), which consisted of either outpatient warfarin titrated to international normalized ratio (INR) of 2 to 3 or intravenous low molecular heparin during periods of hospitalization for disease exacerbation. There was a statistically significant improvement in both survival and mortality associated with acute exacerbation of IPF in the anticoagulant-treated group. Several methodological concerns have been raised about this study. Survival in the control group was much lower than reported in some contemporary IPF clinical trials. Furthermore, 8 out of 31 patients randomized to the anticoagulant group withdrew consent before receiving the study drug, but an intent-to-treat analysis of the whole randomized patient cohort was not conducted. This study, however, suggested a potential role for anticoagulation as a treatment strategy for IPF and informed the Anticoagulant Effectiveness in Idiopathic Pulmonary Fibrosis (ACE-IPF) trial of the IPFnet. ACE-IPF was a randomized, double-blind, controlled study of patients with progressive IPF that were randomized to either placebo or warfarin targeting an INR of 2 to 3 in a 1:1 ratio. The primary end point of ACE-IPF was a composite of time to death, nonbleeding/nonelective hospitalization, or a 10% or greater reduction in FVC. The planned treatment duration was 48 weeks, but after 145 of the planned 245 patients had been enrolled, the data safety monitoring board recommended stopping the study because of a low probability of benefit and, more importantly, a statistically significant increase in mortality among patients randomized to warfarin.[51] The results of both PANTHER-IPF and ACE-IPF illustrate the importance to confirm promising preliminary results with adequately powered placebo-controlled, randomized, clinical trials.

Pirfenidone is a molecule that has been demonstrated to have antifibrotic properties in preclinical studies using animal models of pulmonary fibrosis. In 2005, Azuma and collaborators[52] published a study conducted in Japan in which 107 patients with IPF were randomized to either placebo or pirfenidone. This study largely failed to meet its primary end point but was stopped early by the data safety monitoring board because more patients in the placebo group experienced acute exacerbations of IPF. Subsequently, Taniguchi and collaborators[53] conducted a 3-arm trial of 275 patients with IPF randomized to 2 different doses of pirfenidone (1800 mg or 1200 mg) or placebo. Patients randomized to the higher-dose group had a significant reduction in the rate of decline in vital capacity and improved progression-free survival, which was a secondary end point. Although these results were largely encouraging, it is concerning that the primary end point was changed after the trial was started and that the method chosen to handle missing data might have magnified the treatment effect of pirfenidone. More recently, Noble and colleagues[54] reported the results of 2 concomitant, large, placebo-controlled, randomized trials of pirfenidone that recruited most patients with IPF from centers in the United States. The primary end point of both studies was a change in predicted FVC at week 72. Study 004 randomized 435 patients in a 2:2:1 model to a higher-dose group, a placebo group, or a lower-dose group. Study 006 enrolled 334 patients in a 1:1 model to either a high dose of pirfenidone or placebo. Study 004 met its primary end point but study 006 did not. Overall, both studies demonstrated that pirfenidone has a very good safety profile, but questions remain regarding its efficacy. Pirfenidone is not yet approved for use in the United States but has been approved for the treatment of IPF in the European Union and in Japan.

MANAGING PATIENTS WITH IPF

Recent clinical trials in IPF have largely failed to identify effective therapies for IPF but have given us much-needed insights into the natural history of the disease. Analysis of the placebo arm of a large, multicenter, randomized, clinical trial of interferon-γ-1b in patients with moderate IPF demonstrated that lung physiology had only a minimal decline during the first 12 months following randomization. Approximately half of the deaths that occurred acutely were preceded by a period of rapid deterioration that did not have an identifiable cause. There was an overall trend toward worsening dyspnea and lung physiology before death, but there was great variability among patients and, more importantly, the initial FVC was not a reliable predictor of outcomes.[55] These findings are significant because they emphasize the fact that the clinical course of IPF is unpredictable.[42]

Lung transplantation is the only option to prolong the life of patients with advanced IPF[56] but it has considerable limitations. It is a costly treatment available to only a very selected few and has a 5-year median survival of only 50%.[57]

Because no effective pharmacologic therapies are available, the management of patients with IPF focuses on measures to preserve quality of life, mobility, and independence. Patients with IPF have diminished exercise capacity, significant fatigue, breathlessness, depression, diminished cognitive function, and diminished quality-of-life measures compared with the general population.[58,59]

Pulmonary rehabilitation has been shown to have a positive impact on those elements in patients with chronic obstructive pulmonary disease and is recommended for patients with IPF.[42] Although well-designed prospective and controlled studies exploring the role of pulmonary rehabilitation in IPF are lacking, retrospective cohort studies have suggested that pulmonary rehabilitation is largely beneficial, especially for patients with more advanced disease.[60]

Hypoxemia is often seen in patients with advanced IPF and may be a harbinger of shorter survival[40]; however, no conclusive studies have been performed on the effects of long-term oxygen therapy on survival or level of breathlessness.[61] A few small studies suggest a favorable impact of oxygen therapy on exercise capacity and quality of life.[62,63]

Severe, nonproductive cough is another problem commonly reported in IPF; it is important to consider that about half the cases of persistent cough in patients with interstitial lung diseases may be related to factors, such as upper airway cough syndrome and gastroesophageal reflux.[64]

Gastroesophageal reflux is prevalent in IPF and it has been suggested that it is involved in the pathogenesis as both the initial insult or later as a promoter of recurrent lung injury.[65–67] Supporting this hypothesis, a recent retrospective cohort study reported that the use of antireflux medications was associated with decreased radiologic fibrotic findings and was an independent predictor of longer survival.[68]

Sleep-disordered breathing has been reported to be common in IPF, causing a negative impact in quality of life.[69,70] No studies have explored the impact of nocturnal noninvasive ventilation for IPF patients with sleep-disordered breathing.

A subset of patients, especially those with a significant smoking history, has disease that is characterized by the simultaneous presence of pulmonary fibrosis and emphysema. This combined pulmonary fibrosis and emphysema phenotype occurs more commonly in men, with a mean age of 65 years. It is associated with a relative preservation of lung volumes and marked reductions in D_LCO on PFTs.[71] Such patients are more likely to require oxygen therapy and develop pulmonary hypertension and may have worse outcomes compared with those with only pulmonary fibrosis.[72]

Pulmonary hypertension is often seen in IPF and may be associated with disease progression and poor survival,[73,74] but the best strategies for the diagnosis and management of pulmonary hypertension in IPF remains to be defined.

IPF is typically a gradually progressive disease, but 5% to 10% of patients experience episodic worsening of symptoms and lung function termed acute exacerbations of IPF. Acute exacerbation of IPF has been defined as an unexplained clinical decline within 30 days associated with new bilateral ground-glass opacities or consolidation on imaging on a background of UIP, lack of evidence for infection and exclusion of heart failure, pulmonary thromboembolism, or other known causes of acute lung injury.[75] Acute exacerbations are associated with a high mortality and poor 6-month prognosis among those who survive the episode. Patients who are experiencing acute exacerbations are often treated with high doses of corticosteroids, but there is no evidence that such strategy impacts outcomes.[76]

In summary, patients with IPF ought to receive aggressive treatment of reflux and be referred for pulmonary rehabilitation. If sleep-disordered breathing is present, noninvasive positive pressure ventilation can be considered if no contraindication is present. Most importantly, patients with IPF should be referred early to tertiary care centers to be evaluated for lung transplantation and to be considered for participation in clinical trials.[42]

REFERENCES

1. Katzenstein AL, Myers JL. Idiopathic pulmonary fibrosis: clinical relevance of pathologic classification. Am J Respir Crit Care Med 1998;157(4 Pt 1):1301–15.
2. Bjoraker JA, Ryu JH, Edwin MK, et al. Prognostic significance of histopathologic subsets in idiopathic pulmonary fibrosis. Am J Respir Crit Care Med 1998;157(1): 199–203.
3. Raghu G, Weycker D, Edelsberg J, et al. Incidence and prevalence of idiopathic pulmonary fibrosis. Am J Respir Crit Care Med 2006;174(7):810–6.
4. de Andrade JA, Daniel N, Wille KM, et al. Racial disparities in idiopathic pulmonary fibrosis. Data from a Southeastern U.S. Center. Proc Am Thorac Soc 2008; 2008:A249.
5. Olson AL, Swigris JJ, Lezotte DC, et al. Mortality from pulmonary fibrosis increased in the United States from 1992 to 2003. Am J Respir Crit Care Med 2007;176(3):277–84.
6. Selman M, King TE, Pardo A. Idiopathic pulmonary fibrosis: prevailing and evolving hypotheses about its pathogenesis and implications for therapy. Ann Intern Med 2001;134(2):136–51.
7. Selman M, Pardo A, Barrera L, et al. Gene expression profiles distinguish idiopathic pulmonary fibrosis from hypersensitivity pneumonitis. Am J Respir Crit Care Med 2006;173(2):188–98.

8. Selman M, Carrillo G, Salas J, et al. Colchicine, D-penicillamine, and prednisone in the treatment of idiopathic pulmonary fibrosis: a controlled clinical trial. Chest 1998;114(2):507–12.

9. Collard HR, Ryu JH, Douglas WW, et al. Combined corticosteroid and cyclophosphamide therapy does not alter survival in idiopathic pulmonary fibrosis. Chest 2004;125(6):2169–74.

10. Douglas WW, Ryu JH, Swensen SJ, et al. Colchicine versus prednisone in the treatment of idiopathic pulmonary fibrosis. A randomized prospective study. Members of the Lung Study Group. Am J Respir Crit Care Med 1998;158(1):220–5.

11. Hodgson U, Laitinen T, Tukiainen P. Nationwide prevalence of sporadic and familial idiopathic pulmonary fibrosis: evidence of founder effect among multiplex families in Finland. Thorax 2002;57(4):338–42.

12. Marshall RP, Puddicombe A, Cookson WO, et al. Adult familial cryptogenic fibrosing alveolitis in the United Kingdom. Thorax 2000;55(2):143–6.

13. Nogee LM, Dunbar AE 3rd, Wert SE, et al. A mutation in the surfactant protein C gene associated with familial interstitial lung disease. N Engl J Med 2001;344(8):573–9.

14. Thomas AQ, Lane K, Phillips J 3rd, et al. Heterozygosity for a surfactant protein C gene mutation associated with usual interstitial pneumonitis and cellular nonspecific interstitial pneumonitis in one kindred. Am J Respir Crit Care Med 2002;165(9):1322–8.

15. Wang Y, Kuan PJ, Xing C, et al. Genetic defects in surfactant protein A2 are associated with pulmonary fibrosis and lung cancer. Am J Hum Genet 2009;84(1):52–9.

16. Lawson WE, Cheng DS, Degryse AL, et al. Endoplasmic reticulum stress enhances fibrotic remodeling in the lungs. Proc Natl Acad Sci U S A 2011;108(26):10562–7.

17. Alder JK, Chen JJ, Lancaster L, et al. Short telomeres are a risk factor for idiopathic pulmonary fibrosis. Proc Natl Acad Sci U S A 2008;105(35):13051–6.

18. Cronkhite JT, Xing C, Raghu G, et al. Telomere shortening in familial and sporadic pulmonary fibrosis. Am J Respir Crit Care Med 2008;178(7):729–37.

19. Tsakiri KD, Cronkhite JT, Kuan PJ, et al. Adult-onset pulmonary fibrosis caused by mutations in telomerase. Proc Natl Acad Sci U S A 2007;104(18):7552–7.

20. Brenner DA. Molecular pathogenesis of liver fibrosis. Trans Am Clin Climatol Assoc 2009;120:361–8.

21. Kinnula VL, Fattman CL, Tan RJ, et al. Oxidative stress in pulmonary fibrosis: a possible role for redox modulatory therapy. Am J Respir Crit Care Med 2005;172(4):417–22.

22. Baek HA, Kim do S, Park HS, et al. Involvement of endoplasmic reticulum stress in myofibroblastic differentiation of lung fibroblasts. Am J Respir Cell Mol Biol 2012;46(6):731–9.

23. Cantin AM, Hubbard RC, Crystal RG. Glutathione deficiency in the epithelial lining fluid of the lower respiratory tract in idiopathic pulmonary fibrosis. Am Rev Respir Dis 1989;139(2):370–2.

24. Kuwano K, Nakashima N, Inoshima I, et al. Oxidative stress in lung epithelial cells from patients with idiopathic interstitial pneumonias. Eur Respir J 2003;21(2):232–40.

25. Dasari A, Bartholomew JN, Volonte D, et al. Oxidative stress induces premature senescence by stimulating caveolin-1 gene transcription through p38 mitogen-activated protein kinase/Sp1-mediated activation of two GC-rich promoter elements. Cancer Res 2006;66(22):10805–14.

26. MacNee W. Accelerated lung aging: a novel pathogenic mechanism of chronic obstructive pulmonary disease (COPD). Biochem Soc Trans 2009;37(Pt 4): 819–23.

27. Toussaint O, Medrano EE, von Zglinicki T. Cellular and molecular mechanisms of stress-induced premature senescence (SIPS) of human diploid fibroblasts and melanocytes. Exp Gerontol 2000;35(8):927–45.

28. Waghray M, Cui Z, Horowitz JC, et al. Hydrogen peroxide is a diffusible paracrine signal for the induction of epithelial cell death by activated myofibroblasts. FASEB J 2005;19(7):854–6.

29. Lin JH, Walter P, Yen TS. Endoplasmic reticulum stress in disease pathogenesis. Annu Rev Pathol 2008;3:399–425.

30. Xu C, Bailly-Maitre B, Reed JC. Endoplasmic reticulum stress: cell life and death decisions. J Clin Invest 2005;115(10):2656–64.

31. Lawson WE, Crossno PF, Polosukhin VV, et al. Endoplasmic reticulum stress in alveolar epithelial cells is prominent in IPF: association with altered surfactant protein processing and herpesvirus infection. Am J Physiol Lung Cell Mol Physiol 2008;294(6):L1119–26.

32. Tanjore H, Blackwell TS, Lawson WE. Emerging evidence for endoplasmic reticulum stress in the pathogenesis of idiopathic pulmonary fibrosis. Am J Physiol Lung Cell Mol Physiol 2012;302(8):L721–9.

33. Croce CM. Causes and consequences of microRNA dysregulation in cancer. Nat Rev Genet 2009;10(10):704–14.

34. Latronico MV, Condorelli G. MicroRNAs and cardiac pathology. Nat Rev Cardiol 2009;6(6):419–29.

35. Thum T, Gross C, Fiedler J, et al. MicroRNA-21 contributes to myocardial disease by stimulating MAP kinase signalling in fibroblasts. Nature 2008;456(7224):980–4.

36. van Rooij E, Sutherland LB, Thatcher JE, et al. Dysregulation of microRNAs after myocardial infarction reveals a role of miR-29 in cardiac fibrosis. Proc Natl Acad Sci U S A 2008;105(35):13027–32.

37. Liu G, Friggeri A, Yang Y, et al. miR-21 mediates fibrogenic activation of pulmonary fibroblasts and lung fibrosis. J Exp Med 2010;207(8):1589–97.

38. Kato M, Zhang J, Wang M, et al. MicroRNA-192 in diabetic kidney glomeruli and its function in TGF-beta-induced collagen expression via inhibition of E-box repressors. Proc Natl Acad Sci U S A 2007;104(9):3432–7.

39. Yang S, Banerjee S, de Freitas A, et al. Participation of miR-200 in pulmonary fibrosis. Am J Pathol 2012;180(2):484–93.

40. King TE Jr, Tooze JA, Schwarz MI, et al. Predicting survival in idiopathic pulmonary fibrosis: scoring system and survival model. Am J Respir Crit Care Med 2001;164(7):1171–81.

41. Fell CD, Liu LX, Motika C, et al. The prognostic value of cardiopulmonary exercise testing in idiopathic pulmonary fibrosis. Am J Respir Crit Care Med 2009;179(5): 402–7.

42. Raghu G, Collard HR, Egan JJ, et al. An official ATS/ERS/JRS/ALAT statement: idiopathic pulmonary fibrosis: evidence-based guidelines for diagnosis and management. Am J Respir Crit Care Med 2011;183(6):788–824.

43. Raghu G, Mageto YN, Lockhart D, et al. The accuracy of the clinical diagnosis of new-onset idiopathic pulmonary fibrosis and other interstitial lung disease: a prospective study. Chest 1999;116(5):1168–74.

44. Hunninghake GW, Zimmerman MB, Schwartz DA, et al. Utility of a lung biopsy for the diagnosis of idiopathic pulmonary fibrosis. Am J Respir Crit Care Med 2001; 164(2):193–6.

45. Flaherty KR, King TE Jr, Raghu G, et al. Idiopathic interstitial pneumonia: what is the effect of a multidisciplinary approach to diagnosis? Am J Respir Crit Care Med 2004;170(8):904–10.

46. Raghu G, Collard HR, Anstrom KJ, et al. Idiopathic pulmonary fibrosis: clinically meaningful primary endpoints in phase 3 clinical trials. Am J Respir Crit Care Med 2012;185(10):1044–8.

47. Demedts M, Behr J, Buhl R, et al. High-dose acetylcysteine in idiopathic pulmonary fibrosis. N Engl J Med 2005;353(21):2229–42.

48. Raghu G, Anstrom KJ, King TE Jr, et al. Prednisone, azathioprine, and N-acetylcysteine for pulmonary fibrosis. N Engl J Med 2012;366(21):1968–77.

49. de Andrade JA, Olman MA. Coagulation and fibrinolysis in the pathogenesis of pulmonary fibrosis. In: Schwarz M, King TE, editors. Interstitial lung disease. 5th edition. Shelton (CT): People's Medical Publishing House; 2011. p. 315–34.

50. Kubo H, Nakayama K, Yanai M, et al. Anticoagulant therapy for idiopathic pulmonary fibrosis. Chest 2005;128(3):1475–82.

51. Noth I, Anstrom KJ, Calvert SB, et al. A placebo-controlled randomized trial of warfarin in idiopathic pulmonary fibrosis. Am J Respir Crit Care Med 2012;186(1):88–95.

52. Azuma A, Nukiwa T, Tsuboi E, et al. Double-blind, placebo-controlled trial of pirfenidone in patients with idiopathic pulmonary fibrosis. Am J Respir Crit Care Med 2005;171(9):1040–7.

53. Taniguchi H, Ebina M, Kondoh Y, et al. Pirfenidone in idiopathic pulmonary fibrosis. Eur Respir J 2010;35(4):821–9.

54. Noble PW, Albera C, Bradford WZ, et al. Pirfenidone in patients with idiopathic pulmonary fibrosis (CAPACITY): two randomised trials. Lancet 2011;377(9779):1760–9.

55. Martinez FJ, Safrin S, Weycker D, et al. The clinical course of patients with idiopathic pulmonary fibrosis. Ann Intern Med 2005;142(12 Pt 1):963–7.

56. Grossman RF, Frost A, Zamel N, et al. Results of single-lung transplantation for bilateral pulmonary fibrosis. The Toronto Lung Transplant Group. N Engl J Med 1990;322(11):727–33.

57. Christie JD, Edwards LB, Kucheryavaya AY, et al. The registry of the international society for heart and lung transplantation: twenty-eighth adult lung and heart-lung transplant report–2011. J Heart Lung Transplant 2011;30(10):1104–22.

58. Adams M, Williams A, Fell J. Exercise in the fight against thrombosis: friend or foe? Semin Thromb Hemost 2009;35(3):261–8.

59. Kaser A, Martinelli M, Feller M, et al. Heart rate response determines long term exercise capacity after heart transplantation. Swiss Med Wkly 2009;139(21–22):308–12.

60. Ferreira A, Garvey C, Connors GL, et al. Pulmonary rehabilitation in interstitial lung disease: benefits and predictors of response. Chest 2009;135(2):442–7.

61. Crockett AJ, Cranston JM, Antic N. Domiciliary oxygen for interstitial lung disease. Cochrane Database Syst Rev 2001;(3):CD002883.

62. Tzanakis N, Samiou M, Lambiri I, et al. Evaluation of health-related quality-of-life and dyspnea scales in patients with idiopathic pulmonary fibrosis. Correlation with pulmonary function tests. Eur J Intern Med 2005;16(2):105–12.

63. Harris-Eze AO, Sridhar G, Clemens RE, et al. Oxygen improves maximal exercise performance in interstitial lung disease. Am J Respir Crit Care Med 1994;150(6 Pt 1):1616–22.

64. Madison JM, Irwin RS. Chronic cough in adults with interstitial lung disease. Curr Opin Pulm Med 2005;11(5):412–6.

65. Tobin RW, Pope CE 2nd, Pellegrini CA, et al. Increased prevalence of gastro-esophageal reflux in patients with idiopathic pulmonary fibrosis. Am J Respir Crit Care Med 1998;158(6):1804–8.
66. Raghu G, Freudenberger TD, Yang S, et al. High prevalence of abnormal acid gastro-oesophageal reflux in idiopathic pulmonary fibrosis. Eur Respir J 2006; 27(1):136–42.
67. Raghu G, Yang ST, Spada C, et al. Sole treatment of acid gastroesophageal reflux in idiopathic pulmonary fibrosis: a case series. Chest 2006;129(3):794–800.
68. Lee JS, Ryu JH, Elicker BM, et al. Gastroesophageal reflux therapy is associated with longer survival in patients with idiopathic pulmonary fibrosis. Am J Respir Crit Care Med 2011;184(12):1390–4.
69. Lancaster LH, Mason WR, Parnell JA, et al. Obstructive sleep apnea is common in idiopathic pulmonary fibrosis. Chest 2009;136(3):772–8.
70. Krishnan V, McCormack MC, Mathai SC, et al. Sleep quality and health-related quality of life in idiopathic pulmonary fibrosis. Chest 2008;134(4):693–8.
71. Jankowich MD, Polsky M, Klein M, et al. Heterogeneity in combined pulmonary fibrosis and emphysema. Respiration 2008;75(4):411–7.
72. Mejia M, Carrillo G, Rojas-Serrano J, et al. Idiopathic pulmonary fibrosis and emphysema: decreased survival associated with severe pulmonary arterial hypertension. Chest 2009;136(1):10–5.
73. Lettieri CJ, Nathan SD, Barnett SD, et al. Prevalence and outcomes of pulmonary arterial hypertension in advanced idiopathic pulmonary fibrosis. Chest 2006; 129(3):746–52.
74. Nadrous HF, Pellikka PA, Krowka MJ, et al. Pulmonary hypertension in patients with idiopathic pulmonary fibrosis. Chest 2005;128(4):2393–9.
75. Collard HR, Moore BB, Flaherty KR, et al. Acute exacerbations of idiopathic pulmonary fibrosis. Am J Respir Crit Care Med 2007;176(7):636–43.
76. Hajari AS, de Andrade JA. Acute exacerbations of interstitial lung disease. Clin Pulm Med 2011;18(3):113.
77. Raghu G, Brown KK, Bradford WZ, et al. A placebo-controlled trial of interferon gamma-1b in patients with idiopathic pulmonary fibrosis. N Engl J Med 2004; 350(2):125–33.
78. King TE Jr, Behr J, Brown KK, et al. BUILD-1: a randomized placebo-controlled trial of bosentan in idiopathic pulmonary fibrosis. Am J Respir Crit Care Med 2008;177(1):75–81.
79. Raghu G, Brown KK, Costabel U, et al. Treatment of idiopathic pulmonary fibrosis with etanercept: an exploratory, placebo-controlled trial. Am J Respir Crit Care Med 2008;178(9):948–55.
80. King TE Jr, Albera C, Bradford WZ, et al. Effect of interferon gamma-1b on survival in patients with idiopathic pulmonary fibrosis (INSPIRE): a multicentre, randomised, placebo-controlled trial. Lancet 2009;374(9685):222–8.
81. Daniels CE, Lasky JA, Limper AH, et al. Imatinib treatment for idiopathic pulmonary fibrosis: randomized placebo-controlled trial results. Am J Respir Crit Care Med 2010;181(6):604–10.
82. Zisman DA, Schwarz M, Anstrom KJ, et al. A controlled trial of sildenafil in advanced idiopathic pulmonary fibrosis. N Engl J Med 2010;363(7):620–8.
83. Richeldi L, Costabel U, Selman M, et al. Efficacy of a tyrosine kinase inhibitor in idiopathic pulmonary fibrosis. N Engl J Med 2011;365(12):1079–87.

Sarcoidosis

Daniel A. Culver, DO

KEYWORDS

- Sarcoidosis • Granulomas • Tumor necrosis factor • HLA • EBUS-TBNA
- Steroid-sparing • Corticosteroids • Infliximab

KEY POINTS

- Sarcoidosis is a diagnosis of exclusion. In most patients, it requires a biopsy demonstrating non-necrotizing granulomas and no exposure to other agents known to induce granulomatous inflammation.
- Asymptomatic organ involvement that is not readily apparent on routine blood tests, electrocardiogram, or ophthalmologic examination is unlikely to be clinically important, and extensive screening tests to "stage" sarcoidosis are not generally necessary.
- Sarcoidosis will spontaneously remit in up to two-thirds of patients within 5 years of onset. There are insufficient data to support the hypothesis that early treatment increases the prospects for resolution to warrant routine empiric therapy in all patients.
- Corticosteroids have been traditionally used to treat acute, severe manifestations of sarcoidosis; for chronic or refractory disease, steroid-sparing alternatives may be considered.

INTRODUCTION

Sarcoidosis is a highly variable multisystem syndrome characterized by granulomatous inflammation in affected organs. The pathogenesis of sarcoidosis involves an interaction between a putative triggering antigen, probably inhaled, and a susceptible host. The exact causative agent or agents remain unknown. The incidence, severity, and clinical phenotypes of sarcoidosis are influenced by race, ethnicity, gender, and age. In the United States, African Americans are afflicted more often and more severely than are whites. However, the manifestations in any single patient are unpredictable, so that clinicians must actively tailor diagnostic testing, follow-up, and therapy for each individual.

EPIDEMIOLOGY

Sarcoidosis occurs worldwide, with the highest ascertained incidence rates reported in northern European and African American females. A survey conducted in a health maintenance organization in the Detroit, Michigan, area reported age-adjusted

Respiratory Institute, Cleveland Clinic, 9500 Euclid Avenue, Cleveland, OH 44195, USA
E-mail address: culverd@ccf.org

Immunol Allergy Clin N Am 32 (2012) 487–511
http://dx.doi.org/10.1016/j.iac.2012.08.005
0889-8561/12/$ – see front matter © 2012 Published by Elsevier Inc.

immunology.theclinics.com

incidence rates of 10.9 per 100,000 white population and 35.5 per 100,000 black population, based on diagnosis during usual health care.[1] Using these data, it has been estimated that the lifetime risk for developing sarcoidosis is 0.85% in US whites and 2.4% in US blacks.[1] A geographically broader study, the Black Women's Health Study, enrolled 59,000 black women in the United States.[2] The annual incidence of sarcoidosis in that group was calculated to be 71 per 100,000, with a peak of 92 per 100,000 in women aged 40 to 49 years. In addition to susceptibility, race influences disease phenotype, with blacks far more likely to exhibit chronic disease, multiple organ involvement, and morbidity.

It is important to note, however, that the reliability of disease incidence or prevalence estimates may be tenuous. For example, in the US military, sarcoidosis is much more common in recruits from the southeastern states and less common in those from the southwest region.[3,4] In Japan, sarcoidosis is more common in the northern part of the country.[5] Therefore, incidence estimates from any given region are unlikely to be generalizable. Second, because many cases are clinically silent, most cases of sarcoidosis are probably not recognized. For example, in an autopsy study from northeast Ohio, the prevalence rate was estimated to be 320 per 100,000, a 10-fold higher rate than that predicted by death certificate data from the same period.[6] In countries with population-based mass chest radiographic (CXR) screening programs, approximately 50% of the diagnoses of sarcoidosis are made in asymptomatic individuals.[7]

CAUSE AND PATHOGENESIS

The cause of sarcoidosis remains unknown. Based on epidemiologic evidence, it is generally believed that development of sarcoidosis requires exposure to an environmental antigen(s). This hypothesis is supported by several observations, including studies of disease incidence, reports of case-clusters in small populations, transmission by organ transplantation, and the worldwide reproducibility of intradermal granulomatous reactions only in patients with sarcoidosis after the injection of sarcoidosis lymph node homogenate (the Kveim-Siltzbach test).[8]

Infectious agents have long been suspected as possible causes of sarcoidosis, but early studies failed to yield convincing support for various organisms. Using molecular techniques, there are now accumulating data suggesting that immune responses to mycobacteria or *Propionibacterium acnes* may contribute to the disease.[9–11] Based on analogy with a similar granulomatous lung disease, chronic beryllium disease, it is tempting to speculate that there may be more than one etiologic agent capable of causing sarcoidosis. Therefore, it seems likely that development of a sarcoidosis reaction to a triggering antigen depends on a combination of genetic polymorphisms, the status of the host immune system, and the exposure itself.

Besides a relevant exposure, there are substantial data delineating a role for genetic polymorphisms in the susceptibility and phenotype of sarcoidosis. This topic was reviewed recently in detail elsewhere.[12] One example of the importance of genetics comes from a registry-based study of 210 affected twin pairs in Denmark and Finland.[13] Monozygotic twins had an 80-fold increased susceptibility for development of sarcoidosis versus population controls, compared with only a 7-fold increased chance in dizygotic pairs. A range of other studies have reported similar increased heritable risk.[14,15]

Much of the data suggest that the genetic effect on disease risk or severity depends on human leukocyte antigen (HLA) genes governing the expression of the type II major histocompatibility complex on antigen-presenting cells.[12,16] These observations fit well with the current concepts of disease pathogenesis, reserving a central role for activation of antigen-specific oligoclonal CD4+ T cells by major histocompatibility complex class II–restricted antigen-presenting cells, which then amplify immune mechanisms that lead to granuloma formation (**Fig. 1**).

A promising candidate gene, butrophylin-like 2 (*BTNL2*), a putative T-cell costimulatory molecule, was found to have a truncating splice site mutation that strongly associated with sarcoidosis in German patients, with a 23% population attributable risk.[17] Several other reports confirmed the association in whites but not African Americans.[18–20] However, questions have been raised about whether the *BTNL2* effect is independent of the closely linked *HLA-DRB1* genotype.[18,21] Several genomewide association studies have also been completed in sarcoidosis. The first of these led to identification of a polymorphism in the annexin *A11* gene, a molecule involved in several functions including cell organization, calcium signaling, and apoptosis.[22] The association has been replicated in at least 2 independent samples.[23,24] More recently, genomewide approaches identified associations within chromosomes 6, 10, and 11, but validation and functional studies remain to be completed.[25–28]

Several other genes, most commonly cytokines or chemokines, have been associated with sarcoidosis susceptibility or phenotype. However, lack of validation studies and difficulties with interpopulation genetic variability have limited progress in elucidating the genetic profiles in sarcoidosis. It is most likely that multiple genes in combination inform susceptibility and phenotype. The responsible genes probably differ in various populations, and possibly depending on the responsible antigen as well.

DIAGNOSIS

The diagnosis of sarcoidosis is made when clinicoradiologic features are compatible with the disease, there is pathologic evidence of granulomas consistent with sarcoidosis, and other causes of granulomatous inflammation are excluded.[29] In certain situations, the requirement for histopathologic confirmation can be waived (**Box 1**). In patients with extrapulmonary granulomas, it is necessary to confirm that there is multisystem disease, because granulomas in a single organ (eg, skin, liver) may be the

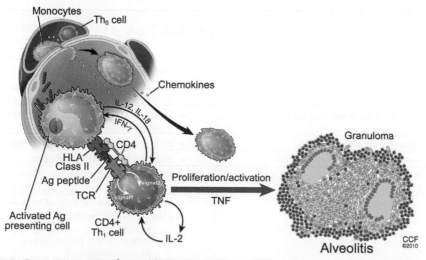

Fig. 1. Current concept of sarcoidosis pathogenesis, centered on an antigen-specific cell-mediated immune response. (*Reprinted with permission* of the American Thoracic Society. Copyright 2012. Baughman RP, Culver DA, Judson MA. A concise review of pulmonary sarcoidosis. Am J Respir Crit Care Med 2011;183(5):573–81.)

Box 1
Situations where sarcoidosis can be confidently diagnosed in the absence of a biopsy

Löfgren syndrome

    Bilateral hilar lymphadenopathy

    Erythema nodosum

    Periarticular inflammation (typically of the ankles, not always present)

    Fever and malaise (usually)

Heerfordt syndrome

    Uveitis

    Parotid swelling

    Fever and malaise (usually)

Asymptomatic bilateral hilar lymphadenopathy

---

result of nonspecific reactions. There are several clinical, radiologic, and laboratory features that influence the likelihood of sarcoidosis (**Table 1**).

Presentation

Sarcoidosis involves the lungs in approximately 90% of patients[30] but causes pulmonary symptoms at presentation in only slightly more than half.[31] The most common symptoms include exertional dyspnea, nonproductive cough, wheezing, and chest pressure. The cough and wheezing may resemble asthma, insofar as they can be triggered by environmental exposures, including dusts, cold air, pollens, and other inhaled agents. The chest pressure associated with sarcoidosis occurs frequently, can be severe, and is often described as squeezing or tightness. It is not related to the size of thoracic lymph nodes.[32] The chest examination is usually unremarkable, so that

Table 1
Selected features influencing the likelihood of sarcoidosis

More Likely	Less Likely
• African American or northern European	• Age <18 • Age >50 in men
• Female	• Smoking
• Symmetric bilateral hilar adenopathy	• Exposure to metal dusts, bioaerosols, organic antigens
• Asymptomatic presentation	• History of exposure to tuberculosis
• Peripheral blood lymphopenia	• History of recurrent infections
• BAL lymphocytes >15% and/or BAL CD4/CD8 ratio >3.5	• Hypogammaglobulinemia

• Multisystem involvement	• Systemic disease capable of inducing granulomatous reactions
	   Malignancy
	   Inflammatory bowel disease
	   Immunodeficiency

• Elevated serum ACE	

Adapted from Judson MA. The diagnosis of sarcoidosis. Clin Chest Med 2008;29:415; with permission from Elsevier.

the presence of rales or clubbing should prompt careful reconsideration of whether sarcoidosis is the correct diagnosis. In patients with airflow obstruction, wheezing may be heard; sometimes the wheezing is focal, representing large airways obstruction from extrinsic compression, architectural distortion, or endobronchial sarcoidosis.

The frequency of abnormal pulmonary function tests (PFTs) correlates loosely with more severe radiologic involvement. For example, abnormal PFTs are found in approximately 20% of patients with Scadding stage I radiographs but are present in 40% to 80% of those with more advanced radiographic stages.[33] Although restrictive physiology is widely assumed to be typical for sarcoidosis, obstructive lung disease is seen as often. At the time of diagnosis, it is present in up to 63% of patients.[34] Bronchoprovocation testing may be positive as well,[35] but exhaled nitric oxide is usually in the normal range.[36]

Chest Imaging

The CXR is abnormal in 85% to 95% of patients with sarcoidosis.[33] Between 30% and 60% of patients present with incidental radiographic abnormalities.[33] The most commonly visible lymph nodes include bilateral hilar, right paratracheal, and aortopulmonary window lymph nodes.[37] The presence of unilateral hilar adenopathy is unusual and should lead to consideration of other diagnoses. When present, infiltrates have a predilection for the mid and upper lung zones. The most common parenchymal findings are reticulonodular infiltrates, but alveolar infiltrates, consolidation, perihilar conglomerate masses, and larger nodules may also be seen.

Chest computed tomography (CT) scanning is now used frequently in diagnosis, but its incremental benefit over CXR has been the subject of controversy.[38] Lymphadenopathy is more commonly noted with CT scan—one pattern that is highly suggestive of sarcoidosis is "frosted" or "icing" calcification in the lymph nodes (**Fig. 2**). With chronic disease, calcifications may become dense or focal but rarely occupy the entire node.

Parenchymal involvement is highly variable. It classically appears as innumerable perilymphatic nodules most concentrated in the mid and upper lung zones (**Fig. 3**). Other CT manifestations include larger nodules, alveolar infiltrates, reticular opacities, septal thickening, and consolidation. Consolidation usually occurs in a perihilar

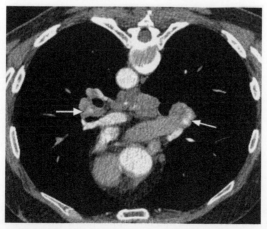

Fig. 2. Faint lymph node calcification characteristic of sarcoidosis on noncontrast chest CT. This pattern has been termed "icing" or "frosting" lymph nodes.

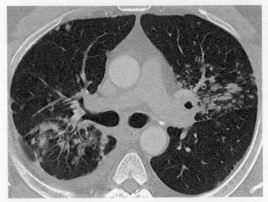

Fig. 3. High-resolution chest CT showing the characteristic micronodular pattern with a bronchovascular distribution seen in many sarcoidosis patients. Chest CT in sarcoidosis is ideally performed without contrast in most situations. (*Courtesy of* Ruchi Yadav, MD.)

distribution in association with fibrosis but does not always imply irreversible disease. Fibrotic sarcoidosis may lead to central or perihilar conglomerate masses, often with architectural distortion or extrinsic compression of the large airways (**Fig. 4**). Other CT features of advanced sarcoidosis include fibrobullous disease and, less frequently, frank honeycombing that may mimic usual interstitial pneumonia.

Sarcoidosis Granulomas

Typically, sarcoidosis granulomas are well-formed clusters of epithelioid histiocytes, together with a few multinucleated giant cells, surrounded by an outer margin of T-lymphocytes (**Fig. 5**). A variable rim of collagen and fibroblasts surrounds the granuloma. Pathologic assessment of sarcoidosis should include stains and cultures for mycobacteria and fungi, which can occasionally cause non-necrotizing granulomas. Sarcoidosis granulomas frequently exhibit focal necrosis,[39] but it is rarely widespread or suppurative. Sarcoidal granulomas contain a variety of inclusion bodies, which were thought in the past to be specific for sarcoidosis but can actually be seen in other

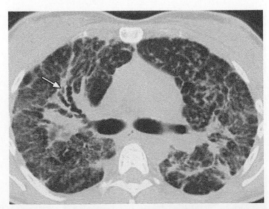

Fig. 4. Fibrobullous sarcoidosis. The pattern of fibrosis in many patients characteristically emanates from the hila, involves the mid and upper lobes, and causes architectural distortion of the airways (*arrow*), often in a curving or arcing pattern that is not seen in other interstitial lung disease.

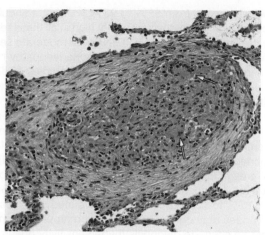

Fig. 5. Pulmonary granuloma from sarcoidosis. A core of epithelioid histiocytes is surrounded by a rim of collagen interspersed with lymphocytes. A few multinucleated giant cells are visible (*arrows*). (*Courtesy of* Carol Farver, MD.)

disorders. These may include calcium bodies (Schaumann bodies, which are made up of calcium carbonate but may contain birefringent calcium oxalate crystals), asteroid bodies within multinucleate giant cells, and Hamazaki-Weisenberg bodies (which may resemble fungal yeast forms).

The granulomas in sarcoidosis tend to be found in the airways submucosa, along the bronchovascular bundle, and in the lymphatics that run along the intralobular septae and pleural surfaces. Besides necrosis, features that suggest alternate diagnoses include loose or poorly formed granulomas, the presence of polarizable material in the granulomas, organizing pneumonia, mononuclear cell infiltrates, and atypical distribution.

Diagnostic Strategy

In most patients with sarcoidosis, a biopsy will be required to confirm the diagnosis. The biopsy site should be selected based on accessibility, procedural morbidity, institutional experience, and patient preference. In general, a physical examination and focused diagnostic testing are adequate to reveal targets for biopsy. Such diagnostic testing in patients with suspected sarcoidosis should include CXR, complete blood count, and liver function testing. High-resolution chest CT is more sensitive than CXR and can be obtained as a second-line test if the CXR is unrevealing. In very difficult cases, whole body PET with flurodeoxyglucose (^{18}F FDG-PET) scan may reveal additional areas of involvement. For example, in a series of 139 scans, unsuspected involvement was revealed in 20 patients (15%), including in the chest in CT-negative patients, peripheral lymph nodes, skin, muscle, and bone.[40] In routine clinical practice, however, FDG-PET is rarely necessary, and its expense is substantial.

The lung is the most frequent site for biopsy confirmation, followed by skin, peripheral lymph nodes, and liver.[41] The approach to diagnosis of pulmonary sarcoidosis changed dramatically with the advent of endobronchial ultrasound (EBUS)-guided transbronchial needle aspiration.[42] A randomized trial in patients with lymphadenopathy suspected to be sarcoidosis comparing EBUS to blind transbronchial needle aspiration (TBNA) found superior sensitivity with EBUS (diagnostic yield of 84% for EBUS vs 54% for standard TBNA).[43] In other series, the yield of EBUS-TBNA for diagnosis of sarcoidosis ranges from 85% to 93%,[44–46] but it should be recognized that the pretest probability of sarcoidosis was very high in all these reports. In a British multicenter prospective study, use of EBUS-TBNA with moderate sedation instead of mediastinoscopy for evaluation of intrathoracic lymphadenopathy reduced costs by 40% ($2117).[47] It is important to recognize that all the studies of diagnostic yield in EBUS-TBNA for sarcoidosis have involved large volume centers with experienced cytopathologists. It is probable that less experienced or less busy cytopathologists will be reluctant to confirm sarcoidosis so that use of EBUS-TBNA as a stand-alone diagnostic mode is still not considered to be the gold standard by many.

Despite the excitement regarding EBUS-TBNA, there are still important roles for standard bronchoscopic techniques. Transbronchial lung biopsy (TBLB) can confirm the diagnosis in 40% to greater than 90% of cases.[48] From 4 to 5 lung biopsies are recommended to maximize the diagnostic yield.[48] When combined with EBUS-TBNA, sensitivity improved from 85% to 93% in one prospective study.[46] Occasionally, reactive intrathoracic lymph nodes may demonstrate granulomatous inflammation consistent with sarcoidosis, but an alternate diagnosis (hypersensitivity pneumonitis, histoplasmosis, malignancy) is made when the lung parenchyma is examined. Therefore, except in classic presentations, it is our practice to routinely obtain TBLB in addition to TBNA specimens.

TBLB is more likely to be diagnostic in patients with parenchymal disease evident on CXR (radiographic stage II or III) than in those with a normal lung parenchyma (radiographic stage 0 or I).[48] Endobronchial biopsy can be performed with the TBLB and has been shown to increase the diagnostic yield for sarcoidosis greater than that by using TBLB alone. The yield of transbronchial lung biopsy for the diagnosis of sarcoidosis is approximately 30% to 50% in patients with hilar adenopathy and no parenchymal infiltrates (CXR stage I).[49]

Bronchoalveolar lavage (BAL) with examination of cell count and lymphocyte populations (CD4/CD8 ratio) is sometimes used as a complementary test for the diagnosis of sarcoidosis. The result of greater than 15% lymphocytes in BAL fluid has a sensitivity of 90% for the diagnosis of sarcoidosis, although the specificity is low.[50] In one study, a lymphocyte CD4/CD8 ratio of greater than 3.5 had a sensitivity of 53%, specificity of 94%, positive predictive value of 76%, and negative predictive value of 85% for the diagnosis of sarcoidosis.[50] The American Thoracic Society recommends routine assessment of cell count and targeted assessment of CD4/CD8 ratio in patients with interstitial lung disease undergoing bronchoscopy.[51]

Diagnostic Pitfalls

Diagnosis is often overlooked as a challenge in sarcoidosis, because many patients exhibit textbook manifestations. However, there is no single test to diagnose sarcoidosis; it relies instead on the clinical acumen of the physician, who must consider the entirety of clinical, radiologic, and pathologic features. Failure to stop and reconsider the diagnosis in situations with incongruent data not infrequently lead to misdiagnosis. Second, because the symptoms and signs of sarcoidosis are very nonspecific, the diagnosis is often not considered at initial presentation. In a multicenter US study, patients with pulmonary symptoms required an average of nearly 5 physician visits before the diagnosis was made.[31]

A common situation in which the diagnosis of pulmonary sarcoidosis is delayed is when the symptoms and signs overlap with other pulmonary diseases, such as asthma. When the presenting CXR has infiltrates but no lymphadenopathy (Scadding stage 3 or 4), the diagnosis is delayed, likely because other interstitial lung diseases or infections are considered first.[31] Certain extrapulmonary organs are often diagnosed very slowly, including neurosarcoidosis (often mistaken for multiple sclerosis), cardiac sarcoidosis (often mistaken for idiopathic cardiomyopathy), ocular sarcoidosis, and sarcoidosis of the upper respiratory tract. When sarcoidosis is in the differential diagnosis for extrapulmonary organs, chest imaging is often helpful.[52]

Sarcoidosis is a systemic disease. When granulomas are found only in extrathoracic organs, a firm diagnosis of sarcoidosis requires evidence of an abnormality consistent with sarcoidosis in a second organ.[41,53] There is no requirement for a biopsy of the second organ—radiologic or other clinical features are typically sufficient. The rationale for this approach is to exclude patients with isolated granulomatous reactions, which are most commonly noted in the skin and liver (**Fig. 6**). A difficulty with this approach is that certain organs, such as the heart and eyes, not infrequently exhibit isolated sarcoidosis.[54,55]

A second major pitfall in the diagnosis of sarcoidosis is failure to identify other causes of granulomatous reactions. These granulomatous reactions may be histopathologically identical to sarcoidosis. For example, in surveys of 2 large sarcoidosis clinics in Germany and Israel, 6% of referred patients were found to have chronic beryllium disease.[56,57] A subsequent Canadian study failed to confirm the association.[58] Other common causes of granulomatous reactions that can be misconstrued as sarcoidosis are listed in **Table 2**. In many cases, the granulomas may be less compact than is typical for sarcoidosis, which should prompt reconsideration of the diagnosis.

A third consideration is exclusion of alternate systemic granulomatous disorders. These are uncommon. Granulomatous reactions may occur in patients with dysregulated immune responses, notably common variable immune deficiency (CVID).[59] The granulomas in CVID tend to be less well formed than in sarcoidosis, and there are often nonspecific inflammatory cell infiltrates in affected tissues. A history of recurring bona fide infections or multiple autoimmune diseases is often a key diagnostic clue; splenomegaly is a common feature as well. When present, therapy may require a combination of immune globulin replacement and immunosuppressive drugs.

Another example is granulomatous lesions of undetermined significance, a syndrome characterized by fevers; granulomas in the liver, bone marrow, spleen, and peripheral lymph nodes; and a nonaggressive course.[60] It is thought to differ from sarcoidosis because (1) the lung is never involved; (2) the serum angiotensin-converting enzyme (ACE) level is normal; (3) when done, the Kveim test result is negative; and (4) it does

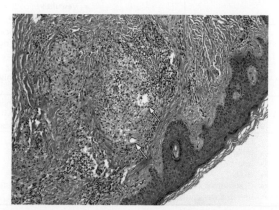

Fig. 6. Nonspecific cutaneous granulomatous reaction to residual foreign material (*arrow*) at the site of a prior trauma decades earlier. The patient had been erroneously labeled as having sarcoidosis.

Table 2
Common or significant major differential diagnosis of sarcoidosis by organ

Organ	Granulomatous Histopathology	Other Mimics
Lung[a]	• Infection (*Mycobacteria*, fungi, Pneumocystis jirovecii) • Hypersensitivity pneumonitis • Metal exposure (beryllium, aluminum, titanium, zirconium) • Granulomatous tumor reactions • Medication reactions • GLILD • Foreign body granulomas (inhaled particulates or aspiration)	• Interstitial lung disease (RBILD, NSIP) • Asthma • Malignancy (lymphoma, metastatic malignancy, adenocarcinoma) • Granulomatosis and polyangiitis (Wegener)
Lymph node	• Infection (*Mycobacteria*, fungi, *Bartonella*, toxoplasmosis, *Brucella*) • Granulomatous tumor reactions • Granulomas associated with immune dysregulation syndromes • GLUS • Foreign body reactions	• Viral (mononucleosis, human immunodeficiency virus, herpes simplex virus) • Lymphoma or other malignancies • Castleman disease • Medication reactions • Lupus erythematosus • Histiocystic necrotizing lymphadenitis (Kikuchi disease) • IgG4-related disease
Skin	• Infections (*Mycobacteria*, fungi) • Foreign body reaction (debris, metals, inflammation) • Rheumatoid nodule/Granuloma annulare • Elastolytic granuloma • Crohn's disease • Nodular vasculitis • Lymphoma	• Prurigo nodularis • Drug eruptions • Vasculitis
Liver	• Infections (tuberculosis, *Brucella*, schistosomiasis) • Primary biliary cirrhosis • Isolated hepatic granulomatosis • Inflammatory bowel disease • GLUS • Lymphoma • Foreign material (e.g mineral oil) • Medications	• Steatohepatitis • Viral hepatitis • Primary sclerosing cholangitis
Eye		• Infections (mycobacterial, syphilis) • Vasculitis • Idiopathic uveitis
Heart	• Giant cell myocarditis	• Eosinophilic myocarditis • Arrhythmogenic right ventricular dysplasia • Amyloidosis • Ischemic and nonischemic cardiomyopathy
Central nervous system	• Infections (tuberculosis, histoplasmosis, cryptococcosis) • Granulomatous tumor reactions	• Malignancy (lymphoma, glioblastoma) • Multiple sclerosis • Neuromyelitis optica (Devic disease)
Spleen	• Granulomatous tumor reactions • Inflammatory bowel disease • Infections (*Mycobacteria*, fungi) • GLUS • Granulomas associated with immune dysregulation syndromes	

Abbreviations: GLILD, granulomatous lymphocytic interstitial lung disease; GLUS, granulomatous lesions of undetermined significance; NSIP, nonspecific interstitial pneumonitis; RBILD, respiratory bronchiolitis interstitial lung disease.

[a] Including intrathoracic lymph nodes.

not cause hypercalcemia.[53] A third multisystem granulomatous disorder is Blau syndrome, a very rare disorder caused by autosomal dominant mutations in the *CARD15/NOD2* gene.[61] Characteristically, Blau syndrome causes uveitis, symmetric polyarticular arthritis, and granulomatous dermatitis.

Assessment of Sarcoidosis

The work-up for routine assessment of organ involvement in sarcoidosis should be parsimonious. The goal of testing is to establish baseline values for commonly involved organs (lungs, liver) and to uncover potentially important occult involvement (eyes, heart). **Box 2** lists the recommended routine studies. When symptoms or physical examination suggest other organ involvement, additional targeted testing may be indicated. However, it is important to consider whether demonstrating organ involvement in a given location will change management in any fashion. A general principle in sarcoidosis is that asymptomatic organ involvement is far more widespread than initially suspected but rarely leads to management changes or affects outcome.

Two organs that may require routine screening even for asymptomatic patients are the eyes and the heart. There is widespread agreement that routine ophthalmologic evaluation, including slit lamp and dilated retinal examinations, is indicated, because unsuspected uveitis may lead to irreversible vision loss.[29] It is less clear whether repeated routine ophthalmologic examinations in asymptomatic patients are useful. Of note, in a US population with sarcoidosis, 23% of patients had developed new organ involvement organ in the interval between diagnosis and 2-year follow-up,[62] including 3% with new ocular inflammation.

Routine screening for cardiac involvement is more controversial. The American Thoracic Society/European Respiratory Society/World Association of Sarcoidosis and Other Granulomatous Disorders consensus statement recommends a baseline electrocardiogram and close follow-up of any consistent symptoms.[29] This is the strategy the author uses at his clinic. However, there is widespread disagreement among sarcoidosis experts, with nearly half suggesting a role for routine echocardiogram and Holter monitoring.[63] In one report, routine use of cardiac magnetic resonance (MR) imaging in a population with chronic sarcoidosis outperformed clinical criteria by a small margin for predicting adverse outcomes.[64] This topic will likely continue to be controversial, as clinicians grapple with balancing the large proportion of patients with clinically irrelevant cardiac involvement ($\sim$80% of those with cardiac

---

Box 2
Suggested initial evaluation of patients with sarcoidosis

Complete history with emphasis on occupational and environmental exposure

Physical examination

    Complete blood count, comprehensive metabolic panel

    Posteroanterior CXR

    Spirometry, carbon monoxide–diffusing capacity

Electrocardiogram

Ophthalmologic examination (with slit lamp)

PPD or interferon-γ release assay for tuberculosis

Urinalysis (if clinically indicated)

involvement) versus the feared complications of sudden cardiac death or advanced cardiomyopathy.

Disease Activity Markers

There is no adequate marker for disease activity in sarcoidosis. Although the serum ACE level is popular and loosely correlates with the total body granuloma burden,[65] it is not sensitive or specific enough to use as a screening test or a basis for diagnosis.[42] As a confounder, the ACE gene has a common insertion-deletion polymorphism that influences serum levels.[66] As a tool for prognosis or for following disease activity, ACE is also very limited. In a cohort of 144 treated and untreated Dutch patients, baseline serum ACE levels were poor predictors of requirement for therapy or of future deterioration in both patients with acute and chronic sarcoidosis.[67] During treatment with corticosteroids, ACE levels fluctuate in an unpredictable fashion that frequently does not correlate with the severity of organ involvement.[68,69] Other serum markers, such as soluble interleukin 2 receptor level, have been inadequately evaluated to recommend widespread adoption at the current time but may outperform ACE.[67,70]

Chest Imaging for Assessment of Sarcoidosis

The baseline CXR confers a loose estimate of the likelihood of spontaneous resolution at 5 years, based on the Scadding stage.[71] The modified Scadding staging system consists of stage 0: no abnormality; stage 1: lymphadenopathy only; stage 2: lymphadenopathy and parenchymal infiltrates; stage 3, parenchymal infiltrates without lymphadenopathy; and stage 4, predominant fibrosis. The staging system has been demonstrated to have approximately equivalent value in European, North American, and Japanese populations. Patients with a baseline stage 1 radiograph have greater than 90% likelihood of disease resolution at 5 years, versus approximately 60% for stage 2 and less than one-third for stage 3. It is important to inform patients that resolution may require several years, a feature that has led some investigators to define chronic disease as 5 years instead of as 2 years (**Fig. 7**).[72,73]

Unfortunately, there are limitations for CXRs in the prognosis and management of sarcoidosis. One study found only fair ($\kappa = 0.43$) agreement between 2 expert readers for defining the Scadding stage of CXRs obtained during a clinical trial.[74] The definition

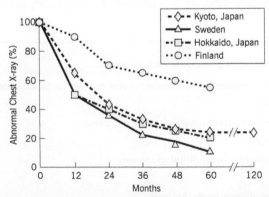

Fig. 7. Rate of CXR resolution. Image used with permission, showing continuous resolution of chest roentgenogram over 5 years with stable findings between 5 and 10 years. (*Reprinted with permission from* Lazar CA, Culver DA. Treatment of sarcoidosis. Semin Respir Crit Care Med 2010;31(4):501–18.)

of stage 4 was the most frequent area of disagreement. Similarly, the readers had only somewhat better concordance ($\kappa = .61$) for global assessment of change with therapy. These data accord with a prospective trial of 36 patients who had exacerbations of pulmonary sarcoidosis.[75] In that study, the 2 readers again had only moderate agreement about whether the radiograph had worsened, and half of the radiographs were interpreted as unchanged or improved during the exacerbation. Based on these data, the role for routine CXR in the follow-up of sarcoidosis has been questioned, unless there are new symptoms or deterioration of PFTs and then only to look for alternate explanations.

Pulmonary Function Testing

Baseline PFTs should be performed for all patients at the time of diagnosis, regardless of the presence of pulmonary sarcoidosis (see **Box 2**). The most commonly used single parameter is the forced vital capacity (FVC), but the diffusing capacity for carbon monoxide independently provides additional useful clinical information.[76] The FVC has been the main endpoint for clinical trials,[77] in large part because it is reproducible, easy to measure, and not influenced by the presence of pulmonary vascular disease. However, the minimal clinically important difference for FVC in sarcoidosis has not been defined. In general, most patients with worsening sarcoidosis will not demonstrate conventionally defined deterioration of greater than 10% to 15% of FVC before seeking treatment. Other tests of pulmonary physiology, such as the 6-minute walk test, plethysmography, cardiopulmonary exercise testing, or measurements of respiratory muscle strength, can be considered in the appropriate clinical context.[78]

EXTRAPULMONARY SARCOIDOSIS

A comprehensive review of extrapulmonary sarcoidosis is beyond the scope of this article. However, sarcoidosis usually involves more than 1 organ. In the ACCESS (A Case Control Etiologic Study of Sarcoidosis) study, approximately half of patients had more than 1 organ involved at presentation.[30] It is not uncommon that health care for these individuals is fragmented among subspecialists, based on which organs are affected. Therefore, it is useful to have an understanding of some of the more common or substantial organs involved with extrapulmonary sarcoidosis. A discussion of the therapeutic approach to these manifestations can be found elsewhere.[73,79]

Skin

Cutaneous sarcoidosis can be divided into 2 categories: specific reactions that are characteristic of the disease in the right setting and a variety of nonspecific lesions that may require a biopsy to confirm the diagnosis. The specific reactions include erythema nodosum (a nongranulomatous panniculitis) and lupus pernio (which does contain granulomas). Ultimately, one-quarter of patients will develop at least 1 dermatologic feature.[80] Erythema nodosum is associated with acute onset of disease and confers a good prognosis for most patients. Tender erythematous raised lesions, usually on the shins, often with associated regional arthritis or periarthritis, are characteristic. Lupus pernio is a chronic plaquelike induration of the face, usually appearing with violacious discoloration of the cheeks, lips, nose, and ears. It may erode into cartilage or bone, causing permanent disfigurement; it is commonly associated with sinonasal sarcoidosis. Lupus pernio generally portends chronic, multisystem sarcoidosis; is more common in older African American or West Indian women; and is notoriously difficult to treat. Other skin lesions include plaques, maculopapular eruptions, hypopigmented or hyperpigmented patches, subcutaneous nodules, and alopecia. Often, the lesions arise in scars or tattoos.

Eyes

Any ocular structure may be affected. In acute disease, anterior uveitis causes photophobia, conjunctivitis, tearing, pain, or blurred vision. It often responds to topical therapy and may be self-limiting. Intermediate or posterior uveitis may be asymptomatic yet lead to significant vision loss over time. Any structure can be involved. Retinal involvement, with characteristic "candle-wax dripping" exudates, multifocal choroiditis, macular edema, and neovascularization, may be asymptomatic but generally requires treatment.

Nervous System

Clinically apparent neurologic disease occurs in 5% to 13% of patients, often in the absence of symptomatic disease in other organs.[81,82] Any neurologic structure may be involved. Central nervous system disease has a predilection for the base of the brain and may cause cranial nerve palsies, especially of the optic or facial nerves. Central nervous system involvement may also cause weakness, ataxia, seizures, headaches, hypopituitarism, and cognitive dysfunction. Peripheral nerve involvement caused by granulomatous neuritis is rare. However, small fiber neuropathy, as a result of nongranulomatous loss of unmeylinated cutaneous sensory and autonomic fibers, is common in chronic sarcoidosis.[83] It responds poorly or not at all to immunosuppressive medications.

MR imaging with gadolinium can be useful, especially when there is leptomeningeal enhancement, which correlates with reversibility.[84] Lumbar puncture should be performed in the appropriate clinical context to exclude mycobacterial or fungal infections or to help monitor disease activity. Cerebrospinal fluid analysis may reveal lymphocytosis, elevated protein, oligoclonal bands, elevated IgG synthesis, and, rarely, elevated ACE levels.[85] As a diagnostic aid, chest imaging should be obtained in patients with suspected neurologic disease, because asymptomatic intrathoracic disease is present in up to 30% of cases.[85]

Heart

In necropsy studies, the prevalence of cardiac disease among US sarcoid patients ranges from 20% to 76%, but clinical disease manifests in only 2% to 7%.[86] In Japan, cardiac involvement is both more frequent and more severe. Because early aggressive treatment improves the prognosis, a high index of suspicion is warranted. Disease manifestations may be caused by active granulomatous inflammation or fibrosis; any cardiac structure may be affected. The most frequent diagnoses include electrophysiologic abnormalities (heart block, dysrhythmias, sudden death) and infiltrative cardiomyopathy.

Imaging of myocardial involvement has evolved in the past decade. Cardiac MR imaging and FDG-PET scanning are more sensitive than perfusion-based modalities such as scintigraphy.[87,88] In a series of consecutive US patients with chronic sarcoidosis, cardiac MR imaging results suggested the possibility of myocardial involvement in 21 (26%) of 81 patients.[64] Metabolism-perfusion PET scanning may be useful to predict response to therapy,[89] although it is limited by expense. Electrocardiography, Holter monitoring, and event monitoring may identify patients with dysrhythmias, and baseline electrocardiography is recommended for all newly diagnosed patients. Endomyocardial biopsy is rarely useful, because of poor sensitivity.[90]

Liver

Biopsies reveal granulomas in 30% to 50% of cases and mild elevations of transaminases or alkaline phosphatase are common, but such findings are rarely of clinical importance.[91] Differentiation from primary biliary cirrhosis can be difficult. Occasionally, liver disease can progress to portal hypertension or cirrhosis. Therapy is not indicated in asymptomatic patients or for mild elevations of liver enzymes.

Spleen and Lymph Nodes

In addition to the high frequency of intrathoracic lymphadenopathy (90%), approximately one-third of patients have palpable peripheral nodes.[29] Palpable splenomegaly, usually asymptomatic, occurs in 14% of cases,[92] whereas histologic disease is present in approximately 50%.

Endocrine System and Calcium Metabolism

Autonomous uncontrolled conversion of 25-hydroxy-vitamin D to 1,25-dihydroxy-vitamin D by activated sarcoid macrophages accounts for the presence of hypercalcemia or hypercalciuria in up to 11% and 20% of patients, respectively.[93] Ectopic vitamin D production usually responds easily to moderate doses of oral corticosteroids or antimalarial agents.

Upper Airway Disease

Involvement of the upper airway occurred in 7% of patients in a referral center but less than 5% of unselected patients.[94] It can be challenging to diagnose, owing to the frequency of nasal symptoms in the general population. The granulomas in upper airways sarcoidosis exhibit necrosis more commonly than in other organs, for unclear reasons.

Besides the typical features of chronic rhinitis, the nasal mucosa may be very friable with crusting or bleeding, and there may be nodularity or marked thickening (**Fig. 8**). Other manifestations include otitis media, vestibular symptoms, hearing loss, exocrine gland swelling, xerostomia, chronic sinusitis, oral ulcerations, and oronasal fistulas. First-line management of all except the most advanced cases should include nasal

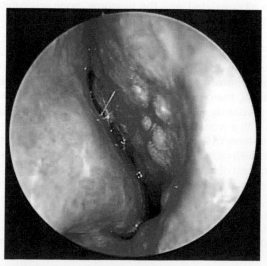

Fig. 8. Cobblestoning appearance of nasal sarcoidosis.

saline spray and saline irrigation. Topical corticosteroids are often only marginally useful. In the author's experience, as well as that of clinicians at other centers, control of upper airways sarcoidosis often requires unusually aggressive therapy.[94]

NATURAL HISTORY AND THERAPY OF SARCOIDOSIS

Although sarcoidosis is usually regarded as a benign disease, it can lead to death; historical estimates placed the attributable mortality risk at 1% to 5%.[29] More recent data from a British population survey spanning 1991–2003 revealed a mortality rate of 5% and 7% at 3 and 5 years, respectively, compared with age- and gender-matched controls for whom mortality was 2% and 4%.[95] An analysis of age-adjusted sarcoidosis mortality based on death certificates suggested that it has increased 51% in women and 30% in men in the United States in the 2 decades from 1988 to 2007.[96] In the United States and Europe, deaths are most commonly a result of progressive pulmonary fibrosis leading to respiratory failure, followed by advanced myocardial or neurologic involvement.[29] In Japan, cardiac involvement has historically been the leading cause of death.[97]

Perhaps more significantly, sarcoidosis causes substantial morbidity because it may lead to persistent symptoms and organ damage in up to one-third of affected individuals.[98,99] Its impact on quality of life is similar to that of other chronic diseases such as acquired immune dysfunction syndrome and moderate to severe chronic obstructive pulmonary disease.[73] Thus, although the course is benign for most afflicted individuals, the true impact of sarcoidosis has likely been underrecognized. Preventing or ameliorating these outcomes is an obvious goal of treatment, but it is complicated by the variable clinical behavior of sarcoidosis.

No single study has comprehensively ascertained which factors most strongly influence the likelihood of spontaneous remission or of clinically bothersome organ involvement. For example, in the US ACCESS study, which was skewed to include a high proportion of patients with pulmonary sarcoidosis, the only independent variables predicting a requirement for ongoing therapy at 2 years after diagnosis were higher dyspnea scores and a requirement for therapy within the first 6 months.[100] **Box 3** lists some features that are most commonly associated with the prognosis. Although these are all correlated with the outcome, none are sufficiently specific to be the sole determinant guiding therapeutic decisions.

Effect of Therapy on Natural History

The bulk of data available do not support the contention that early institution of treatment alters the likelihood of spontaneous remission.[73] For most scenarios, notably pulmonary sarcoidosis, there does not seem to be a worse outcome when therapy is delayed.[101] As previously stated, a requirement for early institution of systemic therapy correlates with a worse prognosis, but it is unclear whether that observation is the result of the severity of the disease or an adverse effect of treatment. In a cohort of Swedish patients with Löfgren syndrome, 80% of *HLA-DRB1*03*-negative patients treated with steroids had disease persistence at 2 years, versus only 37% of untreated patients.[102] Similarly, in a series of primarily African American patients, those individuals who received steroids to control their disease had a 74% likelihood of relapse when therapy was tapered.[103]

There are some controlled trials suggesting the opposite—modest durable improvements of CXR, pulmonary function, and dyspnea with early institution of therapy for up to 18 months.[104–106] However, the effect size in those trials was small and of unclear clinical benefit. At present, there are insufficient data to definitively recommend routine

---

Box 3
Characteristics associated with worse prognosis

Age >40 at onset

African American race

Requirement for steroids

Extrapulmonary involvement

    Cardiac

    Neurologic (except isolated cranial nerve palsy)

    Lupus pernio

    Splenomegaly

    Hypercalcemia

    Osseous disease

Pulmonary involvement

    Stage 3–4 CXR

    Pulmonary hypertension

    Significant lung function impairment

    Moderate to severe dyspnea on presentation

    BAL neutrophilia at presentation

---

institution of empiric therapy for the purpose of improving the natural history for all patients with sarcoidosis, even those with persistent disease.

Indications for Treatment

There are several scenarios that generally require treatment to prevent poor outcomes: posterior or intermediate uveitis, or anterior uveitis refractory to topical therapy; disfiguring cutaneous disease (eg, lupus pernio); cardiac sarcoidosis when it causes cardiomyopathy, dysrhythmias, or atrioventricular block; brain or spinal cord sarcoidosis, except for isolated cranial nerve 7 palsy or mild acute aseptic meningitis; symptomatic hepatosplenic sarcoidosis (ie, pain, consumptive cytopenia, nausea); and significant hypercalcemia.

Therapy

Topical therapy should be considered when possible, including steroid creams, eye drops, nasal corticosteroids, and steroid inhalers. When topical therapy is insufficient, corticosteroids are commonly used as first-line therapy. However, when they are used for maintenance therapy, corticosteroids commonly cause toxicities. As a result, steroid-sparing therapies are used more frequently.

Fig. 9 presents a general algorithm for the management of pulmonary involvement in sarcoidosis. Some organs may require a different approach. For example, cutaneous involvement and hypercalcemia often respond to antimalarial agents or lower doses of steroids. Cardiac sarcoidosis typically requires prolonged treatment before responses are evident. Some authors advocate higher starting doses of corticosteroids for certain organs (eg, cardiac, neurologic), but there are no controlled data on which to base dosing.

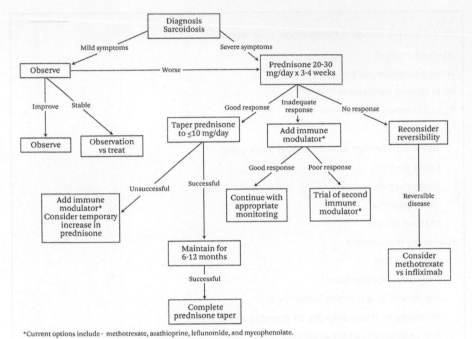

*Current options include - methotrexate, azathioprine, leflunomide, and mycophenolate.

Fig. 9. Algorithm for the management of pulmonary sarcoidosis. (*Reproduced with* Lazar CA, Culver DA. Treatment of sarcoidosis. Semin Respir Crit Care Med 2010;31(4):501–18; with permission.)

A range of alternative therapies are available when there is a poor response to corticosteroids, or when toxicities of corticosteroids occur. The most commonly touted second-line agents include hydroxychloroquine, methotrexate, leflunomide, azathioprine, and mycophenolate mofetil. There have been no head-to-head comparisons of these options. In a 2008 Delphi consensus study among primarily North American sarcoidosis experts, methotrexate was the overwhelming choice for second-line therapy.[107] Since that publication, more data have emerged supporting the use of leflunomide and mycophenolate.[108–110]

The newest widely used medications for sarcoidosis are monoclonal antibody antagonists of tumor necrosis factor (TNF). A randomized, double-blind, placebo-controlled trial of 138 subjects demonstrated the effectiveness of infliximab in chronic treatment–requiring pulmonary disease.[77] In that trial, the mean FVC increased by 2.5% compared with placebo. Patients with FVC less than 70%, higher dyspnea scores and reticulonodular changes on CXR were more likely to respond.[74,77] Although the magnitude of the FVC change has been criticized as small, the effects in the more severe group were similar to those reported in controlled trials of corticosteroids in untreated patients. A secondary endpoint in that study was the effect on extrapulmonary sarcoidosis measured with a novel severity tool; there was a statistically significant improvement in the extrapulmonary manifestations of sarcoidosis in the patients receiving infliximab compared with placebo.[111] Case series have shown that infliximab can also be effective for neurologic, ocular, cutaneous, and bone sarcoidosis.[111–116]

Adalimumab is an alternate monoclonal TNF antagonist with the advantage of subcutaneous administration. It seems to be effective in sarcoidosis in uncontrolled series.[117–119] However, its effect is less rapid than that of infliximab. Potential toxicities from use of TNF antagonists include infection, especially atypical reactivation syndromes from granulomatous organisms, risks of malignancy, and worsening of cardiomyopathy. Given the toxicity concerns and expense of TNF antagonists, their use is generally reserved for patients with moderate to severe disease for whom conventional therapy has failed.

SUMMARY

Sarcoidosis is a protean syndrome that will be encountered by physicians from all specialties. Although it is most common in younger African Americans and northern Europeans, it can occur in adult patients of any age, race, or ethnicity. The pathogenesis remains unclear, but recent data indicate an important role for environmental exposures, possibly from infectious agents, and several genes that are important for immune responses.

The diagnosis of sarcoidosis is challenging, because it is one of exclusion. Finding a granuloma in a pathologic specimen is inadequate to confirm the diagnosis. The astute clinician will consider alternate causes of granulomatous inflammation, search for evidence of multisystem disease, and consider the weight of evidence that weighs for and against the diagnosis.

In most circumstances, assessment of sarcoidosis relies on history, examination, and basic laboratory tools. It is unnecessary to document all possible sites of involvement, because clinically silent disease rarely leads to important sequelae. A noteworthy exception is ocular, and possibly cardiac, sarcoidosis.

Treatment is generally reserved for patients with progressive disease, bothersome symptoms, or organ-threatening involvement. Immunosuppressive drugs are generally titrated to the lowest dose necessary to control the disease. Currently, a range of steroid-sparing agents are used in patients who develop substantial toxicities as a result of corticosteroids or those with refractory disease.

REFERENCES

1. Rybicki BA, Major M, Popovich J Jr, et al. Racial differences in sarcoidosis incidence: a 5-year study in a health maintenance organization. Am J Epidemiol 1997;145(3):234–41.
2. Cozier YC, Berman JS, Palmer JR, et al. Sarcoidosis in black women in the United States: data from the Black Women's Health Study. Chest 2011;139(1): 144–50.
3. McDonough C, Gray GC. Risk factors for sarcoidosis hospitalization among U.S. Navy and Marine Corps personnel, 1981 to 1995. Mil Med 2000;165(8):630–2.
4. Gentry JT, Nitowsky HM, Michael M Jr. Studies on the epidemiology of sarcoidosis in the United States: the relationship to soil areas and to urban-rural residence. J Clin Invest 1955;34(12):1839–56.
5. Yamaguchi M, Hosoda Y, Sasaki R, et al. Epidemiological study on sarcoidosis in Japan. Recent trends in incidence and prevalence rates and changes in epidemiological features. Sarcoidosis 1989;6(2):138–46.
6. Reid JD. Sarcoidosis in coroner's autopsies: a critical evaluation of diagnosis and prevalence from Cuyahoga County, Ohio. Sarcoidosis Vasc Diffuse Lung Dis 1998;15(1):44–51.
7. Hosoda Y, Yamaguchi M, Hiraga Y. Global epidemiology of sarcoidosis. What story do prevalence and incidence tell us? Clin Chest Med 1997;18(4):681–94.
8. Culver DA, Thomassen MJ, Kavuru MS. Pulmonary sarcoidosis: new genetic clues and ongoing treatment controversies. Cleve Clin J Med 2004;71(2):88–90, 2 passim.

9. Ishige I, Usui Y, Takemura T, et al. Quantitative PCR of mycobacterial and propionibacterial DNA in lymph nodes of Japanese patients with sarcoidosis. Lancet 1999;354(9173):120–3.

10. Song Z, Marzilli L, Greenlee BM, et al. Mycobacterial catalase-peroxidase is a tissue antigen and target of the adaptive immune response in systemic sarcoidosis. J Exp Med 2005;201(5):755–67.

11. Oswald-Richter KA, Culver DA, Hawkins C, et al. Cellular responses to mycobacterial antigens are present in bronchoalveolar lavage fluid used in the diagnosis of sarcoidosis. Infect Immun 2009;77(9):3740–8.

12. Grunewald J. Review: role of genetics in susceptibility and outcome of sarcoidosis. Semin Respir Crit Care Med 2010;31(4):380–9.

13. Sverrild A, Backer V, Kyvik KO, et al. Heredity in sarcoidosis: a registry-based twin study. Thorax 2008;63(10):894–6.

14. Rybicki BA, Iannuzzi MC, Frederick MM, et al. Familial aggregation of sarcoidosis. A case-control etiologic study of sarcoidosis (ACCESS). Am J Respir Crit Care Med 2001;164(11):2085–91.

15. McGrath DS, Daniil Z, Foley P, et al. Epidemiology of familial sarcoidosis in the UK. Thorax 2000;55(9):751–4.

16. Rossman MD, Thompson B, Frederick M, et al. HLA-DRB1*1101: a significant risk factor for sarcoidosis in blacks and whites. Am J Hum Genet 2003;73(4):720–35.

17. Valentonyte R, Hampe J, Huse K, et al. Sarcoidosis is associated with a truncating splice site mutation in BTNL2. Nat Genet 2005;37(4):357–64.

18. Wijnen PA, Voorter CE, Nelemans PJ, et al. Butyrophilin-like 2 in pulmonary sarcoidosis: a factor for susceptibility and progression? Hum Immunol 2011; 72(4):342–7.

19. Rybicki BA, Walewski JL, Maliarik MJ, et al. The BTNL2 gene and sarcoidosis susceptibility in African Americans and whites. Am J Hum Genet 2005;77(3): 491–9.

20. Li Y, Wollnik B, Pabst S, et al. BTNL2 gene variant and sarcoidosis. Thorax 2006; 61(3):273–4.

21. Spagnolo P, Sato H, Grutters JC, et al. Analysis of BTNL2 genetic polymorphisms in British and Dutch patients with sarcoidosis. Tissue Antigens 2007; 70(3):219–27.

22. Hofmann S, Franke A, Fischer A, et al. Genome-wide association study identifies ANXA11 as a new susceptibility locus for sarcoidosis. Nat Genet 2008;40(9): 1103–6.

23. Li Y, Pabst S, Kubisch C, et al. First independent replication study confirms the strong genetic association of ANXA11 with sarcoidosis. Thorax 2010;65(10): 939–40.

24. Mrazek F, Stahelova A, Kriegova E, et al. Functional variant ANXA11 R230C: true marker of protection and candidate disease modifier in sarcoidosis. Genes Immun 2011;12(6):490–4.

25. Franke A, Fischer A, Nothnagel M, et al. Genome-wide association analysis in sarcoidosis and Crohn's disease unravels a common susceptibility locus on 10p12.2. Gastroenterology 2008;135(4):1207–15.

26. Fischer A, Schmid B, Ellinghaus D, et al. A novel sarcoidosis risk locus for Europeans on chromosome 11q13.1. Am J Respir Crit Care Med 2012. [Epub ahead of print].

27. Hofmann S, Fischer A, Till A, et al. A genome-wide association study reveals evidence of association with sarcoidosis at 6p12.1. Eur Respir J 2011;38(5): 1127–35.

28. Rybicki BA, Levin AM, McKeigue P, et al. A genome-wide admixture scan for ancestry-linked genes predisposing to sarcoidosis in African-Americans. Genes Immun 2011;12(2):67–77.
29. Hunninghake GW, Costabel U, Ando M, et al. ATS/ERS/WASOG statement on sarcoidosis. American Thoracic Society/European Respiratory Society/World Association of Sarcoidosis and Other Granulomatous Disorders. Sarcoidosis Vasc Diffuse Lung Dis 1999;16(2):149–73.
30. Baughman RP, Teirstein AS, Judson MA, et al. Clinical characteristics of patients in a case control study of sarcoidosis. Am J Respir Crit Care Med 2001;164(10 Pt 1):1885–9.
31. Judson MA, Thompson BW, Rabin DL, et al. The diagnostic pathway to sarcoidosis. Chest 2003;123(2):406–12.
32. Highland KB, Retalis P, Coppage L, et al. Is there an anatomic explanation for chest pain in patients with pulmonary sarcoidosis? South Med J 1997;90(9): 911–4.
33. Lynch JP 3rd, Ma YL, Koss MN, et al. Pulmonary sarcoidosis. Semin Respir Crit Care Med 2007;28(1):53–74.
34. Sharma OP, Johnson R. Airway obstruction in sarcoidosis. A study of 123 nonsmoking black American patients with sarcoidosis. Chest 1988;94(2): 343–6.
35. Shorr AF, Torrington KG, Hnatiuk OW. Endobronchial involvement and airway hyperreactivity in patients with sarcoidosis. Chest 2001;120(3):881–6.
36. Wilsher ML, Fergusson W, Milne D, et al. Exhaled nitric oxide in sarcoidosis. Thorax 2005;60(11):967–70.
37. Bein ME, Putman CE, McLoud TC, et al. A reevaluation of intrathoracic lymphadenopathy in sarcoidosis. AJR Am J Roentgenol 1978;131(3):409–15.
38. Nunes H, Uzunhan Y, Gille T, et al. Imaging of sarcoidosis of the airways and lung parenchyma with correlation with lung function. Eur Respir J 2012;40(3): 750–65.
39. Rosen Y, Vuletin JC, Pertschuk LP, et al. Sarcoidosis: from the pathologist's vantage point. Pathol Annu 1979;14(Pt 1):405–39.
40. Teirstein AS, Machac J, Almeida O, et al. Results of 188 whole-body fluorodeoxyglucose positron emission tomography scans in 137 patients with sarcoidosis. Chest 2007;132(6):1949–53.
41. Teirstein AS, Judson MA, Baughman RP, et al. The spectrum of biopsy sites for the diagnosis of sarcoidosis. Sarcoidosis Vasc Diffuse Lung Dis 2005;22(2): 139–46.
42. Baughman RP, Culver DA, Judson MA. A concise review of pulmonary sarcoidosis. Am J Respir Crit Care Med 2011;183(5):573–81.
43. Tremblay A, Stather DR, Maceachern P, et al. A randomized controlled trial of standard vs endobronchial ultrasonography-guided transbronchial needle aspiration in patients with suspected sarcoidosis. Chest 2009;136(2):340–6.
44. Oki M, Saka H, Kitagawa C, et al. Real-time endobronchial ultrasound-guided transbronchial needle aspiration is useful for diagnosing sarcoidosis. Respirology 2007;12(6):863–8.
45. Garwood S, Judson MA, Silvestri G, et al. Endobronchial ultrasound for the diagnosis of pulmonary sarcoidosis. Chest 2007;132(4):1298–304.
46. Navani N, Booth HL, Kocjan G, et al. Combination of endobronchial ultrasound-guided transbronchial needle aspiration with standard bronchoscopic techniques for the diagnosis of stage I and stage II pulmonary sarcoidosis. Respirology 2011; 16(3):467–72.

47. Navani N, Lawrence DR, Kolvekar S, et al. EBUS-TBNA prevents mediastinoscopies in the diagnosis of isolated mediastinal lymphadenopathy: a prospective trial. Am J Respir Crit Care Med 2012;186(3):255–60.
48. Gilman MJ, Wang KP. Transbronchial lung biopsy in sarcoidosis. An approach to determine the optimal number of biopsies. Am Rev Respir Dis 1980;122(5): 721–4.
49. Koonitz CH, Joyner LR, Nelson RA. Transbronchial lung biopsy via the fiberoptic bronchoscope in sarcoidosis. Ann Intern Med 1976;85(1):64–6.
50. Nagai S, Izumi T. Bronchoalveolar lavage. Still useful in diagnosing sarcoidosis? Clin Chest Med 1997;18(4):787–97.
51. Meyer KC, Raghu G, Baughman RP, et al. An official American Thoracic Society clinical practice guideline: the clinical utility of bronchoalveolar lavage cellular analysis in interstitial lung disease. Am J Respir Crit Care Med 2012;185(9): 1004–14.
52. Kaiser PK, Lowder CY, Sullivan P, et al. Chest computerized tomography in the evaluation of uveitis in elderly women. Am J Ophthalmol 2002;133(4):499–505.
53. Judson MA. The diagnosis of sarcoidosis. Clin Chest Med 2008;29(3):415–27, viii.
54. Wakefield D, Zierhut M. Controversy: ocular sarcoidosis. Ocul Immunol Inflamm 2010;18(1):5–9.
55. Kandolin R, Lehtonen J, Graner M, et al. Diagnosing isolated cardiac sarcoidosis. J Intern Med 2011;270(5):461–8.
56. Muller-Quernheim J, Gaede KI, Fireman E, et al. Diagnoses of chronic beryllium disease within cohorts of sarcoidosis patients. Eur Respir J 2006;27(6):1190–5.
57. Fireman E, Haimsky E, Noiderfer M, et al. Misdiagnosis of sarcoidosis in patients with chronic beryllium disease. Sarcoidosis Vasc Diffuse Lung Dis 2003;20(2): 144–8.
58. Ribeiro M, Fritscher LG, Al-Musaed AM, et al. Search for chronic beryllium disease among sarcoidosis patients in Ontario, Canada. Lung 2011;189(3): 233–41.
59. Morimoto Y, Routes JM. Granulomatous disease in common variable immunodeficiency. Curr Allergy Asthma Rep 2005;5(5):370–5.
60. Brincker H. Granulomatous lesions of unknown significance: the GLUS syndrome. In: James D, editor. Sarcoidosis and other granulomatous disorders. New York: Marcel Dekker; 1994. p. 69–76.
61. Rose CD, Martin TM, Wouters CH. Blau syndrome revisited. Curr Opin Rheumatol 2011;23(5):411–8.
62. Judson MA, Baughman RP, Thompson BW, et al. Two year prognosis of sarcoidosis: the ACCESS experience. Sarcoidosis Vasc Diffuse Lung Dis 2003;20(3): 204–11.
63. Hamzeh NY, Wamboldt FS, Weinberger HD. Management of cardiac sarcoidosis in the United States: a Delphi study. Chest 2012;141(1):154–62.
64. Patel MR, Cawley PJ, Heitner JF, et al. Detection of myocardial damage in patients with sarcoidosis. Circulation 2009;120(20):1969–77.
65. Studdy PR, Bird R, Neville E, et al. Biochemical findings in sarcoidosis. J Clin Pathol 1980;33(6):528–33.
66. Tomita H, Ina Y, Sugiura Y, et al. Polymorphism in the angiotensin-converting enzyme (ACE) gene and sarcoidosis. Am J Respir Crit Care Med 1997; 156(1):255–9.
67. Rothkrantz-Kos S, van Dieijen-Visser MP, Mulder PG, et al. Potential usefulness of inflammatory markers to monitor respiratory functional impairment in sarcoidosis. Clin Chem 2003;49(9):1510–7.

68. Baughman RP, Ploysongsang Y, Roberts RD, et al. Effects of sarcoid and steroids on angiotensin-converting enzyme. Am Rev Respir Dis 1983;128(4): 631–3.
69. Gronhagen-Riska C, Selroos O, Niemisto M. Angiotensin converting enzyme. V. Serum levels as monitors of disease activity in corticosteroid-treated sarcoidosis. Eur J Respir Dis 1980;61(2):113–22.
70. Ziegenhagen MW, Rothe ME, Schlaak M, et al. Bronchoalveolar and serological parameters reflecting the severity of sarcoidosis. Eur Respir J 2003;21(3): 407–13.
71. Scadding JG. Prognosis of intrathoracic sarcoidosis in England. A review of 136 cases after five years' observation. Br Med J 1961;5261:1165–72.
72. Baughman RP, Costabel U, du Bois RM. Treatment of sarcoidosis. Clin Chest Med 2008;29(3):533–48, ix–x.
73. Lazar CA, Culver DA. Treatment of sarcoidosis. Semin Respir Crit Care Med 2010;31(4):501–18.
74. Baughman RP, Shipley R, Desai S, et al. Changes in chest roentgenogram of sarcoidosis patients during a clinical trial of infliximab therapy: comparison of different methods of evaluation. Chest 2009;136(2):526–35.
75. Judson MA, Gilbert GE, Rodgers JK, et al. The utility of the chest radiograph in diagnosing exacerbations of pulmonary sarcoidosis. Respirology 2008;13(1): 97–102.
76. Barros WG, Neder JA, Pereira CA, et al. Clinical, radiographic and functional predictors of pulmonary gas exchange impairment at moderate exercise in patients with sarcoidosis. Respiration 2004;71(4):367–73.
77. Baughman RP, Drent M, Kavuru M, et al. Infliximab therapy in patients with chronic sarcoidosis and pulmonary involvement. Am J Respir Crit Care Med 2006;174(7):795–802.
78. Lynch JP 3rd, Kazerooni EA, Gay SE. Pulmonary sarcoidosis. Clin Chest Med 1997;18(4):755–85.
79. Judson MA. Extrapulmonary sarcoidosis. Semin Respir Crit Care Med 2007; 28(1):83–101.
80. Sharma OP. Cutaneous sarcoidosis: clinical features and management. Chest 1972;61(4):320–5.
81. Stern BJ, Krumholz A, Johns C, et al. Sarcoidosis and its neurological manifestations. Arch Neurol 1985;42(9):909–17.
82. Lower EE, Broderick JP, Brott TG, et al. Diagnosis and management of neurological sarcoidosis. Arch Intern Med 1997;157(16):1864–8.
83. Tavee J, Culver D. Sarcoidosis and small-fiber neuropathy. Curr Pain Headache Rep 2011;15(3):201–6.
84. Dumas JL, Valeyre D, Chapelon-Abric C, et al. Central nervous system sarcoidosis: follow-up at MR imaging during steroid therapy. Radiology 2000;214(2): 411–20.
85. Zajicek JP, Scolding NJ, Foster O, et al. Central nervous system sarcoidosis—diagnosis and management. QJM 1999;92(2):103–17.
86. Deng JC, Baughman RP, Lynch JP. Cardiac involvement in sarcoidosis. Semin Respir Crit Care Med 2002;23(6):513–27.
87. Tadamura E, Yamamuro M, Kubo S, et al. Effectiveness of delayed enhanced MRI for identification of cardiac sarcoidosis: comparison with radionuclide imaging. AJR Am J Roentgenol 2005;185(1):110–5.
88. Yamagishi H, Shirai N, Takagi M, et al. Identification of cardiac sarcoidosis with (13)N-NH(3)/(18)F-FDG PET. J Nucl Med 2003;44(7):1030–6.

89. Isiguzo M, Brunken R, Tchou P, et al. Metabolism-perfusion imaging to predict disease activity in cardiac sarcoidosis. Sarcoidosis Vasc Diffuse Lung Dis 2011;28(1):50–5.

90. Uemura A, Morimoto S, Hiramitsu S, et al. Histologic diagnostic rate of cardiac sarcoidosis: evaluation of endomyocardial biopsies. Am Heart J 1999;138(2 Pt 1): 299–302.

91. Vatti R, Sharma OP. Course of asymptomatic liver involvement in sarcoidosis: role of therapy in selected cases. Sarcoidosis Vasc Diffuse Lung Dis 1997; 14(1):73–6.

92. Kataria YP, Whitcomb ME. Splenomegaly in sarcoidosis. Arch Intern Med 1980; 140(1):35–7.

93. James DG, Neville E, Siltzbach LE. A worldwide review of sarcoidosis. Ann N Y Acad Sci 1976;278:321–34.

94. Panselinas E, Halstead L, Schlosser RJ, et al. Clinical manifestations, radiographic findings, treatment options, and outcome in sarcoidosis patients with upper respiratory tract involvement. South Med J 2010;103(9):870–5.

95. Gribbin J, Hubbard RB, Le Jeune I, et al. Incidence and mortality of idiopathic pulmonary fibrosis and sarcoidosis in the UK. Thorax 2006;61(11):980–5.

96. Swigris JJ, Olson AL, Huie TJ, et al. Sarcoidosis-related mortality in the United States from 1988 to 2007. Am J Respir Crit Care Med 2011;183(11):1524–30.

97. Sekiguchi M, Yazaki Y, Isobe M, et al. Cardiac sarcoidosis: diagnostic, prognostic, and therapeutic considerations. Cardiovasc Drugs Ther 1996;10(5): 495–510.

98. Iannuzzi MC, Rybicki BA, Teirstein AS. Sarcoidosis. N Engl J Med 2007;357(21): 2153–65.

99. Siltzbach LE, James DG, Neville E, et al. Course and prognosis of sarcoidosis around the world. Am J Med 1974;57(6):847–52.

100. Baughman RP, Judson MA, Teirstein A, et al. Presenting characteristics as predictors of duration of treatment in sarcoidosis. QJM 2006;99(5):307–15.

101. Hunninghake GW, Gilbert S, Pueringer R, et al. Outcome of the treatment for sarcoidosis. Am J Respir Crit Care Med 1994;149(4 Pt 1):893–8.

102. Grunewald J, Eklund A. Lofgren's syndrome: human leukocyte antigen strongly influences the disease course. Am J Respir Crit Care Med 2009;179(4):307–12.

103. Gottlieb JE, Israel HL, Steiner RM, et al. Outcome in sarcoidosis. The relationship of relapse to corticosteroid therapy. Chest 1997;111(3):623–31.

104. Pietinalho A, Tukiainen P, Haahtela T, et al. Early treatment of stage II sarcoidosis improves 5-year pulmonary function. Chest 2002;121(1):24–31.

105. Culver DA. Pro: the treatment of the granulomatous response is beneficial in acute sarcoidosis. Respir Med 2010;104(12):1775–7.

106. Gibson GJ, Prescott RJ, Muers MF, et al. British Thoracic Society Sarcoidosis study: effects of long term corticosteroid treatment. Thorax 1996;51(3):238–47.

107. Schutt AC, Bullington WM, Judson MA. Pharmacotherapy for pulmonary sarcoidosis: a Delphi consensus study. Respir Med 2010;104(5):717–23.

108. Sahoo DH, Bandyopadhyay D, Xu M, et al. Effectiveness and safety of leflunomide for pulmonary and extrapulmonary sarcoidosis. Eur Respir J 2011;38(5): 1145–50.

109. Androdias G, Maillet D, Marignier R, et al. Mycophenolate mofetil may be effective in CNS sarcoidosis but not in sarcoid myopathy. Neurology 2011;76(13):1168–72.

110. Bhat P, Cervantes-Castaneda RA, Doctor PP, et al. Mycophenolate mofetil therapy for sarcoidosis-associated uveitis. Ocul Immunol Inflamm 2009;17(3): 185–90.

111. Judson MA, Baughman RP, Costabel U, et al. Efficacy of infliximab in extrapulmonary sarcoidosis: results from a randomised trial. Eur Respir J 2008;31(6): 1189–96.
112. Carter JD, Valeriano J, Vasey FB, et al. Refractory neurosarcoidosis: a dramatic response to infliximab. Am J Med 2004;117(4):277–9.
113. Doty JD, Mazur JE, Judson MA. Treatment of sarcoidosis with infliximab. Chest 2005;127(3):1064–71.
114. Moravan M, Segal BM. Treatment of CNS sarcoidosis with infliximab and mycophenolate mofetil. Neurology 2009;72(4):337–40.
115. Saleh S, Ghodsian S, Yakimova V, et al. Effectiveness of infliximab in treating selected patients with sarcoidosis. Respir Med 2006;100(11):2053–9.
116. Sodhi M, Pearson K, White ES, et al. Infliximab therapy rescues cyclophosphamide failure in severe central nervous system sarcoidosis. Respir Med 2009; 103(2):268–73.
117. Erckens RJ, Mostard RL, Wijnen PA, et al. Adalimumab successful in sarcoidosis patients with refractory chronic non-infectious uveitis. Graefes Arch Clin Exp Ophthalmol 2012;250(5):713–20.
118. Kamphuis LS, Lam-Tse WK, Dik WA, et al. Efficacy of adalimumab in chronically active and symptomatic patients with sarcoidosis. Am J Respir Crit Care Med 2011;184(10):1214–6.
119. Milman N, Graudal N, Loft A, et al. Effect of the TNF-alpha inhibitor adalimumab in patients with recalcitrant sarcoidosis: a prospective observational study using FDG-PET. Clin Respir J 2011. http://dx.doi.org/10.1111/j.1752-699X.2011.00276.x.

Connective Tissue Disease–Associated Lung Disease

Amy L. Olson, MD[a], Kevin K. Brown, MD[a], Aryeh Fischer, MD[a,b],*

KEYWORDS

- Connective tissue disease • Interstitial lung disease • Collagen vascular disease

KEY POINTS

- Patients with CTDs are at high risk for a number of pulmonary complications.
- A multidisciplinary, comprehensive evaluation is indicated for CTD patients with respiratory symptoms to explore a broad differential diagnosis that often includes respiratory infection, medication-associated lung toxicity, and autoimmune mediated lung injury.
- CTD-associated lung disease is often characterized by multi-compartment involvement: airways, lung parenchyma, pleura, and vascular.
- Lung disease may present at any time in the course of a CTD – and may even be the presenting manifestation of a CTD.
- Heightened surveillance for respiratory illness is indicated in the care of all patients with CTD.

INTRODUCTION

The designations of "connective tissue disease" (CTD) or "collagen vascular disease" are used interchangeably and refer to the spectrum of systemic autoimmune diseases characterized by autoimmune phenomena (eg, circulating autoantibodies) and autoimmune-mediated organ damage. Even though these disorders are grouped together, it is important to recognize that there is significant heterogeneity of clinical features associated with each specific CTD. The CTDs include rheumatoid arthritis (RA), systemic lupus erythematosus (SLE), systemic sclerosis (SSc, scleroderma), poly-/dermatomyositis (PM/DM), primary Sjögren syndrome (SjS), mixed CTD (MCTD), and undifferentiated CTD (UCTD) (**Box 1**).

The lungs are a frequent target of autoimmune mediated injury in patients with CTD. There are multiple pulmonary manifestations; essentially every component of the respiratory tract is at risk and certain CTDs are associated with specific patterns of lung involvement (**Box 2 and Table 1**).[1–4] As an example, some CTDs are more likely to be associated with airways disease or interstitial lung disease (ILD) than are others, but all patients with CTD are at risk for multicompartment lung involvement.

[a] Autoimmune and Interstitial Lung Disease Program, National Jewish Health, 1400 Jackson Street, Denver, CO 80206, USA; [b] Division of Rheumatology, National Jewish Health, 1400 Jackson Street, Denver, CO 80206, USA
* Corresponding author. Division of Rheumatology, 1400 Jackson Street, Denver, CO 80206.
E-mail address: fischera@njhealth.org

Immunol Allergy Clin N Am 32 (2012) 513–536
http://dx.doi.org/10.1016/j.iac.2012.09.002
0889-8561/12/$ – see front matter © 2012 Elsevier Inc. All rights reserved.

Box 1
CTDs and other rheumatologic diseases associated with lung disease

Connective Tissue Diseases

Rheumatoid arthritis

Systemic lupus erythematosus

Systemic sclerosis (scleroderma)

Primary Sjogren's syndrome

Poly-/dermatomyositis (Anti-synthetase syndrome)

Mixed connective tissue disease

Undifferentiated connective tissue disease

Other "rheumatologic" disorders

Systemic vasculitis

  Polyangiitis with granulomatosis (Wegener's)

  Microscopic polyangiitis

  Churg-Strauss vasculitis

Spondyloarthropathy

Relapsing polychondritis

Behçet's disease

Antiphospholipid syndrome

Thus, the intersection of lung disease and CTD is complex because of the myriad pulmonary manifestations that can occur with any of these disorders. Furthermore, although many of the lung manifestations occur within the first few years of the CTD diagnosis, their development much later is not unusual, and they may even be the presenting feature of an underlying CTD.[5–11] In the following sections, we review the characteristics and impact of CTD-associated lung disease.

CATEGORIES OF LUNG INVOLVEMENT

It is important to consider several diagnostic possibilities when a patient with CTD presents with new respiratory symptoms (see **Box 2**). A wide range of differential diagnostic possibilities exist, and these may be grouped into the following categories: infection, drug-induced lung toxicity, direct pulmonary complications (eg, ILD); indirect complications (eg, hypoventilation secondary to myopathy); cardiovascular complications (eg, coronary artery disease or cardiomyopathy); and unrelated disease.[4] In particular, because cardiovascular complications are responsible for a significant proportion of the mortality seen in patients with CTD,[12] it is also important to consider ischemia and cardiomyopathy.

Respiratory Infection

Respiratory infections are common in CTD and account for significant morbidity and mortality. Predisposing risk factors for respiratory infection in patients with CTD include intrinsic abnormalities such as respiratory muscle weakness, airways disease, and underlying immune dysfunction. Furthermore, and perhaps most significant, many of these patients are on potent immunosuppressive medications.[13] Thus, patients with CTD are at increased risk for the development of infection, and when respiratory

Box 2
Primary and secondary pulmonary manifestations of CTDs

Primary manifestations

Pleural

    Pleurisy

    Effusion/thickening

Airways

    Upper

        Cricoarytenoid disease

        Tracheal disease

    Lower

        Bronchiectasis

        Bronchiolitis

Vascular

    Pulmonary arterial hypertension

    Vasculitis

Parenchymal

    ILD

    Diffuse alveolar hemorrhage

    Acute pneumonitis

Rheumatoid nodules

Secondary manifestations

Infections

Drug toxicity

Malignancy

Thromboembolism

Table 1
Most common CTD-associated pulmonary manifestations

	SSc	RA	Primary SjS	MCTD	PM/DM	SLE
Airways	–	++	++	+	–	+
ILD	+++	++	++	++	+++	+
Pleural	–	++	+	+	–	+++
Vascular	+++	–	+	++	+	+
DAH	–	–	–	–	–	++

The number of + signs indicates relative prevalence of each manifestation.
Data from Fischer A, du Bois R. Interstitial lung disease in connective tissue disorders. Lancet 2012;380(9842):689–98.

symptoms develop, thorough evaluation to exclude the presence of routine and opportunistic infections should be undertaken.[13–15]

Medication-Induced Lung Toxicity

Many of the anti-inflammatory and immunosuppressive medications used to treat CTD have been associated with the development of lung toxicity. These include aspirin, nonsteroidal anti-inflammatory drugs, sulfasalazine, methotrexate (MTX), cyclophosphamide, azathioprine, mycophenolate mofetil, D-penicillamine, leflunomide, and anti–tumor necrosis factor (TNF)α antagonists.[2,4,14–17] However, a diagnosis of drug-induced lung disease can be challenging – because the clinical presentation and radiographic and histologic patterns are nonspecific and frequently mimic either infection or primary CTD-associated pulmonary involvement. A comprehensive and updated list of medications with their reported pulmonary toxicities can be found online at www.pneumotox.com.

Of all the immunosuppressive medications used to treat patients with CTD, MTX is generally considered to have the most potential for pulmonary toxicity. Symptomatically, it is characterized by the subacute (during several weeks) onset of dyspnea, cough, and fever. However, acute (occurring over days), chronic (occurring over months), and a delayed reaction occurring after the discontinuation of MTX have all been described. Radiographically, a pattern of interstitial (with or without alveolar) infiltrates in the lower lung fields may be present, whereas the histopathologic patterns seen on surgical lung biopsy sample include a cellular (lymphoplasmacytic) interstitial infiltrate with or without granulomata and acute and organizing diffuse alveolar damage (DAD). Neither the duration nor the dose predicts MTX pulmonary toxicity, although underlying RA and male sex may be risk factors to its development.[4,16] Therapy includes the discontinuation of MTX and the initiation of steroids; mortality ranges from 13% to 22%.[16,18,19]

Cyclophosphamide, an alkylating agent often used in SSc-associated ILD, has rarely been associated with both early and delayed pulmonary toxicity.[20] Early toxicity typically occurs after 1 to 6 months of exposure, may result in nonspecific reticulonodular infiltrates on imaging, and is potentially reversible after withdrawal of the agent and initiation of glucocorticoid therapy. Delayed pulmonary toxicity occurs after months to years of therapy and is difficult to distinguish from ILD associated with the underlying CTD. Characteristic radiographic manifestations are reported to include lung fibrosis with bilateral pleural thickening. This form of toxicity is typically irreversible and may be progressive despite the cessation of drug.[4,20] Both azathioprine and mycophenolate mofetil are commonly used in the management of various forms of CTD – including CTD-associated ILD (CTD-ILD).[21] It is important that each has also been rarely associated with pulmonary toxicity ranging from DAD to lung fibrosis, and these effects have been reported to be dose related.[22–24]

During the past 15 years, the management of the rheumatic diseases has been revolutionized by the advent of targeted biologic therapy. In particular, the anti-TNFα antagonists have demonstrated a high degree of efficacy for RA, inflammatory bowel disease, psoriasis, ankylosing spondylitis, and miscellaneous other autoinflammatory diseases.[25] There have been numerous case reports describing the new development of diffuse parenchymal lung disease in patients being treated with each of these agents, suggesting a component of direct pulmonary toxicity associated with their use.[14,15,17,26–30] Even more significant than their potential for pulmonary toxicity, the class of anti-TNFα antagonists is highly immunosuppressive and patients treated with these agents are at high risk for typical and atypical respiratory infections.

Pulmonary Manifestations

The lung itself is a frequent target of autoimmune-mediated damage in patients with CTD, although the incidence of any particular complication varies by individual CTD (see **Box 2**). Within the lung, each of the unique anatomic compartments can be involved by 1 or more pathologic processes that adversely affects its ability to function normally, including cellular infiltration (inflammation), fibrosis, and architectural distortion. The airway, from the larynx to the bronchiole; the parenchyma; the vasculature; and the pleural can also be involved either individually or in some combination.[3,4] For example, in SSc, isolated pulmonary arterial hypertension, sole fibrosing ILD, or a combination of these processes is responsible for most associated deaths.[31]

ILD is a frequently identified entity in preexisting CTD; recent studies of CTD cohorts have shown radiographic prevalence rates of subclinical ILD ranging from 33% to 57%.[31–36] ILD is particularly common in patients who have SSc, PM/DM, RA, primary SjS, and MCTD. However, just because ILD is identified in a patient with CTD does not mean the 2 are necessarily related. For example, the presence of preexisting RA does not preclude, and may predispose toward, the development of lung injury as a result of other causes (eg, infection and drug-induced pneumonitis). In this regard, just as with any other patient who presents with diffuse parenchymal lung disease, a comprehensive evaluation is needed to explore all potential causes (eg, infection, drug-toxicity, environmental and occupational exposures, familial disease, smoking-related lung disease, and malignancy). Determining whether the ILD is associated with the preexisting CTD is decided through a process of elimination.[2]

Indirect Pulmonary Complications

Because of the systemic nature of CTD, virtually all organ systems are impacted. Indirect pulmonary complications are the result of abnormalities in extrathoracic aspects that have a direct bearing on lung function but not through a primary alteration of the underlying lung architecture per se. Such manifestations may include musculoskeletal abnormalities (eg, respiratory muscle weakness caused by myopathy in PM/DM), gastrointestinal diseases (eg, gastroesophageal reflux with aspiration in SSc), or immunologic (eg, immunodeficiency secondary to complement abnormalities in SLE), hematologic (eg, antiphospholipid antibody positivity), or cardiovascular dysfunction (eg, cardiomyopathy in PM/DM). Abnormalities in 1 or more of these systems often leads to clinically significant respiratory compromise even in the absence of underlying structural lung disease and further highlights the need for comprehensive assessments in the patient with CTD with respiratory symptoms.[2,4]

SPECIFIC CTDS
SSc (Scleroderma)

SSc is a systemic autoimmune disease characterized by autoimmunity, fibrosis, and widespread small-vessel vasculopathy. Lung disease is identified in most patients with SSc; indeed, ILD and pulmonary arterial hypertension (PAH) are the leading causes of mortality.[31,37] One of the cardinal features of SSc is thickening of the skin, and the extent of skin involvement defines its various subtypes. Limited cutaneous systemic sclerosis (LcSSc) is defined by skin thickening limited to body surface areas below the elbows and knees and not involving the trunk (chest or abdominal wall).[38] In contrast, diffuse cutaneous systemic sclerosis (DcSSc) is defined by more proximal and extensive skin thickening that includes sclerodermatous skin changes proximal to the elbows or knees or involving the trunk.[38] In addition, some patients have characteristic clinical features of SSc without overt evidence of skin thickening, and these patients may be considered to represent a subset of LcSSc or are more accurately characterized as having SSc sine scleroderma (ssSSc).[39] Distinguishing these subtypes of SSc is important because they often have different clinical courses and have different patterns of lung involvement.[31,40]

LcSSc and ssSSc typically present insidiously and are characterized by minimal skin-associated symptoms. Raynaud phenomenon is seen in virtually all of these patients and may predate any subsequent manifestations by 10 to 15 years. Digital edema (puffy hands), palmar and facial telangiectasia, and gastroesophageal reflux disease are also identified in nearly all of these patients. SSc-specific autoantibodies provide particular insights into the type of lung disease that occur with LcSSc and ssSSc.[40] Those with anticentromere antibodies have the highest risk for PAH and are at much less risk for progressive ILD. In contrast, those with anti–Scl-70 antibodies are at highest risk for progressive ILD and a lower risk for PAH. An in-between category is composed of patients with SSc with positive nucleolar staining antinuclear antibodies (ANA) with a negative anti–Scl-70. These patients are considered to have an "isolated nucleolar" ANA and are at high risk for developing both progressive ILD and PAH.[31,40]

Patients with DcSSc present more acutely with a variety of symptoms. Active and diffuse skin thickening is often a prominent early feature. Digital edema, inflammatory arthritis, and symptoms of carpal tunnel syndrome also may be early findings. Constitutional symptoms of fatigue, malaise, weight loss, and low-grade fevers are common. Patients with DcSSc are at high risk for early progressive ILD and scleroderma renal crisis. As a group, DcSSc is associated with a worse prognosis than is LcSSc or ssSSc.

The 2 most common pulmonary manifestations of SSc are ILD and PAH – and these manifestations alone account for 60% of SSc-related deaths.[31,41] As a general rule, PAH tends to be a later manifestation in SSc and is most strongly associated with LcSSc, and either a positive anticentromere or isolated nucleolar ANA. Progressive ILD tends to be an earlier manifestation (within the first 5–7 years) and is most strongly associated with the presence of a positive anti–Scl-70 antibody or those with nucleolar-pattern ANA – in either LcSSc, DcSSc, or ssSSc subtype.[31,37] It is important to recognize that although these descriptions can be helpful to better understand and risk stratify patients based on precise clinical phenotype, both progressive ILD and PAH have been described in each of the subsets of disease and as early or late manifestations.

Airways Disease and Pleural Disease

Although evidence of airways disease on pulmonary function testing may be identified, clinically significant airways disease is rare.[42] These subtle abnormalities may be related to prior tobacco exposure or possible subclinical follicular bronchiolitis.[43,44]

Unlike other CTDs such as RA and SLE, symptomatic pleuritis and/or pleural effusions are uncommon in SSc.[4]

Vascular Disease

SSc-associated PAH may result from primary arteriopathy (histologically similar to idiopathic PAH with either plexiform lesions and/or concentric intimal obliteration of pulmonary vessels).[45] The true prevalence of PAH in SSc is unknown, but it is estimated that right-heart catheter-proved PAH has a prevalence of about 10%.[46] Risk factors for the development of SSc-PAH includes limited cutaneous disease, long-standing Raynaud phenomenon, extensive telangiectasia, positive anticentromere antibody or isolated nucleolar ANA, or isolated reduction in diffusing capacity for carbon monoxide (DLco).[46] The introduction of PAH-specific therapies has favorably impacted survival in SSc-PAH. Before the discovery and use of these agents in SSc- PAH, the 1-year survival rate in SSc-PAH was 45%.[47] However, recent reported 1- and 3-year survival rates for patients with SSc-PAH are 78% and 47%, respectively.[48]

ILD

Proportionally, ILD is identified more often in SSc than in any other CTD; evidence of radiographic findings of ILD occurs in nearly all patients with SSc and clinically significant disease occurs in approximately 40% of patients (**Fig. 1**).[49] The most prevalent histologic pattern identified in SSc is fibrotic nonspecific interstitial pneumonia (NSIP) followed by the usual interstitial pneumonia (UIP) lung injury pattern.[50–53]

Aspiration/Gastroesophageal Reflux Disease

Esophageal dysmotility and gastroesophageal reflux disease are quite common in patients with SSc. Medication therapy with proton-pump inhibitors for gastroesophageal reflux disease and a proactive approach to prevent aspiration are usually advised.

Bronchogenic Carcinoma

The true risk of bronchogenic carcinoma in patients with SSc is unknown and the available data are conflicting.[54] Several large population-based epidemiologic studies have reported a significant increase in risk.[54] In a Swedish study from 1965 to 1983, the standardized incidence ratio for lung cancer in patients with DcSSc was 7.8 (95% confidence interval, 2.5–18.2).[55] Similar results were reported from an epidemiologic study in South Australia.[56] However, these results are tempered by 2 recent epidemiologic investigations conducted in the United States that did not show increases in the risk of lung cancer in patients with SSc.[57,58]

PM/DM

PM/DM are classified as idiopathic inflammatory myopathies. Both diseases are characterized by inflammatory muscle disease involving the proximal muscle groups, and DM is further defined by its characteristic cutaneous involvement.[59,60] Both are associated with underlying malignancy, with higher malignancy rates identified in DM.[61] Both are rare with an estimated annual incidence of less than 10 per 1 million population per year.[4,62] These diseases can affect any age group but have a bimodal incidence pattern with a peak in childhood (10–15 years of age) and a second peak

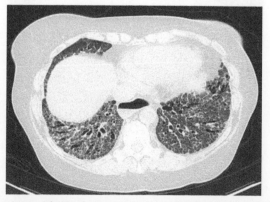

Fig. 1. HRCT of a patient with SSc demonstrating moderate bibasilar predominant ground-glass opacifications, reticulation, and traction bronchiectasis suggestive of fibrotic NSIP. Note the markedly dilated, fluid-filled esophagus characteristic of SSc.

between 35 and 65 years of age. Women are more commonly affected than men.[4,62] Some form of pulmonary involvement occurs in more than 50% of patients, and ILD is the most common and potentially most devastating pulmonary manifestation of PM/DM.[4,62] A subset of PM/DM is the antisynthetase syndrome, which is characterized by a combination of several clinical features that include inflammatory myopathy, ILD, fever, inflammatory arthritis, Raynaud phenomenon, "mechanic's hands," esophageal dysmotility, and the presence of an anti–transfer RNA–synthetase antibody (eg, anti–Jo-1, anti–PL-7, anti–PL-12).[9,63] Many patients with the antisynthetase syndrome may only with present partial features of the syndrome and inflammatory muscle disease may be absent or subclinical in nature.[9,63]

Airways Disease, Pleural Disease, and Vascular Disease

Both airway and pleural disease are rare.[62] Clinically evident pulmonary arterial hypertension is rare in PM/DM. If PAH is diagnosed, secondary causes should be thoroughly evaluated including respiratory muscle weakness resulting in hypoventilation, significant ILD, and underlying PM/DM-associated cardiomyopathy.[4]

ILD

ILD is the most common pulmonary manifestation of PM/DM, and its presence has been associated with increased morbidity and mortality (**Fig. 2**).[62,64,65] Clinically significant disease seems to occur in approximately 30%, whereas high-resolution computed tomography (HRCT) evidence of ILD may be present in more than 70% of patients with PM/DM.[62,64,65] Women with PM/DM are more likely to develop ILD, and the mean age at presentation is 50 years. ILD may be the presenting manifestation in many patients and is particularly common in those with the antisynthetase syndrome or in those who have a positive anti–transfer RNA–synthetase antibody.[63–65]

Based on the findings of histopathologic studies, NSIP is the most common pattern seen on surgical lung biopsy followed by UIP and organizing pneumonia.[66,67] An acute interstitial pneumonia-like disease occurs with an underlying histopathologic pattern of DAD. Similar to idiopathic acute interstitial pneumonia, the prognosis is poor.[68] The antisynthetase syndrome often has a characteristic HRCT pattern suggesting NSIP with overlapping organizing pneumonia with extreme bibasilar predominance

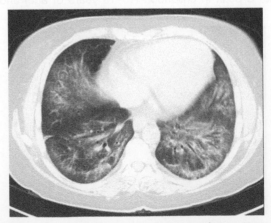

Fig. 2. HRCT image of a patient with the antisynthetase syndrome. Note the bibasilar distribution of ground-glass opacifications suggestive of nonspecific interstitial pneumonia and the consolidative features suggesting organizing pneumonia.

and reticular and ground-glass opacifications that to seem hug or "pancake" the diaphragm (see **Fig. 2**).[9]

Aspiration/Gastroesophageal Reflux Disease

Similar to SSc, esophageal dysmotility and gastroesophageal reflux disease are quite common in PM/DM. Medication therapy with proton-pump inhibitors for gastroesophageal reflux disease and a proactive approach to prevent aspiration are usually advised.

Complications of Muscle Weakness

Respiratory muscle weakness resulting in alveolar hypoventilation is a less common manifestation of PM/DM occurring in approximately 7% of patients.[4] Involvement of the hypopharyngeal and upper esophageal muscles results in dysphagia and aspiration. Aspiration pneumonia and repeated infections are frequent, occurring in as many as 20% of patients with PM/DM.[4]

RA

RA is a systemic autoimmune disease characterized by a symmetric, progressive, destructive, and chronic inflammatory polyarthritis.[69] It is the most common CTD and affects approximately 1% of the population worldwide. Women are twice as likely as men to be affected, and although it can occur at any age, the peak incidence is between the fourth and sixth decades.[4] Its extra-articular manifestations are frequent and may occur in virtually all organ systems. Pulmonary complications are common, may be the presenting manifestation of the disease, can impact every component of the respiratory tract, and account for 10% to 20% of deaths.[70–73]

Airways Disease

Upper airways
When assessed by direct laryngoscopy, the cricoarytenoid joint is affected in as many as 75% of patients with RA.[74] Symptoms of upper airways disease include hoarseness, sore throat, odynophagia, dysphagia, and globus.[4] Although the clinical importance of mild laryngoscopic changes are of uncertain significance, true cricoarytenoid arthritis can lead to life-threatening airway compromise – particularly in the setting of endotracheal intubation.[4] Less common upper airway complications include vocal cord paralysis (from involvement of the occipito-atlanto-axial joint with cervicomedullary compression), laryngeal rheumatoid nodules, secondary amyloidosis, and secondary SjS manifestations of xerostomia and xerotrachea.[4]

Lower airways
HRCT evidence of bronchiectasis is common; it has been noted in up to 58% of patients,[75] although the prevalence of clinically significant disease is considerably lower.[76] Symptoms (including dyspnea, cough, hemoptysis, and recurrent infections) and physiologic airway obstruction (including a reduced forced expiratory volume in 1 second [FEV_1], forced vital capacity [FVC], and forced expiratory flow 25%–75%) have been associated with its presence.[4] It is more common in long-standing RA, and fatalities from resultant recurrent infections and respiratory failure have been reported. Furthermore, the presence of bronchiectasis in a patient with RA being treated with anti-TNFα antagonist therapy may be an additional risk factor for the development of tuberculous and nontuberculous mycobacterial respiratory infection.

Similar to bronchiectasis, the prevalence of small airways inflammatory disease (bronchiolitis) in RA is unknown, but physiologic evidence of its presence occurs in 16% to 68% of patients.[77] HRCT seems to be more sensitive than pulmonary function tests in its detection; in patients with RA with normal physiology, HRCT evidence of bronchiolitis (including air-trapping, heterogeneity in lung attenuation, and centrilobular nodules) has been reported in up to two-thirds of patients.[78] Symptomatic bronchiolitis classically presents with dyspnea and cough. Pulmonary physiology often reveals a reduced FEV_1, FEV_1/FVC ratio, and DL_{CO}; reduced airflow at low lung volumes; and an increased RV and RV/TLC ratio.[4] On surgical lung biopsy, either a cellular or fibrosing bronchiolar process is typically identified.[79] Cellular bronchiolar diseases include follicular bronchiolitis (more commonly) and, rarely, diffuse panbronchiolitis. Follicular bronchiolitis may be responsive to corticosteroids, whereas diffuse panbronchiolitis may respond to chronic macrolide therapy.[80] Fibrosing bronchiolar disease, termed obliterative bronchiolitis or constrictive bronchiolitis, is poorly responsive to immunomodulatory therapy and frequently leads to respiratory failure and death.[81]

Pleural Disease

Pleuritis and pleural effusions are common in men with established disease, high rheumatoid factor (RF) titers, and rheumatoid nodules.[4] Asymptomatic pleural effusion may be present in as many as 70% of patients, whereas symptomatic effusions occur in approximately 5%.[4] Because several other pleural diseases can occur in RA, including infection/empyema, sterile empyema, chylothorax, and malignancy, the cause of an unidentified effusion should be pursued. Biochemical characteristics of RA pleural effusions include (1) an exudative process; (2) a low pH (<7.3); (3) a decreased glucose level (<50% of the serum glucose level); (4) an elevated lactated dehydrogenase (>700 IU/L); and (5) an elevated RF titer.[4]

Parenchymal Disease

Rheumatoid nodules

Rheumatoid nodules are present in as many as 20% of patients with RA on HRCT and are the most common finding on surgical lung pathologic examination, occurring in as high as 33% of specimens.[82–84] Radiographically, they range in size from 1 millimeter to several centimeters. Multiple nodules may be present, and central cavitation occurs in approximately 50% of these lesions.[83,84] Histopathologically, these nodules comprise central fibrinoid necrosis with surrounding granulomatous inflammation. Although most often asymptomatic, they can result in symptoms secondary to complications (including pneumothorax, hydropneumothorax, and hemoptysis) and must be distinguished from infection and malignancy.[4,83,84]

Eosinophilic lung disease

Several case reports of eosinophilic pneumonia occurring in patients with RA have been published. Clinically, RA-associated eosinophilic pneumonia seems to be identical to idiopathic chronic eosinophilic pneumonia. The clinical features include fever, cough, dyspnea, weight loss, and a peripheral blood eosinophilia. Thoracic imaging demonstrates peripheral infiltrates, and bronchoalveolar lavage has an eosinophilic predominance.[4]

ILD

The reported prevalence of RA-associated fibrosing ILD (RA-ILD) varies significantly depending on the method of detection and the population examined. Using HRCT, ILD may be seen in more than 50% of all patients with RA.[4,32] However, clinically significant disease is less common and estimated to occur in approximately 10% of patients.[85] Unlike articular RA, which is more common in women, RA-ILD is more common in men.[4]

Although the nonspecific interstitial pneumonia NSIP pattern is the most common in the CTDs as a whole,[53] in RA, UIP seems to be the most common pattern.[53,86,87] Organizing pneumonia, DAD, lymphocytic interstitial pneumonia, and desquamative interstitial pneumonia histologic patterns have also been described. In patients with RA, DAD has been reported to occur both in those without preexisting ILD and in those with preexisting fibrotic ILD.[4] Recent studies have highlighted that ILD may be the first clinically apparent manifestation of RA and that patients without arthritis but with a positive anti-cyclic citrullinated peptide (anti-CCP) antibody and airways or parenchymal lung disease may represent a prearticular RA phenotype.[7,88]

SLE

SLE is the prototypic systemic autoimmune disorder, affects approximately 1 per 2000 persons, and occurs 6 times more often in women than in men.[4,89] It is characterized by autoantibody positivity and immune-mediated damage to virtually every organ system. Constitutional symptoms, serositis, mucocutaneous disease, musculoskeletal, renal, neurologic, and hematologic involvement are all common. Some form of pulmonary abnormality occurs in nearly all patients with SLE.[4,89]

Airways Disease

Laryngeal involvement in SLE is generally benign and includes laryngeal ulcerations, edema, and vocal cord paralysis, which is typically responsive to corticosteroid therapy. However, life-threatening airway complications including necrotizing vasculitis, subglottic stenosis, and epiglottis have been reported.[4,89] Although lower airways disease is identified on HRCT in approximately 20% of patients with SLE, clinically important airways disease is rare.[90,91] Bronchiolitis seems to occur more often in those with SLE along with secondary SjS.[72,89]

Pleural Disease

Pleuritis is the most common pulmonary manifestation of SLE. Pleuritic chest pain occurs in 35% to 60% of patients during the course of disease and may be the initial manifestation in 5% of patients.[72,89] Clinically evident pleural effusions are identified in nearly half of patients with pleurisy. Autopsy studies report pleural involvement in almost all and pleural effusions in approximately two-thirds of subjects. Pleural effusions are likely to be bilateral, small to moderate in size, and exudative. In comparison to RA, SLE effusions are more likely have a normal glucose and pH and lower lactated dehydrogenase levels. However, a diagnostic evaluation is indicated when a new effusion is seen because other causes must be excluded including infection (parapneumonic effusions/empyema), pulmonary embolism, and congestive heart failure. Symptomatic pleurisy typically responds to nonsteroid anti-inflammatory agents, and more severe disease may require immunosuppressive agents.[72,89]

Vascular Disease

Pulmonary hypertension may be the result of a primary vascular abnormality with histopathologic features similar to those in idiopathic PAH or SSc-PAH or as a result of a variety of cardiopulmonary disorders including ILD, thromboembolic disease, Libman-Sacks endocarditis, cardiomyopathy, diastolic dysfunction, or obstructive sleep apnea.[72]

Thromboembolic Disease

Antiphospholipid antibodies (aPL) are common in SLE, occurring in approximately one-third of patients. Their presence is associated with an increased risk of vascular thrombosis and fetal loss. In patients with SLE with aPL, the risk of thrombosis is approximately 6 times that of patients without aPL.[92] In addition to the thrombotic complications of disease including pulmonary emboli, aPL has been associated with PAH, diffuse alveolar hemorrhage (DAH), and DAD.[93]

Parenchymal Disease

Interstitial lung disease

Clinically significant ILD is less common in SLE than in the other CTDs. A longitudinal cohort study of 626 patients with SLE found that only 4% developed clinical or plain chest radiographic evidence of pulmonary fibrosis after a mean disease duration of 5.3 years. Like other CTDs-ILDs, the histologic patterns of SLE-associated ILDs mirror the patterns described for the idiopathic interstitial pneumonias, most commonly NSIP.[53,94]

DAH

DAH is one of the life-threatening pleuropulmonary manifestations of SLE. DAH is uncommon, occurring in less than 4% of tertiary hospital admissions for SLE, and is more likely to occur in patients with an established diagnosis of SLE.[95,96] At presentation, symptoms include the acute onset of dyspnea and cough, imaging studies may reveal new alveolar infiltrates, and laboratory data may confirm a declining hematocrit. The absence of hemoptysis should not exclude the diagnosis; approximately half of patients do not present with it, although it typically appears during the hospital course.[95,96] Further, the presence of hemoptysis in a patient with SLE does not always imply a diagnosis of DAH as it can occur in both pulmonary infections and acute lupus pneumonitis. Commonly patients with DAH will have evidence of active concurrent extrapulmonary disease with the most common being lupus nephritis.[95,96] The diagnosis can be confirmed with sequential bronchoalveolar lavage samples revealing an increasing red blood cell count.

The most common underlying histologic pattern on surgical lung biopsy is capillaritis, although patterns of both bland pulmonary hemorrhage and diffuse alveolar damage have been described.[95–97]

Acute lupus pneumonitis

The classically described clinical characteristics of acute lupus pneumonitis include the acute onset of fever, dyspnea/tachypnea, cough, and hypoxemia with radiographic evidence of bilateral patchy or diffuse infiltrates, typically with a basilar predominance and often resulting in acute respiratory failure.[4,89] The most frequent histologic pattern is DAD, although some have described a capillaritis. There has been debate about whether acute lupus pneumonitis is a distinct syndrome or whether it is actually representative of either diffuse alveolar hemorrhage (with or without capillaritis) or DAD/acute respiratory distress syndrome resulting from a specific cause (eg, infection).[4,89]

Shrinking lung syndrome

Shrinking lung syndrome (SLS) is a rare complication of SLE that results in unexplained dyspnea and restrictive physiology with low lung volumes in the absence of significant underlying pleuroparenchymal disease.[98] Although the cause of SLS is unknown, theories regarding its pathogenesis speculate about some degree of diaphragmatic dysfunction either caused by neuromuscular myopathy with respiratory muscle weakness or limited diaphragmatic excursion caused by chronic pleural inflammation. The prognosis is favorable because most patients either improve or stabilize with therapy and death from SLS has rarely been reported.[98]

Syndrome of Acute Reversible Hypoxemia

The syndrome of acute reversible hypoxemia presents clinically with the acute onset of hypoxemia and a widened alveolar-arterial gradient with normal radiographic imaging studies. The pathophysiology of this syndrome is unknown, but one proposed mechanism is complement activation resulting in neutrophil aggregation within the pulmonary vasculature. A rapid and dramatic response to glucocorticoids is a characteristic finding in this syndrome[4,89]

PRIMARY SJÖGREN SYNDROME (SJS)

SjS is a systemic autoimmune disorder characterized by lymphocytic infiltration of the exocrine glands. The salivary and lacrimal glands are most often involved leading to the characteristic symptoms of disease including dry eyes (keratoconjunctivitis sicca) and dry mouth (xerostomia). The prevalence of primary SjS is estimated to be 0.5% to 1% in the population, whereas the prevalence of secondary SjS (ie, occurring in the setting of another CTD) is as high as 30%. Women are more commonly affected and most patients with SjS will have some form of pulmonary involvement.[4,99,100]

Airways Disease

Large airways

As many as 50% of patients with SjS develop a dry cough.[4] It is thought to result from xerotrachea – or desiccation of the tracheobronchial tree. Xerotrachea has been associated with reduced mucociliary clearance – which may result in obstructive physiology and predispose patients with SjS to recurrent infection and bronchiectasis.[4,100,101]

Small airways

Small airways disease, defined by the presence of reduced maximal expiratory flows at 25% and 50% of FVC, is the most common pulmonary abnormality, occurring in more than half of patients with SjS.[4] These physiologic abnormalities are typically mild and tend to remain stable. Histopathology studies of lung tissue from patients with SjS with more severe obstructive lung disease have revealed evidence of lymphocytic or follicular bronchiolitis.[102,103]

Pleural and pulmonary vascular disease complications are quite rare in patients with primary SjS and their presence should highlight the need for evaluation of alternative causes.

ILD

Clinically significant ILD is estimated to occur in 8% to 38% of patients with SjSs (Fig. 3).[4,104] A higher proportion of patients have subclinical ILD.[32] The most common histopathologic pattern identified in SjS is NSIP, but it is not uncommon to find the lung injury patterns of lymphocytic interstitial pneumonia, OP, or UIP in patients with SjS.[102,103,105]

Non-Hodgkin Lymphoma and Other Malignancies

The most serious complication of SjS is non-Hodgkin lymphoma (NHL): 1 in 5 SjS deaths are attributable to this malignancy.[4,106,107] The risk of NHL in SjS has been reported to be 16 to 44 times higher than matched control populations, with an estimated lifetime risk of 5% to 10%. Risk factors for the development of NHL include

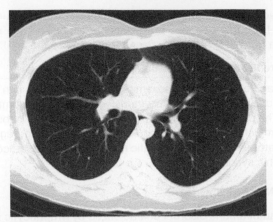

Fig. 3. HRCT image of a patient with primary SjS. This patient had the incidental finding of subclinical cystic lung disease most suggestive lymphocytic interstitial pneumonia.

a decreased CD4+/CD8[+] T-lymphocyte ratio, hypocomplementemia, and vasculitis of the skin. It arises most often in the salivary glands, but lymph nodes, bone marrow, solid organs (including the spleen, liver, and kidney), and mucosal sites including the stomach, skin, and lung are all at risk.[4,106,107] In patients with systemic NHL, lung involvement is estimated to occur in approximately 20%.[4,106,107]

MCTD

MCTD is a specific CTD that often resembles either SSc or SLE. It is characterized clinically by SLE or SSc-type symptoms but is distinguished from these and other CTDs by its serologic profile of a positive ANA along with an isolated positive anti-ribonucleoprotein antibody.[108,109] This means that patients are not classified as having MCTD if other autoantibodies are present along with the ribonucleoprotein antibody (eg, RF, anti-Smith, anti-dsDNA, anti-SSA, or anti-SSB). MCTD is often associated with similar pulmonary manifestations as SSc and these patients are thus incorporated into the concept of representing a "scleroderma spectrum" of disease. Practically speaking, patients with MCTD have similar pulmonary manifestations as SSc and as such require heightened surveillance for clinically significant ILD and recommended to undergo PAH screening similar to those with SSc.[46]

SUGGESTIVE FORMS OF CTD-ILD
Undifferentiated CTD

In addition to well-characterized forms of CTD, it is common to encounter patients who have partial or incomplete forms of CTD and these cases are often considered to have UCTD (**Table 2**).[110,111] UCTD has been generally defined as a condition manifesting with signs and symptoms suggestive of a CTD, along with ANA positivity, but not fulfilling existing rheumatologic classification criteria for any specific CTD.[110,111] Mosca and colleagues[110,111] have reported that about 60% of patients with UCTD will remain undifferentiated, and that when evolution to defined CTD occurs, it usually does so within the first 5 years of disease. UCTD may evolve into any of the CTDs but most often evolves into SLE. Patients with UCTD who do not develop a characterizable CTD are considered to have a mild clinical picture – or "stable" UCTD – characterized by the presence of arthralgias or arthritis, Raynaud phenomenon, leukopenia, anemia, and dry eyes or dry mouth. An important distinguishing characteristic of UCTD is that *no major organ involvement* (eg, lung disease) has been described.[110–114]

A recent expert review on UCTD distinguishes "monosymptomatic UCTD" composed of single organ-dominant diseases (eg, ILD) that do not fulfill specific CTD criteria from that of stable, mild "oligosymptomatic UCTD."[111] The authors acknowledge that the concept of UCTD includes a wide spectrum of diseases ranging from "organ-dominant" conditions to "stable UCTD" to early CTDs or mild forms of CTDs.[111] They suggest that only persistently oligosymptomatic conditions–and not "organ dominant" disease–be classified as "UCTD." Mosca and colleagues[111] have proposed the following preliminary classification criteria for UCTD: (i) signs and symptoms suggestive of a CTD, but not fulfilling criteria for defined CTDs, (ii) positive ANAs, and (iii) a disease duration of at least 3 years.

The concept of UCTD has been of interest within the ILD community as well. In 2007, Kinder and colleagues[115] proposed a broader and less specific set of UCTD criteria and applied these criteria to a cohort of patients with idiopathic interstitial pneumonia (IIP). Retrospectively, they identified 28 subjects with an IIP who met their proposed criteria for UCTD and compared these subjects with a control group of 47 subjects with an IIP that did not meet their criteria. Interestingly, those whom they defined as having UCTD were more likely to be female, younger, and nonsmokers and were more likely to have ground-glass opacities on HRCT and NSIP on surgical lung biopsy. In all, 88% of those with idiopathic NSIP met their definition for UCTD and led the authors to conclude that most patients previously classified as having idiopathic NSIP have clinical, serologic, radiographic, and pathologic characteristics of autoimmune disease, and they proposed that idiopathic NSIP is the lung manifestation of UCTD.[115] The accompanying editorial pointed out several limitations of the Kinder study and argued against accepting the conclusion that idiopathic NSIP is UCTD.[116] Corte and colleagues[117] also recently called into question the clinical relevance of defining ILD patients as having UCTD and specifically called into question the application of the broader, less-specific UCTD criteria proposed by Kinder and colleagues. They retrospectively studied 45 patients with biopsy-proved NSIP and 56 patients with biopsy-proved UIP. They reported that CTD features are common in patients with IIP, with 31% of patients with NSIP and 13% of patients with IPF fulfilling the stricter, more traditional criteria for UCTD. However, when the broader, less specific, criteria of Kinder and colelagues for UCTD was applied, an astounding 71% of patients with NSIP and 36% of patients with IPF could be reclassified as having UCTD. Because of its lack of specificity, these and other authors have argued against further implementation of the Kinder set of criteria to define UCTD in patients with ILD.[1,10,117]

"Autoimmune-Featured ILD"

Vij and colleagues[118] have described a cohort of UIP-predominant ILD patients retrospectively identified as having a possible form of CTD-ILD (see **Table 2**). Among 200 patients who presented to an ILD referral center, 63 were considered to have "autoimmune- featured ILD" if they had a sign or symptom suggestive of a CTD, but with insufficient features to label as definite CTD, and a serologic test reflective of an autoimmune process. The cohort that met their case definition of autoimmune-featured ILD had a similar demographic profile as IPF: most were older (average age of 66 years) and male. The most common clinical symptoms in the autoimmune-featured ILD cohort were nonspecific symptoms of dry eyes or dry mouth (57%) and gastroesophageal reflux disease (44%). Seventy-five percent of those that met their case definition for autoimmune-featured ILD had a lung injury pattern of UIP. Finally, the survival of

Table 2
Proposed criteria for categories of suggestive forms of CTD-ILD

Proposed Category	Clinical Features	Laboratory or Histopathologic Findings
Undifferentiated CTD (stricter definition) (requires at least 1 clinical feature and 1 laboratory finding)	One or more of the following symptoms: Dry eyes or dry mouth, joint pain or swelling Raynaud phenomenon Proximal muscle weakness Morning stiffness	One or more of these autoantibodies: ANA (*high titer*) RF (high titer) Anti-Smith Anti-ribonucleoprotein Anti-double-strand DNA Anti-Ro Anti-La Anti-Jo-1 Anti-topoisomerase (Scl-70) Anti-centromere
Undifferentiated CTD (broader definition) (requires at least 1 clinical feature and 1 laboratory finding)	One or more of the following symptoms: Dry eyes or dry mouth Gastroesophageal reflux disease Weight loss Recurrent unexplained fever Joint pain or swelling Rash Photosensitivity Dysphagia Nonandrogenic alopecia Mouth ulcers Raynaud phenomenon Morning stiffness Proximal muscle weakness	One or more of these laboratory abnormalities: ANA (*any titer*) RF Anti-Ro Anti-La Anti-Jo-1 Anti-topoisomerase (Scl-70) Erythrocyte sedimentation rate (2× normal) C-reactive protein elevation
Lung-dominant CTD (requires all 3 listed clinical features and either 4a or 4b)	All of the following features: 1. NSIP, UIP, lymphocytic interstitial pneumonia, OP, DAD (or desquamative interstitial pneumonia if no smoking history), as determined by surgical lung biopsy or suggested by HRCT *and*	4a. Any 1 of these autoantibodies: ANA >1:320 titer RF >60 IU/mL Anti-nucleolar ANA (any titer) Anti-centromere Anti-CCP

2. Insufficient extrathoracic features of a definite CTD and
3. No identifiable alternative cause of IP and

- Anti-Ro
- Anti-La
- Anti-double-strand DNA
- Anti-ribonucleoprotein
- Anti-Smith
- Anti-topoisomerase (Scl-70)
- Anti-transfer RNA synthetase
- Anti-PM-Scl

4b. *OR at least 2 of these histopathologic features:*
- Lymphoid aggregates with germinal centers
- Extensive pleuritis
- Prominent plasmacytic infiltration
- Dense perivascular collagen

Autoimmune-featured ILD (requires at least 1 clinical feature and 1 laboratory finding)

One or more of the following symptoms:
- Dry eyes or dry mouth
- Gastroesophageal reflux disease
- Weight loss
- Foot or leg swelling
- Joint pain or swelling
- Rash
- Photosensitivity
- Dysphagia
- Hand ulcers
- Mouth ulcers
- Raynaud phenomenon
- Morning stiffness
- Proximal muscle weakness

One or more of these laboratory abnormalities:
- ANA ≥1:160 titer
- RF
- Anti-Ro
- Anti-La
- Anti-Smith
- Anti-ribonucleoprotein
- Anti-dsDNA
- Anti-topoisomerase (Scl-70)
- Anti-CCP
- Anti-Jo-1
- Aldolase
- Creatine phosphokinase

Data from Fischer A, du Bois R. Interstitial lung disease in connective tissue disorders. Lancet 2012;380(9842):689–98.

those with autoimmune-featured ILD was similar to those with IPF and worse compared with CTD-ILD.[118] Arguing against the inclusion of nonspecific symptoms in the proposed criteria, only the presence of an ANA at greater than 1:1280 titer was associated with improved survival.

"Lung-Dominant CTD"

Fischer and colleagues[10] proposed a set of provisional classification criteria to define the cohort of individuals with suggestive forms of CTD-ILD as having "lung-dominant CTD" (LD-CTD) (see **Table 2**). A classification of LD-CTD would be reserved for those patients in whom the ILD has a "rheumatologic flavor" as supported by specific auto-antibodies or histopathologic features and yet does not meet criteria for a defined CTD based on the lack of adequate extrapulmonary features to confer a diagnosis of definite CTD-ILD. The authors argued that implicit with the concept of LD-CTD is the recognition that specific autoantibodies and/or histopathologic features alone can be sufficient to classify a patient as having CTD-ILD.[10] The presence of objective extrapulmonary features highly suggestive of CTD (eg, Raynaud phenomenon, inflammatory arthritis) are important and will lend further support for an underlying CTD, but their absence should not preclude a classification of LD-CTD. The authors emphasized that their intent was that the concept of LD-CTD and the associated criteria should be viewed as provisional, and that they might serve as a platform for further multidisciplinary, multicenter investigations, including validation via prospective study.[10]

Several potential advantages to the introduction of this novel classification were suggested: (1) The criteria offered are objective and measurable. (2) Nonspecific symptoms (eg, dry eyes, myalgias, arthralgias, or gastroesophageal reflux disease), nonspecific inflammatory markers (eg, erythrocyte sedimentation rate or C-reactive protein), and low-titer ANA or RF are not included because of their high prevalence in patients without CTD. (3) Surveillance for evolution to characterizable forms of CTD is encouraged. (4) The diagnosis isolates them from the (default) category of IIP and provides a framework by which questions regarding this subset's natural history, pathobiology, treatment, and prognosis can be answered. (5) The classification allows their distinction from well-characterized forms of CTD, without attempting to redefine existing CTD categories (eg, UCTD).[10]

SUMMARY

The CTDs represent a heterogeneous spectrum of systemic autoimmune diseases and the lungs are a frequent target of autoimmune-mediated organ damage. Any of the lung compartments are at risk of injury, and multicompartment lung involvement is a frequent finding in the CTDs. The intersection of ILD and CTD is particularly complex: ILD may be present in subclinical forms, may be chronic and slowly progressive in nature, or may present as an acute, fulminant disorder. ILD is known to occur within a context of preexisting CTD, can be the presenting manifestation of a CTD, or can be identified in patients who have suggestive features of a CTD. The clinical care of patients with CTD is often enhanced by an understanding of these complex interactions and a multidisciplinary approach to evaluation and management.

REFERENCES

1. Fischer A, du Bois R. Interstitial lung disease in connective tissue disorders. Lancet 2012;380(9842):689–98.

2. Fischer A, du Bois RM. A practical approach to connective tissue disease-associated lung disease. 2nd edition. New York: Springer; 2012.
3. Frankel SK, Brown KK. Collagen vascular diseases of the lung. Clin Pulm Med 2006;13(1):25–36.
4. Olson AL, Brown KK. Connective tissue disease-associated lung disorders. Eur Resp Mon 2009;46:225–50.
5. Cottin V. Interstitial lung disease: are we missing formes frustes of connective tissue disease? Eur Respir J 2006;28(5):893–6.
6. Fischer A, Meehan RT, Feghali-Bostwick CA, et al. Unique characteristics of systemic sclerosis sine scleroderma-associated interstitial lung disease. Chest 2006;130(4):976–81.
7. Fischer A, Solomon JJ, du Bois RM, et al. Lung disease with anti-CCP antibodies but not rheumatoid arthritis or connective tissue disease. Respir Med 2012;106(7):1040–7.
8. Fischer A, Swigris JJ, du Bois RM, et al. Minor salivary gland biopsy to detect primary Sjogren syndrome in patients with interstitial lung disease. Chest 2009;136(4):1072–8.
9. Fischer A, Swigris JJ, du Bois RM, et al. Anti-synthetase syndrome in ANA and anti-Jo-1 negative patients presenting with idiopathic interstitial pneumonia. Respir Med 2009;103(11):1719–24.
10. Fischer A, West SG, Swigris JJ, et al. Connective tissue disease-associated interstitial lung disease: a call for clarification. Chest 2010;138(2):251–6.
11. Mittoo S, Gelber AC, Christopher-Stine L, et al. Ascertainment of collagen vascular disease in patients presenting with interstitial lung disease. Respir Med 2009;103(8):1152–8.
12. Turesson C, Jacobsson LT, Matteson EL. Cardiovascular co-morbidity in rheumatic diseases. Vasc Health Risk Manag 2008;4(3):605–14.
13. Wolfe F, Caplan L, Michaud K. Treatment for rheumatoid arthritis and the risk of hospitalization for pneumonia: associations with prednisone, disease-modifying antirheumatic drugs, and anti-tumor necrosis factor therapy. Arthritis Rheum 2006;54(2):628–34.
14. Carbone J, Perez-Rojas J, Sarmiento E. Infectious pulmonary complications in patients treated with anti-TNF-alpha monoclonal antibodies and soluble TNF receptor. Curr Infect Dis Rep 2009;11(3):229–36.
15. Furst DE. The risk of infections with biologic therapies for rheumatoid arthritis. Semin Arthritis Rheum 2008;39(5):327–46.
16. Alarcon GS, Kremer JM, Macaluso M, et al. Risk factors for methotrexate-induced lung injury in patients with rheumatoid arthritis. A multicenter, case-control study. Methotrexate-lung study group. Ann Intern Med 1997;127(5):356–64.
17. Camus P. Drug induced infiltrative lung diseases. Fourth edition. Hamilton (Ontario): BC Decker, Inc; 2003.
18. Kremer JM, Alarcon GS, Weinblatt ME, et al. Clinical, laboratory, radiographic, and histopathologic features of methotrexate-associated lung injury in patients with rheumatoid arthritis: a multicenter study with literature review. Arthritis Rheum 1997;40(10):1829–37.
19. Lateef O, Shakoor N, Balk RA. Methotrexate pulmonary toxicity. Expert Opin Drug Saf 2005;4(4):723–30.
20. Malik SW, Myers JL, DeRemee RA, et al. Lung toxicity associated with cyclophosphamide use. Two distinct patterns. Am J Respir Crit Care Med 1996;154(6 Pt 1):1851–6.

21. Fischer A, Brown KK, Frankel SK. Treatment of connective tissue disease related interstitial lung disease. Clin Pulm Med 2009;16(2):74–80.

22. Bedrossian CW, Sussman J, Conklin RH, et al. Azathioprine-associated interstitial pneumonitis. Am J Clin Pathol 1984;82(2):148–54.

23. Morrissey P, Gohh R, Madras P, et al. Pulmonary fibrosis secondary to administration of mycophenolate mofetil. Transplantation 1998;65(10):1414.

24. Shrestha NK, Mossad SB, Braun W. Pneumonitis associated with the use of mycophenolate mofetil. Transplantation 2003;75(10):1762.

25. Koopman WJ. Dawn of the era of biologics in the treatment of the rheumatic diseases. Arthritis Rheum 2008;58(Suppl 2):S75–8.

26. Huggett MT, Armstrong R. Adalimumab-associated pulmonary fibrosis. Rheumatology (Oxford) 2006;45(10):1312–3.

27. Ognenovski VM, Ojo TC, Fox DA. Etanercept-associated pulmonary granulomatous inflammation in patients with rheumatoid arthritis. J Rheumatol 2008;35(11): 2279–82.

28. Peno-Green L, Lluberas G, Kingsley T, et al. Lung injury linked to etanercept therapy. Chest 2002;122(5):1858–60.

29. Villeneuve E, St-Pierre A, Haraoui B. Interstitial pneumonitis associated with infliximab therapy. J Rheumatol 2006;33(6):1189–93.

30. Zimmer C, Beiderlinden M, Peters J. Lethal acute respiratory distress syndrome during anti-TNF-alpha therapy for rheumatoid arthritis. Clin Rheumatol 2006; 25(3):430–2.

31. Steen VD. The lung in systemic sclerosis. J Clin Rheumatol 2005;11(1):40–6.

32. Doyle TJ, Hunninghake GM, Rosas IO. Subclinical interstitial lung disease: why you should care. Am J Respir Crit Care Med 2012;185(11):1147–53.

33. Gabbay E, Tarala R, Will R, et al. Interstitial lung disease in recent onset rheumatoid arthritis. Am J Respir Crit Care Med 1997;156(2 Pt 1):528–35.

34. Gochuico BR, Avila NA, Chow CK, et al. Progressive preclinical interstitial lung disease in rheumatoid arthritis. Arch Intern Med 2008;168(2):159–66.

35. Launay D, Remy-Jardin M, Michon-Pasturel U, et al. High resolution computed tomography in fibrosing alveolitis associated with systemic sclerosis. J Rheumatol 2006;33(9):1789–801.

36. Uffmann M, Kiener HP, Bankier AA, et al. Lung manifestation in asymptomatic patients with primary Sjogren syndrome: assessment with high resolution CT and pulmonary function tests. J Thorac Imaging 2001;16(4):282–9.

37. Steen VD, Conte C, Owens GR, et al. Severe restrictive lung disease in systemic sclerosis. Arthritis Rheum 1994;37(9):1283–9.

38. LeRoy EC, Black C, Fleischmajer R, et al. Scleroderma (systemic sclerosis): classification, subsets and pathogenesis. J Rheumatol 1988;15(2): 202–5.

39. Poormoghim H, Lucas M, Fertig N, et al. Systemic sclerosis sine scleroderma: demographic, clinical, and serologic features and survival in forty-eight patients. Arthritis Rheum 2000;43(2):444–51.

40. Steen VD. Autoantibodies in systemic sclerosis. Semin Arthritis Rheum 2005; 35(1):35–42.

41. Steen VD, Medsger TA. Changes in causes of death in systemic sclerosis, 1972–2002. Ann Rheum Dis 2007;66(7):940–4.

42. Spagnolatti L, Zoia MC, Volpini E, et al. Pulmonary function in patients with systemic sclerosis. Monaldi Arch Chest Dis 1997;52(1):4–8.

43. Bjerke RD, Tashkin DP, Clements PJ, et al. Small airways in progressive systemic sclerosis (PSS). Am J Med 1979;66(2):201–9.

44. Harrison NK, Myers AR, Corrin B, et al. Structural features of interstitial lung disease in systemic sclerosis. Am Rev Respir Dis 1991;144(3 Pt 1):706–13.

45. Cool CD, Kennedy D, Voelkel NF, et al. Pathogenesis and evolution of plexiform lesions in pulmonary hypertension associated with scleroderma and human immunodeficiency virus infection. Hum Pathol 1997;28(4):434–42.

46. Fischer A, Bull TM, Steen VD. Practical approach to screening for scleroderma-associated pulmonary arterial hypertension. Arthritis Care Res (Hoboken) 2012; 64(3):303–10.

47. Koh ET, Lee P, Gladman DD, et al. Pulmonary hypertension in systemic sclerosis: an analysis of 17 patients. Br J Rheumatol 1996;35(10):989–93.

48. Condliffe R, Kiely DG, Peacock AJ, et al. Connective tissue disease-associated pulmonary arterial hypertension in the modern treatment era. Am J Respir Crit Care Med 2009;179(2):151–7.

49. Highland KB, Garin MC, Brown KK. The spectrum of scleroderma lung disease. Semin Respir Crit Care Med 2007;28(4):418–29.

50. Bouros D, Wells AU, Nicholson AG, et al. Histopathologic subsets of fibrosing alveolitis in patients with systemic sclerosis and their relationship to outcome. Am J Respir Crit Care Med 2002;165(12):1581–6.

51. Fischer A, Swigris JJ, Groshong SD, et al. Clinically significant interstitial lung disease in limited scleroderma: histopathology, clinical features, and survival. Chest 2008;134(3):601–5.

52. Kim DS, Yoo B, Lee JS, et al. The major histopathologic pattern of pulmonary fibrosis in scleroderma is nonspecific interstitial pneumonia. Sarcoidosis Vasc Diffuse Lung Dis 2002;19(2):121–7.

53. Park JH, Kim DS, Park IN, et al. Prognosis of fibrotic interstitial pneumonia: idiopathic versus collagen vascular disease-related subtypes. Am J Respir Crit Care Med 2007;175(7):705–11.

54. Wooten M. Systemic sclerosis and malignancy: a review of the literature. South Med J 2008;101(1):59–62.

55. Rosenthal AK, McLaughlin JK, Linet MS, et al. Scleroderma and malignancy: an epidemiological study. Ann Rheum Dis 1993;52(7):531–3.

56. Hill CL, Nguyen AM, Roder D, et al. Risk of cancer in patients with scleroderma: a population based cohort study. Ann Rheum Dis 2003;62(8):728–31.

57. Chatterjee S, Dombi GW, Severson RK, et al. Risk of malignancy in scleroderma: a population-based cohort study. Arthritis Rheum 2005;52(8):2415–24.

58. Derk CT, Rasheed M, Artlett CM, et al. A cohort study of cancer incidence in systemic sclerosis. J Rheumatol 2006;33(6):1113–6.

59. Bohan A, Peter JB. Polymyositis and dermatomyositis (second of two parts). N Engl J Med 1975;292(8):403–7.

60. Bohan A, Peter JB. Polymyositis and dermatomyositis (first of two parts). N Engl J Med 1975;292(7):344–7.

61. Zantos D, Zhang Y, Felson D. The overall and temporal association of cancer with polymyositis and dermatomyositis. J Rheumatol 1994;21(10):1855–9.

62. Schwarz MI. The lung in polymyositis. Clin Chest Med 1998;19(4):701–12, viii.

63. Solomon J, Swigris JJ, Brown KK. Myositis-related interstitial lung disease and anti-synthetase syndrome. J Bras Pneumol 2011;37(1):100–9 [in English, Portuguese].

64. Schnabel A, Hellmich B, Gross WL. Interstitial lung disease in polymyositis and dermatomyositis. Curr Rheumatol Rep 2005;7(2):99–105.

65. Schnabel A, Reuter M, Biederer J, et al. Interstitial lung disease in polymyositis and dermatomyositis: clinical course and response to treatment. Semin Arthritis Rheum 2003;32(5):273–84.

66. Arakawa H, Yamada H, Kurihara Y, et al. Nonspecific interstitial pneumonia associated with polymyositis and dermatomyositis: serial high-resolution CT findings and functional correlation. Chest 2003;123(4):1096–103.

67. Douglas WW, Tazelaar HD, Hartman TE, et al. Polymyositis-dermatomyositis-associated interstitial lung disease. Am J Respir Crit Care Med 2001;164(7): 1182–5.

68. Kang EH, Lee EB, Shin KC, et al. Interstitial lung disease in patients with polymyositis, dermatomyositis and amyopathic dermatomyositis. Rheumatology (Oxford) 2005;44(10):1282–6.

69. Arnett FC, Edworthy SM, Bloch DA, et al. The American rheumatism association 1987 revised criteria for the classification of rheumatoid arthritis. Arthritis Rheum 1988;31(3):315–24.

70. Gabriel SE, Crowson CS, Kremers HM, et al. Survival in rheumatoid arthritis: a population-based analysis of trends over 40 years. Arthritis Rheum 2003; 48(1):54–8.

71. Minaur NJ, Jacoby RK, Cosh JA, et al. Outcome after 40 years with rheumatoid arthritis: a prospective study of function, disease activity, and mortality. J Rheumatol Suppl 2004;69:3–8.

72. Olson AL, Swigris JJ, Sprunger DB, et al. Rheumatoid arthritis-interstitial lung disease-associated mortality. Am J Respir Crit Care Med 2011;183(3):372–8.

73. Sihvonen S, Korpela M, Laippala P, et al. Death rates and causes of death in patients with rheumatoid arthritis: a population-based study. Scand J Rheumatol 2004;33(4):221–7.

74. Lawry GV, Finerman ML, Hanafee WN, et al. Laryngeal involvement in rheumatoid arthritis. A clinical, laryngoscopic, and computerized tomographic study. Arthritis Rheum 1984;27(8):873–82.

75. Metafratzi ZM, Georgiadis AN, Ioannidou CV, et al. Pulmonary involvement in patients with early rheumatoid arthritis. Scand J Rheumatol 2007;36(5): 338–44.

76. Lieberman-Maran L, Orzano IM, Passero MA, et al. Bronchiectasis in rheumatoid arthritis: report of four cases and a review of the literature–implications for management with biologic response modifiers. Semin Arthritis Rheum 2006; 35(6):379–87.

77. White ES, Tazelaar HD, Lynch JP 3rd. Bronchiolar complications of connective tissue diseases. Semin Respir Crit Care Med 2003;24(5):543–66.

78. Perez T, Remy-Jardin M, Cortet B. Airways involvement in rheumatoid arthritis: clinical, functional, and HRCT findings. Am J Respir Crit Care Med 1998; 157(5 Pt 1):1658–65.

79. Hayakawa H, Sato A, Imokawa S, et al. Bronchiolar disease in rheumatoid arthritis. Am J Respir Crit Care Med 1996;154(5):1531–6.

80. Kinoshita M, Higashi T, Tanaka C, et al. Follicular bronchiolitis associated with rheumatoid arthritis. Intern Med 1992;31(5):674–7.

81. Devouassoux G, Cottin V, Liote H, et al. Characterisation of severe obliterative bronchiolitis in rheumatoid arthritis. Eur Respir J 2009;33(5):1053–61.

82. Cortet B, Flipo RM, Remy-Jardin M, et al. Use of high resolution computed tomography of the lungs in patients with rheumatoid arthritis. Ann Rheum Dis 1995;54(10):815–9.

83. Hakala M, Paakko P, Huhti E, et al. Open lung biopsy of patients with rheumatoid arthritis. Clin Rheumatol 1990;9(4):452–60.

84. Yousem SA, Colby TV, Carrington CB. Lung biopsy in rheumatoid arthritis. Am Rev Respir Dis 1985;131(5):770–7.

85. Turesson C, O'Fallon WM, Crowson CS, et al. Extra-articular disease manifestations in rheumatoid arthritis: incidence trends and risk factors over 46 years. Ann Rheum Dis 2003;62(8):722–7.

86. Kim EJ, Elicker BM, Maldonado F, et al. Usual interstitial pneumonia in rheumatoid arthritis-associated interstitial lung disease. Eur Respir J 2010;35(6): 1322–8.

87. Lee HK, Kim DS, Yoo B, et al. Histopathologic pattern and clinical features of rheumatoid arthritis-associated interstitial lung disease. Chest 2005;127(6):2019–27.

88. Gizinski AM, Mascolo M, Loucks JL, et al. Rheumatoid arthritis (RA)-specific autoantibodies in patients with interstitial lung disease and absence of clinically apparent articular RA. Clin Rheumatol 2009;28(5):611–3.

89. Swigris JJ, Fischer A, Gillis J, et al. Pulmonary and thrombotic manifestations of systemic lupus erythematosus. Chest 2008;133(1):271–80.

90. Kinney WW, Angelillo VA. Bronchiolitis in systemic lupus erythematosus. Chest 1982;82(5):646–9.

91. Fenlon HM, Doran M, Sant SM, et al. High-resolution chest CT in systemic lupus erythematosus. AJR Am J Roentgenol 1996;166(2):301–7.

92. Wahl DG, Guillemin F, de Maistre E, et al. Risk for venous thrombosis related to antiphospholipid antibodies in systemic lupus erythematosus–a meta-analysis. Lupus 1997;6(5):467–73.

93. Asherson RA, Cervera R, Shepshelovich D, et al. Nonthrombotic manifestations of the antiphospholipid syndrome: away from thrombosis? J Rheumatol 2006; 33(6):1038–44.

94. Bertoli AM, Vila LM, Apte M, et al. Systemic lupus erythematosus in a multiethnic US Cohort LUMINA XLVIII: factors predictive of pulmonary damage. Lupus 2007;16(6):410–7.

95. Santos-Ocampo AS, Mandell BF, Fessler BJ. Alveolar hemorrhage in systemic lupus erythematosus: presentation and management. Chest 2000;118(4): 1083–90.

96. Zamora MR, Warner ML, Tuder R, et al. Diffuse alveolar hemorrhage and systemic lupus erythematosus. Clinical presentation, histology, survival, and outcome. Medicine (Baltimore) 1997;76(3):192–202.

97. Eagen JW, Memoli VA, Roberts JL, et al. Pulmonary hemorrhage in systemic lupus erythematosus. Medicine (Baltimore) 1978;57(6):545–60.

98. Toya SP, Tzelepis GE. Association of the shrinking lung syndrome in systemic lupus erythematosus with pleurisy: a systematic review. Semin Arthritis Rheum 2009;39(1):30–7.

99. Fox RI, Howell FV, Bone RC, et al. Primary sjogren syndrome: clinical and immunopathologic features. Semin Arthritis Rheum 1984;14(2):77–105.

100. Mialon P, Barthelemy L, Sebert P, et al. A longitudinal study of lung impairment in patients with primary sjogren's syndrome. Clin Exp Rheumatol 1997;15(4): 349–54.

101. Mathieu A, Cauli A, Pala R, et al. Tracheo-bronchial mucociliary clearance in patients with primary and secondary sjogren's syndrome. Scand J Rheumatol 1995;24(5):300–4.

102. Ito I, Nagai S, Kitaichi M, et al. Pulmonary manifestations of primary sjogren's syndrome: a clinical, radiologic, and pathologic study. Am J Respir Crit Care Med 2005;171(6):632–8.

103. Deheinzelin D, Capelozzi VL, Kairalla RA, et al. Interstitial lung disease in primary sjogren's syndrome. Clinical-pathological evaluation and response to treatment. Am J Respir Crit Care Med 1996;154(3 Pt 1):794–9.

104. Papathanasiou MP, Constantopoulos SH, Tsampoulas C, et al. Reappraisal of respiratory abnormalities in primary and secondary sjogren's syndrome. A controlled study. Chest 1986;90(3):370–4.
105. Parambil JG, Myers JL, Lindell RM, et al. Interstitial lung disease in primary sjogren syndrome. Chest 2006;130(5):1489–95.
106. Ioannidis JP, Vassiliou VA, Moutsopoulos HM. Long-term risk of mortality and lymphoproliferative disease and predictive classification of primary sjogren's syndrome. Arthritis Rheum 2002;46(3):741–7.
107. Theander E, Henriksson G, Ljungberg O, et al. Lymphoma and other malignancies in primary sjogren's syndrome: a cohort study on cancer incidence and lymphoma predictors. Ann Rheum Dis 2006;65(6):796–803.
108. Aringer M, Smolen JS. Mixed connective tissue disease: what is behind the curtain? Best Pract Res Clin Rheumatol 2007;21(6):1037–49.
109. Venables PJ. Mixed connective tissue disease. Lupus 2006;15(3):132–7.
110. Mosca M, Neri R, Bombardieri S. Undifferentiated connective tissue diseases (UCTD): a review of the literature and a proposal for preliminary classification criteria. Clin Exp Rheumatol 1999;17(5):615–20.
111. Mosca M, Tani C, Carli L, et al. Undifferentiated CTD: a wide spectrum of autoimmune diseases. Best Pract Res Clin Rheumatol 2012;26(1):73–7.
112. Mosca M, Tani C, Bombardieri S. Undifferentiated connective tissue diseases (UCTD): a new frontier for rheumatology. Best Pract Res Clin Rheumatol 2007; 21(6):1011–23.
113. Mosca M, Tani C, Neri C, et al. Undifferentiated connective tissue diseases (UCTD). Autoimmun Rev 2006;6(1):1–4.
114. Mosca M, Tavoni A, Neri R, et al. Undifferentiated connective tissue diseases: the clinical and serological profiles of 91 patients followed for at least 1 year. Lupus 1998;7(2):95–100.
115. Kinder BW, Collard HR, Koth L, et al. Idiopathic nonspecific interstitial pneumonia: lung manifestation of undifferentiated connective tissue disease? Am J Respir Crit Care Med 2007;176(7):691–7.
116. Nagai S, Kitaichi M, Itoh H, et al. Idiopathic nonspecific interstitial pneumonia/fibrosis: comparison with idiopathic pulmonary fibrosis and BOOP. Eur Respir J 1998;12(5):1010–9.
117. Corte TJ, Copley SJ, Desai SR, et al. Significance of connective tissue disease features in idiopathic interstitial pneumonia. Eur Respir J 2012;39(3):661–8.
118. Vij R, Noth I, Strek ME. Autoimmune-featured interstitial lung disease: a distinct entity. Chest 2011;140(5):1292–9.

Hypersensitivity Pneumonitis

Shinichiro Ohshimo, MD, PhD[a], Francesco Bonella, MD[b],
Josune Guzman, MD, PhD[c], Ulrich Costabel, MD, PhD[b],*

KEYWORDS

- Extrinsic allergic alveolitis • Farmer's lung • Bird fancier's disease • HRCT
- Bronchoalveolar lavage • Prognosis

KEY POINTS

- Clinical manifestations of hypersensitivity pneumonitis may closely mimic other interstitial lung diseases, and the disease onset is usually insidious.
- High-resolution computed tomography and bronchoalveolar lavage are the sensitive and characteristic diagnostic tests for hypersensitivity pneumonitis.
- The relevant antigen to hypersensitivity pneumonitis cannot be identified in up to 20% to 30% of patients.
- Clinicians should be aware that hypersensitivity pneumonitis must be considered in all cases of interstitial lung disease, and a detailed environmental exposure history is mandatory.

INTRODUCTION

Hypersensitivity pneumonitis (HP), synonymous with extrinsic allergic alveolitis (EAA), is a complex syndrome resulting from repeated exposure to a variety of antigenic particles found in the environment.[1] Because the resulting inflammatory response involves not only the alveoli but the terminal bronchioli and the interstitium, the term HP may be more correct.

The prevalence of HP is difficult to determine, because the disease is often unrecognized or misdiagnosed. The estimated prevalence of farmer's lung ranges from 1% to 19% of exposed farmers,[2–4] the prevalence of pigeon breeder's lung is from 6% to 20% of exposed individuals,[5] and the prevalence of budgerigar's lung is from 1% to 8% of

Financial disclosure: This work was supported by Arbeitsgemeinschaft zur Förderung der Pneumologie an der Ruhrlandklinik (AFPR).
[a] Department of Molecular and Internal Medicine, Graduate School of Biomedical Sciences, Hiroshima University, Japan; [b] Department of Pneumology/Allergy, Ruhrlandklinik, University Hospital, Essen, Germany; [c] General and Experimental Pathology, Ruhr-University, Bochum, Germany
* Corresponding author. Department of Pneumology/Allergy, Ruhrlandklinik, University Hospital, Tüschener Weg 40, Essen 45239, Germany.
E-mail address: ulrich.costabel@ruhrlandklinik.uk-essen.de

exposed individuals.[6] The disease may also arise in children. Clinical behavior in children is similar to adult cases.[7,8]

The clinical manifestations have regional characteristics. Farmer's lung and pigeon breeder's lung are more common in cold and wet regions, mainly in Europe, whereas summer-type HP is limited to Japan.

A wide variety of particles sized less than 5 μm can reach the alveoli and may be the pathogens of HP. The causative particles include fungal (ie, *Aspergillus* and *Penicillium* species), bacterial, protozoal, animal (mostly bird) and insect proteins, and low-molecular-weight chemical compounds (ie, isocyanates, zinc, inks, and dyes) (**Table 1**).[9]

More recent studies have suggested that mist from a domestic ultrasonic humidifier,[10] steam iron,[11] dry sausage dust,[12,13] wind instruments including saxophone[14,15] and trombone,[16] colistin,[17] catechin (green tea extract),[18] and methylmethacrylate (in dental technicians)[19] can be the cause of HP. Feather duvet lung has been reported as a rare subgroup of bird fancier's lung.[20,21]

HP may present as acute, subacute, or chronic clinical forms, but these forms frequently overlap. The clinical presentation of HP is influenced by several factors including the nature and the amount of inhaled antigen, the intensity and frequency of exposure, and the host immune response, which is likely determined by a genetic background (**Table 2**).[1]

It is not known why HP develops only in a minority of exposed individuals, or why some cases of chronic HP show progression without further antigen exposure.

CLINICAL FEATURES

The spectrum of clinical features varies and has been conventionally classified into acute, subacute, and chronic forms. The interval between sensitization by antigen inhalation and the symptomatic onset of HP is unknown. It seems to be variable and may range from several months to several years after the antigen exposure.

Acute Form

Acute HP is characterized by an influenzalike syndrome (fever, chills, malaise, myalgia, headache) and respiratory symptoms (dry cough, dyspnea, tachypnea, chest tightness). However, respiratory symptoms in acute HP are sometimes absent. The disease onset is abrupt and usually occurs 4 to 12 hours after antigen exposure. In general, acute HP is nonprogressive and spontaneously improves within a few days after antigen avoidance.[1] The disease often recurs after the reexposure of antigen. The clinical examination shows bibasilar crackles and occasional cyanosis, whereas finger clubbing is rare. Patients with recurrent acute farmer's lung may sometimes develop an obstructive lung disease with centrilobular emphysema instead of fibrosis.[22]

Subacute Form

Subacute HP may be associated with repeated low-level exposure to inhaled antigens.[23] After recurrent acute episodes, this form may also become chronic, resulting in fibrosis. It is characterized by an insidious onset of dyspnea, fatigue, and cough. Because the respiratory symptoms are usually mild or absent in subacute HP, infectious pneumonia or noninfectious interstitial lung disease (ILD) is the important differential diagnosis.

Chronic Form

Chronic HP may result from continuous, low-level exposure to inhaled antigens.[23] Bird antigen exposure is the most common in this form of disease. The onset of chronic HP is insidious with slowly increasing dyspnea, dry cough, fatigue, and weight loss. Digital

Table 1
Environmental exposure and antigens in various types of HP

Disease	Exposure	Antigen
Microorganisms		
Farmer's lung	Moldy hay, grain	*Saccharospora rectivirgula*, *Thermoactinomyces vulgaris*, *Aspergillus* spp
Humidifier lung; air conditioner lung	Contaminated humidifiers and air conditioners	Amoebae, nematodes, yeasts, bacteria
Misting fountain HP	Contaminated water	Bacteria, molds, yeasts
Steam iron HP	Contaminated water reservoir	*Sphingobacterium spiritivorum*
Suberosis	Moldy cork	*Penicillium* spp
Sequoiosis	Moldy redwood dust	*Graphium* spp, *Pullularia* spp, *Trichoderma* spp
Woodworker's lung	Contaminated wood pulp or dust	*Alternaria* spp
Wood-trimmer's lung	Contaminated wood trimmings	*Rhizopus* spp, *Mucor* spp
Maple-bark stripper's lung	Contaminated maple logs	*Cryptostroma corticale*
Domestic allergic alveolitis	Decayed wood	Molds
Sauna-taker's lung	Contaminated sauna water	*Aureobasidium* spp
Basement lung	Contaminated basements	*Cephalosporium* spp, *Penicillium* spp
Hot-tub lung	Mold on ceiling, tub water	*Mycobacterium avium* complex
Swimming pool lung	Mist from pool water, sprays and fountains	*M avium* complex
Thatched roof lung	Dried grasses and leaves	*Saccharomonospora viridis*, *T vulgaris*, *Aspergillus* spp
Bagassosis	Moldy pressed sugar cane (bagasse)	*Thermoactinomyces sacchari*, *T vulgaris*
Mushroom-worker's lung	Moldy compost and mushrooms	*S rectivirgula*, *T vulgaris*, *Aspergillus* spp
Malt-worker's lung	Contaminated barley	*Aspergillus clavatus*
Cheese-washer's lung	Moldy cheese or cheese casings	*Penicillium casei*
Dry sausage worker's lung	Moldy sausage dust	*Penicillium* spp
Paprika slicer's lung	Moldy paprika pods	*Mucor stolonifer*
Compost lung	Compost	*Aspergillus* spp, *T vulgaris*
Wine-maker's lung	Mold on grapes	*Botrytis cinerea*
Tobacco-grower's lung	Mold on tobacco	*Aspergillus* spp
Potato-riddler's lung	Moldy hay around potatoes	Thermophilic actinomycetes, *Aspergillus* spp
Summer-type HP	Contaminated houses	*Trychosporon cutaneum*
Detergent lung, washing powder lung	Detergents (during processing or use)	*Bacillus subtilis* enzymes

(continued on next page)

Table 1
(*continued*)

Disease	Exposure	Antigen
Machine-operator's lung	Contaminated metalworking fluid	*Pseudomonas* spp, nontuberculous mycobacteria *Aspergillus fumigatus*
Stipatosis	Esparto dust	Thermophilic actinomycetes
Peat moss HP	Contaminated peat moss	*Monocillium* spp; *Penicillium citreonigum*
Wind-instrument lung	Contaminated saxophones, trombone	Molds, bacteria
Chiropodist's lung	Foot skin and nail dust	Fungi
Animal proteins		
Bird fancier's lung; pigeon breeder's lung	Parakeets, budgerigars, pigeons, parrots, cockatiels, chickens, turkeys, geese, ducks, lovebirds	Proteins in avian droppings, in serum, and on feathers
Feather duvet lung	Feather beds, pillows, duvets	Avian proteins
Pituitary snuff-taker's lung	Bovine and porcine pituitary powder	Pituitary proteins
Furrier's lung	Animal pelts	Animal fur dust
Animal handler's lung, laboratory worker's lung	Rats, gerbils	Proteins from urine, serum, pelts
Pearl oyster shell HP	Dust of shells	Pearl oyster proteins
Mollusk shell HP	Sea snail shell dust	Sea snail shell protein
Silk production HP	Dust from silkworm larvae and cocoons	Silkworm proteins
Miller's lung	Contaminated grain	*Sitophilius granarius* (wheat weevil)
Chemicals		
Chemical worker's lung	Polyurethane foams, spray paints, elastomers, glues	Diisocyanates, trimellitic anhydride
Epoxy resin lung	Heated epoxy resin	Phthalic anhydride
Unknown		
Mummy-handler's lung	Cloth wrappings of mummies	—
Coffee-worker's lung	Coffee-bean dust	—
Tap water lung	Contaminated tap water	—
Tea-grower's lung	Tea plants	—

Adapted from Costabel U, Bonella F, Guzman J. Chronic hypersensitivity pneumonitis. Clin Chest Med 2012; 33:151–63.

clubbing may be present in 20% to 50% of patients[1,23] and predicts clinical deterioration.[24] Chronic HP often develops progressive fibrosis with cor pulmonale and mimics idiopathic pulmonary fibrosis (IPF) or fibrotic nonspecific interstitial pneumonia (NSIP) in the advanced stage.[25] This form of disease, therefore, often leads the

Table 2
Symptoms and signs in 116 patients with HP

Feature	Frequency (%)
Dyspnea	98
Cough	91
Chills	34
Fever	19
Chest tightness	35
Weight loss	42
Body aches	24
Wheezing	31
Inspiratory crackles	87
Cyanosis	32
Clubbing	21

Adapted from Costabel U, Bonella F, Guzman J. Chronic hypersensitivity pneumonitis. Clin Chest Med 2012; 33:151–63.

physician to mistake the disease for other chronic ILDs. The auscultatory findings include bibasilar crackles and characteristically inspiratory squeaks resulting from the coexisting bronchiolitis.

Acute Exacerbation

Acute exacerbation of chronic HP is an emerging concept showing an accelerated respiratory deterioration with the presence of new bilateral ground-glass opacities on high-resolution computed tomography (HRCT).[26,27] The pathogenesis of acute exacerbations in chronic HP is unknown.

It is likely to occur without further exposure to the inhaled antigens. Low total lung capacity (TLC) and diffusing capacity of the lung for carbon monoxide (D_{LCO}), fewer lymphocytes and increased neutrophils in bronchoalveolar lavage (BAL) fluids, and a UIP-like pattern in histology at the time of diagnosis seem to be the risk factors for acute exacerbation.[26] Pathologic findings include organizing pneumonia (OP) or diffuse alveolar damage.

The definitions of acute exacerbations in chronic HP have been proposed as shown in **Box 1**.[26,27] As in IPF, acute exacerbations predict poor outcome. The 2-year frequency of an acute exacerbation is 11.5%.[26]

IMAGING FINDINGS: CHEST RADIOGRAPHY

On the chest radiograph, combined findings of transient diffuse ground-glass attenuation, airspace consolidation, micronodules, reticular shadows, and honeycombing are

Box 1
Definition of acute exacerbation of HP

1. Prior diagnosis of chronic HP
2. Worsening of dyspnea within 1 to 2 months
3. New radiographic opacities
4. Absence of apparent infection, heart disease, and/or other identifiable cause

prominent according to the clinical subforms of HP. In acute HP, diffuse ground-glass attenuation (GGA) and/or airspace consolidation, associated with some micronodules, may be seen. In subacute HP, micronodules, GGA, and reticular shadows are prominent. In chronic HP, reticular shadows and honeycombing are more predominant. In contrast with IPF, the changes are diffuse or may show upper zone predominance.

Mild enlargement of the mediastinal lymph nodes is occasionally found. Pleural involvement is rare. Clinicians should be aware that the chest radiograph may be normal in up to 30% of patients with HP.

IMAGING FINDINGS: HRCT

HRCT is useful in detecting HP and in separating the clinical subforms of HP. In acute HP, HRCT may be normal.[28] When abnormal, the characteristic findings on HRCT are patchy or diffuse GGA and/or centrilobular poorly defined small nodules; consolidation is rarely seen.[29–34] Mosaic perfusion (air trapping) caused by concomitant bronchiolitis is also observed. This finding represents indirect signs of small airway obstruction. These small nodules are the common characteristics in not only acute but subacute or chronic HP (**Fig. 1**).

In subacute HP, patchy air-trapping areas on expiratory scans become more prominent, often in a lobular distribution.[30,35] Because of the considerable overlap in subacute and chronic HP, the findings in chronic HP may be observed in subacute HP to varying degrees.

In chronic HP, the prominent findings on HRCT are the signs of lung fibrosis combined with GGA and centrilobular small nodules. The signs of lung fibrosis include interlobular septal thickening, lobar volume loss, linear-reticular opacities, traction bronchiectasis, and honeycombing (**Fig. 2**).[29,36]

The reticulation is often distributed in the peribronchovascular area and lacks lower zone or subpleural predominance as in IPF. HRCT seems to be useful to distinguish IPF and NSIP from HP in many cases.[36,37] In 1 study, the most characteristic findings in NSIP compared with chronic HP were the subpleural sparing, absence of lobular areas with GGA, and lack of honeycombing.[37] The most characteristic findings in IPF compared with chronic HP were the basal predominance of honeycombing, absence of relative subpleural sparing, and absence of centrilobular nodules. Honeycombing was seen in 64% of patients with chronic HP, which was as high a frequency as in IPF.[36]

Additional emphysema can be seen in 20% of nonsmoking patients with chronic HP.[32–34] Patients with chronic farmer's lung are more likely to develop emphysema than fibrosis.[22]

Subacute and chronic HP sometimes show thin-walled cysts in areas of ground-glass attenuation, which mimic those observed in lymphocytic interstitial pneumonia.[36,38]

PULMONARY FUNCTION TESTS

Although lung function may be normal in acute HP,[28] abnormal lung function is common in most patients with chronic HP. The most frequent functional abnormalities are a restrictive impairment and/or an impaired gas exchange (decreased diffusing capacity or increased alveolar/arterial oxygen gradient). Only few patients with farmer's lung show obstructive impairment resulting from emphysema.[39] However, these changes are not characteristic for chronic HP but are also found in any type of ILDs. Therefore, these abnormalities are not diagnostic for HP. Although hypoxemia is common in HP, patients with mild to moderate disease may lack this symptom and only present hypoxemia with exercise.

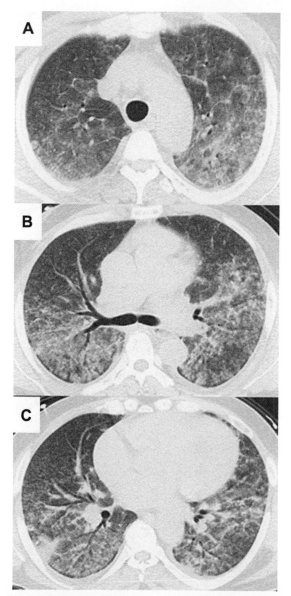

Fig. 1. HRCT of a patient with acute HP showing bilateral ground-glass densities with centrilobular micronodular accentuation and minor consolidation. (*A*) Upper lobes, (*B*) middle lobes, (*C*) lower lobes.

The functional impairment is not well correlated with the severity of radiological abnormalities. The importance of pulmonary function tests is to evaluate the severity of the physiologic impairment at diagnosis and during follow-up.[24]

BAL AND INDUCED SPUTUM

BAL is a highly sensitive method to detect HP. An increase in the total cell count (usually more than 20 million in a total of 100 mL of BAL fluid) with a large increment

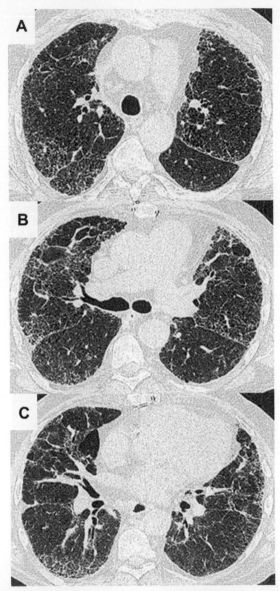

Fig. 2. HRCT of a patient with chronic HP showing bilateral reticular shadowing, traction bronchiectasis, and minor mosaic perfusion along with some micronodules. (*A*) Upper lobes, (*B*) middle lobes, (*C*) lower lobes.

of lymphocytes (usually more than 50%) is characteristic for HP, but not specific.[40] BAL lymphocytes show the highest count in HP of all ILDs. This increase is unusual in other differential diagnoses, including IPF.[41,42] However, in patients with chronic HP or smokers, the increase in BAL lymphocytes may be less prominent.[23,32,43] In contrast, even asymptomatic sensitized individuals may show increased lymphocytes in BAL fluid.[44,45]

The evaluation of CD4+ and CD8+ T-cell subsets usually shows a relative predominance of CD8+ T cells resulting in a low CD4/CD8 ratio with mean values ranging between 0.5 and 1.0. However, the routine evaluation of the CD4/CD8 ratio is not recommended for clinical practice, because the various studies showed no consistent findings in CD4/CD8 ratio. The reasons for this discrepancy are unclear. The possible confounding factors may include the different disease manifestations (eg, the mean value of the CD4/CD8 ratio is higher in chronic HP than in subacute HP[46]), the timing of BAL investigations, the type of inhaled antigen, the intensity of exposure, the smoking habit, and the clinical stage.[24,42,46–48] CD4/CD8 ratios are increased within 24 hours after the last antigen exposure, and become lowest between 7 and 30 days.[49] Persistent BAL abnormalities during the follow-up may indicate incomplete antigen avoidance.

Small numbers of neutrophils, eosinophils, mast cells, and, more characteristically, plasma cells are also found in BAL fluid.[32,49–52] The number of plasma cells in BAL fluid and immunoglobulin levels revealed a positive correlation, suggesting that the local production of immunoglobulins by plasma cells may play a pathogenetic role in susceptible individuals.[51]

Other morphologic features include signs of T-cell and macrophage activation.[53] Activated T cells show folded nuclei and/or broad cytoplasm, and have increased expression of counterligand CD28. Activated macrophages show foamy macrophages, and have increased expression of CD80/CD86.[54]

The proteomic analysis of BAL fluids in HP seems to be useful for differentiating usual interstitial pneumonia (UIP) pattern from NSIP pattern.[55] Surfactant protein A, immunoglobulin heavy chain α, heat shock glycoprotein, haptoglobin β, and immunoglobulin J chain were increased in patients with UIP pattern, whereas glutathione S-transferase, vitamin D–binding protein, and β-actin were increased in patients with NSIP pattern.

In induced sputum from patients with HP, total cells and lymphocytes are also increased.[56] Differential cell counts showed that induced sputum and BAL reflected different compartments of inflammation.[56] A recent study showed that the CD4/CD8 ratio recovered from induced sputum is as useful as that recovered from BAL fluid.[57] Therefore, induced sputum may be complementary, but not an alternative, to BAL. The usefulness of induced sputum in the clinical practice or research use for HP is currently unclear.

LABORATORY TESTS

The presence of specific immunoglobulin (Ig) G antibodies (serum precipitins) to the exposed antigen is evidence of sensitization but not of disease. However, a positive test can be complementary for the diagnosis of HP and give the clinician useful additional information.[58]

Approximately 10% of asymptomatic farmers and 40% of asymptomatic pigeon breeders show positive precipitating antibodies to the exposed antigens.[59–61] Negative precipitating antibodies do not exclude the diagnosis of HP.[62–64]

Various serologic/immunologic techniques including immune-electrophoresis enzyme immunoassay, fluoroenzyme immunoassay, peptide nucleic acid–fluorescence in situ hybridization, and DNA–fluorescence in situ hybridization assays were found to be useful for detecting HP antigens.[65–67] Enzyme-linked immunosorbent assay is usually the preferred method. Increasing IgG antibody titers are correlated with the likelihood of HP, and decreasing titers reflect antigen avoidance.[68]

A recent study enrolling a total of 122 patients with a suspected HP (including 31 cases of true HP) evaluated the diagnostic value of serum precipitins to mold antigens in HP, and showed that negative predictive values varied from 81% to 88% and positive predictive values varied from 71% to 75%.[58] The selection of antigens to be tested needs to be determined based on the local predominant antigens.[69,70]

In acute HP, the neutrophil fraction of the white blood cell count and the levels of C-reactive protein are increased. In chronic HP, polyclonal hypergammaglobulinemia is frequent. The rheumatoid factor may be positive in 50% of patients with pigeon HP.[71]

PROVOCATION TESTS

Inhalative provocation tests with the suspected antigen should only be performed in selected patients, because of the risk of a severe attack and the lack of standard procedure.[24] A natural exposure to the workplace or home seems to be a safer and more reasonable way to provoke symptoms.[72,73]

Positive provocation findings typically include cough, dyspnea, fever, decrease in forced vital capacity and oxygen desaturation 8 to 12 hours after exposure. Because of the severity of the attack, patients should be monitored closely for at least 24 hours.

PATHOGENESIS

The pathogenesis of HP is complex, and the mechanisms involved are poorly understood. The presence of circulating precipitins to the relevant exposed antigens supported the concept that the disease is mediated by the deposition of antigen/antibody complexes within the alveolar walls (type III hypersensitivity).

However, several findings are not consistent with this hypothesis: (1) patients may develop disease but may lack serum precipitins, (2) histopathology does not show vasculitis or prominent neutrophil infiltration, and (3) in animal models passive serum transfer followed by aerosol exposure is not able to induce histologic changes of HP.[62]

Histology of lymphocytic interstitial infiltrates with granuloma formation and signs of macrophage and lymphocyte activation in BAL may suggest a cell-mediated immune reaction (type IV hypersensitivity).[50]

There is evidence for overproduction of Th1 cytokines[74] (interferon-γ, interleukin [IL]-12, and IL-18) along with tumor necrosis factor (TNF) receptors,[75] counterregulators of TNF, by alveolar macrophages from patients with HP.

Although HP is typically defined as Th1 disease, chronic HP evolving to fibrosis seems to be characterized by a switch to a Th2-biased immune response. The BAL fluid analyses from patients with chronic HP show overproduction of a Th2 chemokine family (CXC chemokine receptor [CXCR] 4, thymus and activation-regulated chemokine [TARC]/C-C motif ligand [CCL] 17), and downregulation of a Th1 chemokine family (CXCR3, interferon γ–induced protein [IP]-10, interferon-γ).[46,76]

Although the mechanisms of HP have been partially clarified, it is still unclear why the disease develops only in a minority of exposed individuals. A 2-hit hypothesis suggested that the presence of an inducing factor (inhaled antigen) and a promoting factor (genetic susceptibility) may be essential for the development of HP. Several gene polymorphisms including TNF-α, transporter associated with antigen processing (TAP) genes, and the low-molecular-weight proteasome (LMP) 7 gene have been shown to be involved in the susceptibility HP.[77–80] By contrast, polymorphisms in the tissue inhibitor of metalloproteinase (TIMP)-3 promoter gene may protect against the development of HP.[81,82]

Toll-like receptors (TLRs) are expressed on immune cells and recognize various antigens. When specific TLRs are activated, many proinflammatory cytokines and mediators are released through an intracellular pathway (MyD88 pathway).[83] In experimental models of HP, the expression of TLR-9 and CD34 are essential for the development of a Th1 granulomatous inflammatory response.[84,85]

Despite this progress, it is still not known why some patients show resolution of disease and others progress to fibrosis even without further antigen exposure.

PATHOLOGY

The difficulty in the interpretation of pathology results from the lack of a gold standard defining HP. Pathologic analyses in acute HP are rare. A retrospective study of selected cases of acute HP showed nonspecific diffuse pneumonitis and interstitial inflammation in a peribronchiolar pattern with mononuclear cell and neutrophil infiltration and fibrin deposition.[1] Intra-alveolar fibrin accumulation may be prominent in some selected cases with acute fibrinous and organizing pneumonia (AFOP).

Subacute HP is characterized by a lymphocytic, bronchiolocentric interstitial pneumonitis. The central regions of the secondary lobule are the predominant site to be involved.[86] It is independent of the presence or absence of further antigen exposure. Lymphocytes with fewer plasma cells and histiocytes are the main cells associated with inflammation. The granulomas are typically small, loose, poorly formed, and non-necrotizing, with the exception of hot-tub lung. Granulomatous changes may be absent in approximately 30% of patients with HP.[87] The staining with cathepsin K, a cysteine protease expressed in activated macrophages and epithelioid cells, may be useful for detecting microgranulomas in HP.[86] Cathepsin K staining is negative in patients with desquamative interstitial pneumonia (DIP) and respiratory bronchiolitis-ILD (RB-ILD), in which accumulation of alveolar macrophages is prominent. These findings suggest that cathepsin K may be a sensitive and specific marker to detect granulomas in chronic HP.

Chronic HP is characterized by progressive fibrosis, bronchiolitis obliterans, and architectural distortion in addition to the subacute changes. However, chronic HP may lack typical subacute changes.[43] The pathologic patterns may mimic UIP, NSIP, OP, or peribronchiolar interstitial fibrosis.[9,43] In late chronic stages, the pathologic findings may become more similar to IPF/UIP.

The characteristic pathologic findings supporting HP includes bronchiolocentric inflammation, peribronchiolar fibrosis, bronchiolar epithelial hyperplasia, and the presence of granulomas or multinucleated giant cells.[25] Peribronchiolar metaplasia is frequently observed in HP, but is rare in IPF/UIP.[88] Peribronchiolar (centrilobular) fibrosis often extends to the perilobular areas, and forms the appearance of bridging fibrosis. This pathologic finding can distinguish chronic HP from IPF.[89]

Although pathologic changes in HP are uniform in distribution, lung biopsy specimens sometimes show discordant findings.[88] This observation suggests that biopsy should be taken from at least 2 different lobes, as in IPF.

A recent study reported the coexistence of HP and pulmonary alveolar proteinosis (PAP).[90] Although all patients had typical HRCT findings of PAP to a varying degree, typical HRCT findings of HP were sometimes absent. The linkage between HP and PAP is still unclear.

DIAGNOSTIC CRITERIA

Several diagnostic criteria for HP have been recommended.[91,92] However, none of these criteria has been validated. The diagnosis of HP relies on a high level of clinical suspicion; the recognition of antecedent antigen exposure; and a constellation of clinical, radiologic, laboratory, and pathologic findings.

A large prospective multicenter cohort study (116 patients with HP, 284 control subjects with other ILD) showed that the diagnosis of HP could be made with 6 significant predictors (**Box 2**). If all of the 6 predictors are present, the probability of having HP is 98%.[69] If none of the 6 predictors are present, the probability is 0%.[69]

Careful history taking is mandatory. Clinicians should have specific expertise concerning the relevant antigens to HP. Important factors are hay feeding, bird keeping, feather duvet and pillows in the home, air conditioning or ventilators in the buildings, and formation of mold on room walls or in the cellars. Indirect contact with birds should also be asked for, such as visits to friends or relatives who keep birds in their homes. Improvement on vacation or during hospitalization may also be a clue to the diagnosis.

HRCT is a useful diagnostic test. Although it may be normal in some patients, the sensitivity is more than 95%, and the finding of a centrilobular micronodular ground-glass pattern and evidence of mosaic perfusion (trapped air) is characteristic of HP. The major differential diagnosis in this setting is respiratory bronchiolitis/ILD or *Pneumocystis carinii* infection.

The most sensitive diagnostic test is BAL. In the author's experience and based on literature review, a normal BAL widely excludes the diagnosis of HP. The characteristic finding is a lymphocytosis in the subacute and chronic forms. In asymptomatic sensitized individuals (subclinical alveolitis), BAL lymphocytosis is also apparent. BAL lymphocytosis greater than 30% is recommended as a discriminative factor of chronic HP showing UIP pattern on HRCT from IPF.[41]

BAL analyses have complementary information on HRCT. Lymphocytosis is characteristic for HP, a predominance of smoker's macrophages is characteristic for RB-ILD, and the presence of microorganisms is characteristic for *Pneumocystis carinii* pneumonia.

Pathologic evaluation of lung tissue is usually unnecessary for the diagnosis of HP. If needed, the preferred approach is surgical biopsy rather than transbronchial biopsy.

An important problem in the diagnosis of HP is that the relevant antigen cannot be identified in up to 20% to 30% of patients. In these patients the diagnosis must be suspected based on histopathology, BAL findings, and HRCT characteristics.[93]

DIFFERENTIAL DIAGNOSIS

The differential diagnoses include the wide spectrum of ILD, mainly idiopathic interstitial pneumonias (IIPs) and sarcoidosis.[69] Frequent misdiagnosis is pneumonia in acute forms and chronic bronchitis in chronic forms with normal chest radiograph, which may occur in 20%. Chronic HP, especially the insidious form of bird fancier's lung, may closely mimic IPF or idiopathic fibrotic NSIP.[94]

Clinicians should be aware that HP must be considered in all cases of ILD, and a detailed environmental exposure history is mandatory. **Fig. 3** shows the diagnostic algorithm for HP.

Box 2
Diagnosis of HP

1. Exposure to a known offending antigen
2. Positive precipitating antibodies
3. Recurrent episodes of symptoms
4. Inspiratory crackles
5. Symptoms 4 to 8 hours after exposure
6. Weight loss

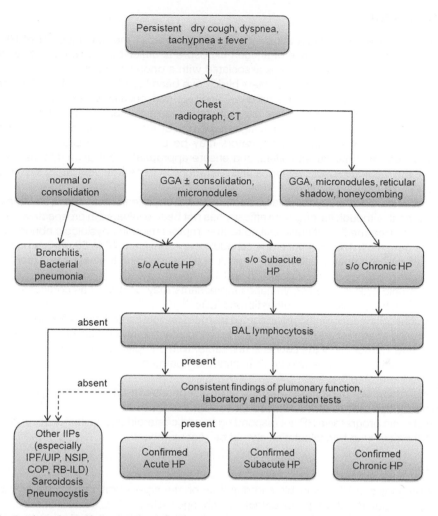

Fig. 3. Flow chart of diagnostic algorithm for HP. BAL, bronchoalveolar lavage; COP, cryptogenic organizing pneumonia; CT, computed tomography; NSIP, nonspecific interstitial pneumonia; RB-ILD, respiratory bronchiolitis-interstitial lung disease.

PITFALLS: EFFECT OF CIGARETTE SMOKING

HP is less frequent in smokers than in nonsmokers under the same exposure.[24] Cigarette smoking seems to protect against the development of HP. When exposed to high levels of antigens, smokers have lower levels of specific antibodies to the causative antigen compared with nonsmokers.

Although the mechanisms of the protective effect of smoking against HP are unclear, nicotine seems to be one of the key factors.[95] Nicotine inhibits macrophage activation, decreases lymphocyte proliferation, and impairs T-cell function.[95,96]

Although HP develops more frequently in nonsmokers, when HP occurs in smokers, the patients may develop a chronic clinical course with more recurrent episodes and a significantly poorer survival compared with nonsmoker patients.[97]

MANAGEMENT

Early diagnosis and antigen avoidance are key factors in the management of HP. Although complete avoidance of antigen exposure is difficult in some patients with HP, sustained antigen inhalation is associated with a poorer outcome.

Antigens may persist in rooms where birds have been kept for a long time. Feather pillows and blankets should be removed. Indirect and occasional exposure in the homes of friends or relatives where birds are kept should also be avoided. It is important to minimize microbial or avian antigen exposure by having a clean environment at home. The use of air-purifying respirators may be useful in some cases. Farmers should wear dust masks with filters, and ensure appropriate ventilation. Mechanization of the feeding process on farms and alterations in forced-air ventilatory systems may also be useful.

Corticosteroid therapy is usually recommended in patients who show functional impairment, although its long-term efficacy has not been evaluated in prospective clinical trials. Treatment continues until no further improvement in physiologic abnormalities is observed. An empiric therapy schedule may consist of 40 to 50 mg per day of prednisone for a month, followed by a gradual tapering during the next 2 to 3 months and a maintenance dose between 7.5 and 15 mg per day.

In chronic progressive HP, immunosuppressants may be added as corticosteroid sparing agents, as is done in other fibrotic ILDs.[94]

Routine follow-up investigations should be more narrow immediately after diagnosis and during treatment (1–3 months is appropriate); later the interval can be extended to every 6 to 12 months. If the course is favorable, with complete remission after avoidance of further exposure and/or corticosteroid treatment, routine follow-up can be stopped after 2 to 3 years.

Inhaled steroids or pentoxifylline may be other options of treatment[98]; however, their efficiency has not yet been validated.

In chronic progressive HP not responding to corticosteroid and/or immunosuppressant therapy, lung transplantation should be recommended.

PROGNOSIS

The prognosis of HP is variable and depends on the type, duration, and intensity of antigen exposure; the type of pathologic changes (UIP, NSIP, OP-like fibrosis, or emphysema); and possibly genetic background.[9] The findings of fibrosis at lung biopsy or HRCT are associated with poor prognosis in patients with chronic HP and may serve as a useful prognostic indicator.[93]

Patients with OP-like or cellular NSIP-like fibrosis have a more favorable outcome than those with fibrotic NSIP-like and UIP-like fibrosis.[94] The UIP-like and fibrotic NSIP-like fibrosis are associated with decreased survival.[99]

Some patients may experience progression, despite avoiding exposure and undergoing treatment. There is no good explanation for the mechanism. Acute exacerbation of chronic HP is associated with a poor prognosis.[26] In a previous study enrolling 100 consecutive patients with chronic bird farmer's lung, 14 patients developed an acute exacerbation, and 12 of them died of this episode.[26]

A previous surveillance in the United States showed that overall age-adjusted death rates in HP increased significantly ($P<.0001$) between 1980 and 2002, from 0.09 to 0.29 per million, although it is unclear what factors were associated with this increase.[100] By contrast, another surveillance in England and Wales showed that the mortality in HP was almost stable between 1968 and 2008, from 0.04 to 0.08 per million.[101]

In general, acute HP seems to have a favorable prognosis. After acute attacks, if correctly and timely diagnosed and treated, patients usually have a complete remission. If acute attacks occur frequently, such as in some patients with farmer's lung, the outcome may be the development of emphysema.

Patients with farmer's lung who experienced recurrent attacks tend to have emphysema more frequently and lower diffusing capacity than patients who experienced only a single attack.[102]

Complications of lung cancer may affect the prognosis in HP. A recent retrospective review on 104 patients with chronic HP showed that the prevalence of lung cancer in chronic HP seems to be increased (10.6%), as seen in IPF.[103]

Pulmonary hypertension occurs in approximately 20% of patients with chronic HP, and is associated with a greater risk of death (see **Box 2**).[104]

SUMMARY

HP is a complex syndrome caused by repeated inhalation of environmental and occupational antigens. Clinical manifestations of HP may closely mimic other ILDs, including IPF or NSIP, and the disease onset is usually insidious; diagnosis of HP is therefore sometimes difficult. An appropriate removal of antigen exposure is essential for treatment of HP, otherwise the disease results in poor outcomes. Therefore, clinicians should be aware that HP must be considered in all cases of ILD, and should start the appropriate management as soon as possible.

REFERENCES

1. Costabel U, Bonella F, Guzman J. Chronic hypersensitivity pneumonitis. Clin Chest Med 2012;33:151-63.
2. Gruchow HW, Hoffmann RG, Marx JJ Jr, et al. Precipitating antibodies to farmer's lung antigens in a Wisconsin farming population. Am Rev Respir Dis 1981;124:411-5.
3. Terho EO, Heinonen OP, Lammi S, et al. Incidence of clinically confirmed farmer's lung in Finland and its relation to meteorological factors. Eur J Respir Dis Suppl 1987;152:47-56.
4. Depierre A, Dalphin JC, Pernet D, et al. Epidemiological study of farmer's lung in five districts of the French Doubs province. Thorax 1988;43:429-35.
5. Rodríguez de Castro F, Carrillo T, Castillo R, et al. Relationships between characteristics of exposure to pigeon antigens. Clinical manifestations and humoral immune response. Chest 1993;103:1059-63.
6. Hendrick DJ, Faux JA, Marshall R. Budgerigar-fancier's lung: the commonest variety of allergic alveolitis in Britain. Br Med J 1978;2:81-4.
7. Grech V, Vella C, Lenicker H. Pigeon breeder's lung in childhood: varied clinical picture at presentation. Pediatr Pulmonol 2000;30:145-8.
8. Ratjen F, Costabel U, Griese M, et al. Bronchoalveolar lavage fluid findings in children with hypersensitivity pneumonitis. Eur Respir J 2003;21:144-8.
9. Lacasse Y, Girard M, Cormier Y. Recent advances in hypersensitivity pneumonitis. Chest 2012;142:208-17.
10. Koschel D, Stark W, Karmann F, et al. Extrinsic allergic alveolitis caused by misting fountains. Respir Med 2005;99:943-7.
11. Kämpfer P, Engelhart S, Rolke M, et al. Extrinsic allergic alveolitis (hypersensitivity pneumonitis) caused by *Sphingobacterium spiritivorum* from the water reservoir of a steam iron. J Clin Microbiol 2005;43:4908-10.

12. Morell F, Cruz MJ, Gómez FP, et al. Chacinero's lung - hypersensitivity pneumonitis due to dry sausage dust. Scand J Work Environ Health 2011;37:349–56.

13. Rouzaud P, Soulat JM, Trela C, et al. Symptoms and serum precipitins in workers exposed to dry sausage mould: consequences of exposure to sausage mould. Int Arch Occup Environ Health 2001;74:371–4.

14. Metzger F, Haccuria A, Reboux G, et al. Hypersensitivity pneumonitis due to molds in a saxophone player. Chest 2010;138:724–6.

15. Lodha S, Sharma OP. Hypersensitivity pneumonitis in a saxophone player. Chest 1988;93:1322.

16. Metersky ML, Bean SB, Meyer JD, et al. Trombone player's lung: a probable new cause of hypersensitivity pneumonitis. Chest 2010;138:754–6.

17. Leong KW, Ong S, Chee HL, et al. Hypersensitivity pneumonitis due to high-dose colistin aerosol therapy. Int J Infect Dis 2010;14:e1018–9.

18. Otera H, Tada K, Sakurai T, et al. Hypersensitivity pneumonitis associated with inhalation of catechin-rich green tea extracts. Respiration 2011;82:388–92.

19. Scherpereel A, Tillie-Leblond I, Pommier de Santi P, et al. Exposure to methyl methacrylate and hypersensitivity pneumonitis in dental technicians. Allergy 2004;59:890–2.

20. Koschel D, Lützkendorf L, Wiedemann B, et al. Antigen-specific IgG antibodies in feather duvet lung. Eur J Clin Invest 2010;40:797–802.

21. Koschel D, Wittstruck H, Renck T, et al. Presenting features of feather duvet lung. Int Arch Allergy Immunol 2010;152:264–70.

22. Malinen AP, Erkinjuntti-Pekkanen RA, Partanen PL, et al. Long-term sequelae of farmer's lung disease in HRCT: a 14-year follow-up study of 88 patients and 83 matched control farmers. Eur Radiol 2003;13:2212–21.

23. Ohtani Y, Saiki S, Sumi Y, et al. Clinical features of recurrent and insidious chronic bird fancier's lung. Ann Allergy Asthma Immunol 2003;90:604–10.

24. Selman M, Pardo A, King TE Jr. Hypersensitivity pneumonitis: insights in diagnosis and pathobiology. Am J Respir Crit Care Med 2012;186(4):314–24.

25. Churg A, Muller NL, Flint J, et al. Chronic hypersensitivity pneumonitis. Am J Surg Pathol 2006;30:201–8.

26. Miyazaki Y, Tateishi T, Akashi T, et al. Clinical predictors and histologic appearance of acute exacerbations in chronic hypersensitivity pneumonitis. Chest 2008;134:1265–70.

27. Olson AL, Huie TJ, Groshong SD, et al. Acute exacerbations of fibrotic hypersensitivity pneumonitis: a case series. Chest 2008;134:844–50.

28. Lynch DA, Rose CS, Way D, et al. Hypersensitivity pneumonitis: sensitivity of high-resolution CT in a population-based study. AJR Am J Roentgenol 1992;159:469–72.

29. Tateishi T, Ohtani Y, Takemura T, et al. Serial high-resolution computed tomography findings of acute and chronic hypersensitivity pneumonitis induced by avian antigen. J Comput Assist Tomogr 2011;35:272–9.

30. Patel RA, Sellami D, Gotway MB, et al. Hypersensitivity pneumonitis: patterns on high-resolution CT. J Comput Assist Tomogr 2000;24:965–70.

31. Adler BD, Padley SP, Müller NL, et al. Chronic hypersensitivity pneumonitis: high-resolution CT and radiographic features in 16 patients. Radiology 1992;185:91–5.

32. Remy-Jardin M, Remy J, Wallaert B, et al. Subacute and chronic bird breeder hypersensitivity pneumonitis: sequential evaluation with CT and correlation with lung function tests and bronchoalveolar lavage. Radiology 1993;189:111–8.

33. Erkinjuntti-Pekkanen R, Rytkonen H, Kokkarinen JI, et al. Long-term risk of emphysema in patients with farmer's lung and matched control farmers. Am J Respir Crit Care Med 1998;158:662–5.
34. Cormier Y, Brown M, Worthy S, et al. High-resolution computed tomographic characteristics in acute farmer's lung and in its follow-up. Eur Respir J 2000; 16:56–60.
35. Hansell DM, Wells AU, Padley SP, et al. Hypersensitivity pneumonitis: correlation of individual CT patterns with functional abnormalities. Radiology 1996;199:123–8.
36. Silva CI, Müller NL, Lynch DA, et al. Chronic hypersensitivity pneumonitis: differentiation from idiopathic pulmonary fibrosis and nonspecific interstitial pneumonia by using thin-section CT. Radiology 2008;246:288–97.
37. Lynch DA, Newell JD, Logan PM, et al. Can CT distinguish hypersensitivity pneumonitis from idiopathic pulmonary fibrosis? AJR Am J Roentgenol 1995; 165:807–11.
38. Franquet T, Hansell DM, Senbanjo T, et al. Lung cysts in subacute hypersensitivity pneumonitis. J Comput Assist Tomogr 2003;27:475–8.
39. Lalancette M, Carrier G, Laviolette M, et al. Farmer's lung. Long-term outcome and lack of predictive value of bronchoalveolar lavage fibrosing factors. Am Rev Respir Dis 1993;148:216–21.
40. Semenzato G, Bjermer L, Costabel U, et al. Clinical guidelines and indications for bronchoalveolar lavage (BAL): extrinsic allergic alveolitis. Eur Respir J 1990;3:945–6.
41. Ohshimo S, Bonella F, Cui A, et al. Significance of bronchoalveolar lavage for the diagnosis of idiopathic pulmonary fibrosis. Am J Respir Crit Care Med 2009;179: 1043–7.
42. Meyer KC, Raghu G, Baughman RP, et al. An official American Thoracic Society clinical practice guideline: the clinical utility of bronchoalveolar lavage cellular analysis in interstitial lung disease. Am J Respir Crit Care Med 2012;185:1004–14.
43. Gaxiola M, Buendía-Roldán I, Mejía M, et al. Morphologic diversity of chronic pigeon breeder's disease: clinical features and survival. Respir Med 2011; 105:608–14.
44. Cormier Y, Bélanger J, Laviolette M. Persistent bronchoalveolar lymphocytosis in asymptomatic farmers. Am Rev Respir Dis 1986;133:843–7.
45. Cormier Y, Létourneau L, Racine G. Significance of precipitins and asymptomatic lymphocytic alveolitis: a 20-yr follow-up. Eur Respir J 2004;23:523–5.
46. Barrera L, Mendoza F, Zuñiga J, et al. Functional diversity of T-cell subpopulations in subacute and chronic hypersensitivity pneumonitis. Am J Respir Crit Care Med 2008;177:44–55.
47. Ando M, Konishi K, Yoneda R, et al. Difference in the phenotypes of bronchoalveolar lavage lymphocytes in patients with summer-type hypersensitivity pneumonitis, farmer's lung, ventilation pneumonitis, and bird fancier's lung: report of a nationwide epidemiologic study in Japan. J Allergy Clin Immunol 1991;87:1002–9.
48. Wahlström J, Berlin M, Lundgren R, et al. Lung and blood T-cell receptor repertoire in extrinsic allergic alveolitis. Eur Respir J 1997;10:772–9.
49. Drent M, van Velzen-Blad H, Diamant M, et al. Bronchoalveolar lavage in extrinsic allergic alveolitis: effect of time elapsed since antigen exposure. Eur Respir J 1993;6:1276–81.
50. Costabel U. The alveolitis of hypersensitivity pneumonitis. Eur Respir J 1988;1:5–9.
51. Drent M, Wagenaar S, van Velzen-Blad H, et al. Relationship between plasma cell levels and profile of bronchoalveolar lavage fluid in patients with subacute extrinsic allergic alveolitis. Thorax 1993;48:835–9.

52. Groot Kormelink T, Pardo A, Knipping K, et al. Immunoglobulin free light chains are increased in hypersensitivity pneumonitis and idiopathic pulmonary fibrosis. PLoS One 2011;6:e25392.

53. Costabel U, Bross KJ, Rühle KH, et al. Ia-like antigens on T-cells and their subpopulations in pulmonary sarcoidosis and in hypersensitivity pneumonitis. Analysis of bronchoalveolar and blood lymphocytes. Am Rev Respir Dis 1985; 131:337–42.

54. Blatman KH, Grammer LC. Chapter 19: hypersensitivity pneumonitis. Allergy Asthma Proc 2012;33(Suppl 1):64–6.

55. Okamoto T, Miyazaki Y, Shirahama R, et al. Proteome analysis of bronchoalveolar lavage fluid in chronic hypersensitivity pneumonitis. Allergol Int 2012;61:83–92.

56. D'Ippolito R, Chetta A, Foresi A, et al. Induced sputum and bronchoalveolar lavage from patients with hypersensitivity pneumonitis. Respir Med 2004;98: 977–83.

57. Economidou F, Samara KD, Antoniou KM, et al. Induced sputum in interstitial lung diseases: novel insights in the diagnosis, evaluation and research. Respiration 2009;77:351–8.

58. Fenoglio CM, Reboux G, Sudre B, et al. Diagnostic value of serum precipitins to mould antigens in active hypersensitivity pneumonitis. Eur Respir J 2007;29: 706–12.

59. Cormier Y, Bélanger J, Durand P. Factors influencing the development of serum precipitins to farmer's lung antigen in Quebec dairy farmers. Thorax 1985;40: 138–42.

60. Fink JN. Epidemiologic aspects of hypersensitivity pneumonitis. Monogr Allergy 1987;21:59–69.

61. Dalphin JC, Toson B, Monnet E, et al. Farmer's lung precipitins in Doubs (a department of France): prevalence and diagnostic value. Allergy 1994;49: 744–50.

62. Sennekamp J, Niese D, Stroehmann I, et al. Pigeon breeders' lung lacking detectable antibodies. Clin Allergy 1978;8:305–10.

63. Cormier Y, Bélanger J. The fluctuant nature of precipitating antibodies in dairy farmers. Thorax 1989;44:469–73.

64. Erkinjuntti-Pekkanen R, Reiman M, Kokkarinen JI, et al. IgG antibodies, chronic bronchitis, and pulmonary function values in farmer's lung patients and matched controls. Allergy 1999;54:1181–7.

65. Rodrigo MJ, Postigo I, Wangensteen O, et al. A new application of Streptavidin ImmunoCAP for measuring IgG antibodies against non-available commercial antigens. Clin Chim Acta 2010;411:1675–8.

66. Reboux G, Piarroux R, Roussel S, et al. Assessment of four serological techniques in the immunological diagnosis of farmers' lung disease. J Med Microbiol 2007;56:1317–21.

67. Selvaraju SB, Kapoor R, Yadav JS. Peptide nucleic acid-fluorescence in situ hybridization (PNA-FISH) assay for specific detection of mycobacterium immunogenum and DNA-FISH assay for analysis of pseudomonads in metalworking fluids and sputum. Mol Cell Probes 2008;22:273–80.

68. McSharry C, Dye GM, Ismail T, et al. Quantifying serum antibody in bird fanciers' hypersensitivity pneumonitis. BMC Pulm Med 2006;6:16.

69. Lacasse Y, Selman M, Costabel U, et al. Clinical diagnosis of hypersensitivity pneumonitis. Am J Respir Crit Care Med 2003;168:952–8.

70. Ojanen T. Class specific antibodies in serodiagnosis of farmer's lung. Br J Ind Med 1992;49:332–6.

71. Aguilar León DE, Novelo Retana V, Martínez-Cordero E. Anti-avian antibodies and rheumatoid factor in pigeon hypersensitivity pneumonitis. Clin Exp Allergy 2003;33:226–32.

72. Ramírez-Venegas A, Sansores RH, Pérez-Padilla R, et al. Utility of a provocation test for diagnosis of chronic pigeon breeder's disease. Am J Respir Crit Care Med 1998;158:862–9.

73. Ohtani Y, Kojima K, Sumi Y, et al. Inhalation provocation tests in chronic bird fancier's lung. Chest 2000;118:1382–9.

74. Yamasaki H, Ando M, Brazer W, et al. Polarized type 1 cytokine profile in bronchoalveolar lavage T cells of patients with hypersensitivity pneumonitis. J Immunol 1999;163:3516–23.

75. Dai H, Guzman J, Chen B, et al. Production of soluble tumor necrosis factor receptors and tumor necrosis factor-alpha by alveolar macrophages in sarcoidosis and extrinsic allergic alveolitis. Chest 2005;127:251–6.

76. Kishi M, Miyazaki Y, Jinta T, et al. Pathogenesis of cBFL in common with IPF? Correlation of IP-10/TARC ratio with histological patterns. Thorax 2008;63:810–6.

77. Camarena A, Juarez A, Mejia M, et al. Major histocompatibility complex and tumor necrosis factor-alpha polymorphisms in pigeon breeder's disease. Am J Respir Crit Care Med 2001;163:1528–33.

78. Schaaf BM, Seitzer U, Pravica V, et al. Tumor necrosis factor-alpha-308 promoter gene polymorphism and increased tumor necrosis factor serum bioactivity in farmer's lung patients. Am J Respir Crit Care Med 2001;163:379–82.

79. Aquino-Galvez A, Camarena A, Montano M, et al. Transporter associated with antigen processing (TAP) 1 gene polymorphisms in patients with hypersensitivity pneumonitis. Exp Mol Pathol 2008;84:173–7.

80. Camarena A, Aquino-Galvez A, Falfan-Valencia R, et al. PSMB8 (LMP7) but not PSMB9 (LMP2) gene polymorphisms are associated to pigeon breeder's hypersensitivity pneumonitis. Respir Med 2010;104:889–94.

81. Hill MR, Briggs L, Montano MM, et al. Promoter variants in tissue inhibitor of metalloproteinase-3 (TIMP-3) protect against susceptibility in pigeon breeders' disease. Thorax 2004;59:586–90.

82. Janssen R, Kruit A, Grutters JC, et al. TIMP-3 promoter gene polymorphisms in BFL. Thorax 2005;60:974.

83. Nance SC, Yi AK, Re FC, et al. MyD88 is necessary for neutrophil recruitment in hypersensitivity pneumonitis. J Leukoc Biol 2008;83:1207–17.

84. Bhan U, Newstead MJ, Zeng X, et al. Stachybotrys chartarum-induced hypersensitivity pneumonitis is TLR9 dependent. Am J Pathol 2011;179: 2779–87.

85. Blanchet MR, Bennett JL, Gold MJ, et al. CD34 is required for dendritic cell trafficking and pathology in murine hypersensitivity pneumonitis. Am J Respir Crit Care Med 2011;184:687–98.

86. Reghellin D, Poletti V, Tomassett S, et al. Cathepsin-K is a sensitive immunohistochemical marker for detection of micro-granulomas in hypersensitivity pneumonitis. Sarcoidosis Vasc Diffuse Lung Dis 2010;27:57–63.

87. Myers JL. Hypersensitivity pneumonia: the role of lung biopsy in diagnosis and management. Mod Pathol 2012;25:S58–67.

88. Trahan S, Hanak V, Ryu JH, et al. Role of surgical lung biopsy in separating chronic hypersensitivity pneumonia from usual interstitial pneumonia/idiopathic pulmonary fibrosis: analysis of 31 biopsies from 15 patients. Chest 2008;134:126–32.

89. Akashi T, Takemura T, Ando N, et al. Histopathologic analysis of sixteen autopsy cases of chronic hypersensitivity pneumonitis and comparison with idiopathic

pulmonary fibrosis/usual interstitial pneumonia. Am J Clin Pathol 2009;131: 405–15.

90. Verma H, Nicholson AG, Kerr KM, et al. Alveolar proteinosis with hypersensitivity pneumonitis: a new clinical phenotype. Respirology 2010;15:1197–202.

91. Terho EO. Diagnostic criteria for farmer's lung disease. Am J Ind Med 1986; 10:329.

92. Schuyler M, Cormier Y. The diagnosis of hypersensitivity pneumonitis. Chest 1997;111:534–6.

93. Hanak V, Golbin JM, Hartman TE, et al. High-resolution CT findings of parenchymal fibrosis correlate with prognosis in hypersensitivity pneumonitis. Chest 2008;134:133–8.

94. Ohtani Y, Saiki S, Kitaichi M, et al. Chronic bird fancier's lung: histopathological and clinical correlation. An application of the 2002 ATS/ERS consensus classification of the idiopathic interstitial pneumonias. Thorax 2005;60:665–71.

95. Blanchet MR, Israël-Assayag E, Cormier Y. Inhibitory effect of nicotine on experimental hypersensitivity pneumonitis in vivo and in vitro. Am J Respir Crit Care Med 2004;169:903–9.

96. Nizri E, Irony-Tur-Sinai M, Lory O, et al. Activation of the cholinergic anti-inflammatory system by nicotine attenuates neuroinflammation via suppression of Th1 and Th17 responses. J Immunol 2009;183:6681–8.

97. Ohtsuka Y, Munakata M, Tanimura K, et al. Smoking promotes insidious and chronic farmer's lung disease, and deteriorates the clinical outcome. Intern Med 1995;34:966–71.

98. Tanaka H, Tsunematsu K, Nakamura N, et al. Successful treatment of hypersensitivity pneumonitis caused by *Grifola frondosa* (Maitake) mushroom using a HFA-BDP extra-fine aerosol. Intern Med 2004;43:737–40.

99. Vourlekis JS, Schwarz MI, Cherniack RM, et al. The effect of pulmonary fibrosis on survival in patients with hypersensitivity pneumonitis. Am J Med 2004;116: 662–8.

100. Bang KM, Weissman DN, Pinheiro GA, et al. Twenty-three years of hypersensitivity pneumonitis mortality surveillance in the United States. Am J Ind Med 2006;49:997–1004.

101. Hanley A, Hubbard RB, Navaratnam V. Mortality trends in asbestosis, extrinsic allergic alveolitis and sarcoidosis in England and Wales. Respir Med 2011; 105:1373–9.

102. Erkinjuntti-Pekkanen R, Kokkarinen JI, Tukiainen HO, et al. Long-term outcome of pulmonary function in farmer's lung: a 14 year follow-up with matched controls. Eur Respir J 1997;10:2046–50.

103. Kuramochi J, Inase N, Miyazaki Y, et al. Lung cancer in chronic hypersensitivity pneumonitis. Respiration 2011;82:263–7.

104. Koschel DS, Cardoso C, Wiedemann B, et al. Pulmonary hypertension in chronic hypersensitivity pneumonitis. Lung 2012;190(3):295–302.

Eosinophilic Lung Diseases

Vincent Cottin, MD, PhD[a,b,*], Jean-François Cordier, MD[a,b]

KEYWORDS

- Eosinophil • Eosinophilic pneumonia • Interstitial lung disease
- Churg-Strauss syndrome • Aspergillus

KEY POINTS

- Eosinophilic lung diseases may present as eosinophilic pneumonia with chronic or acute onset, or as Löffler syndrome.
- The diagnosis of eosinophilic pneumonia is based on characteristic clinical-imaging features and the demonstration of alveolar eosinophilia (>25% eosinophils at bronchoalveolar lavage, and preferably >40%). Lung biopsy is generally not necessary.
- Peripheral blood eosinophilia (>1000/mm^3 and preferably >1500/mm^3) may be absent at presentation especially in idiopathic acute eosinophilic pneumonia and in patients receiving corticosteroid treatment.
- Idiopathic chronic eosinophilic pneumonia is the most frequent eosinophilic lung disease in Europe and North America. Idiopathic acute eosinophilic pneumonia may be misdiagnosed as severe infectious pneumonia.
- Possible causes of eosinophilia (especially fungus or parasitic infection, drug or toxic exposure) must be thoroughly investigated.
- Clues that should raise the suspicion of allergic bronchopulmonary aspergillosis in asthmatics include poor asthma control, expectoration of mucous plugs, peripheral eosinophilia, serum immunoglobulin E levels greater than1000 ng/mL, positive skin prick tests to *Aspergillus fumigatus*, and central bronchiectasis, centrilobular nodules, tree-in-bud pattern, and finger-in-glove pattern at chest imaging.
- Extrathoracic manifestations with eosinophilic lung disease suggest the diagnosis of Churg-Strauss syndrome. Cardiac involvement must be investigated systematically especially in the eosinophilic tissular subtype of Churg-Strauss syndrome. Management is adapted to five prognostic factors.

Financial support: Hospices Civils de Lyon, Université Lyon I.
Conflicts of interest: None.

[a] Service de pneumologie, Hospices Civils de Lyon, Centre de référence national des maladies pulmonaires rares, Hôpital Louis Pradel, Lyon Cedex 69677, France; [b] Université de Lyon, Université Lyon I, INRA, UMR754 INRA-Vetagrosup EPHE IFR 128, Lyon, France
* Corresponding author.
E-mail address: vincent.cottin@chu-lyon.fr

Immunol Allergy Clin N Am 32 (2012) 557–586
http://dx.doi.org/10.1016/j.iac.2012.08.007
0889-8561/12/$ – see front matter © 2012 Elsevier Inc. All rights reserved.

immunology.theclinics.com

INTRODUCTION
Definition

Eosinophilic lung diseases are a group of diffuse parenchymal lung diseases[1,2] characterized by the prominent infiltration by polymorphonuclear eosinophils of the lung interstitium and the alveolar spaces, with conservation of the lung architecture. As a consequence, a common denominator of eosinophilic lung diseases is represented by a dramatic response to systemic corticosteroid therapy and healing without any sequelae in almost all cases, despite frequent impressive impairment of lung function at presentation.

Alveolar eosinophilia is defined by differential cell count greater than 25% (preferably >40%) eosinophils at bronchoalveolar lavage (BAL) and peripheral blood eosinophilia by eosinophil count greater than 1000/mm^3 (preferably >1500/mm^3).

Classification

Eosinophilic lung disorders may present as acute or chronic pneumonia (ie, with symptoms present for <1 month or >1 month, respectively), or as the transient Löffler syndrome mostly of parasitic origin (**Box 1**). Eosinophilic pneumonia may remain idiopathic or be related to a known cause, especially drug or toxic exposure or fungus infection. They may occur as solitary pulmonary disorders or in the context of systemic conditions, such as Churg-Strauss syndrome (CSS) or the idiopathic hypereosinophilic syndromes.

PATHOPHYSIOLOGY
Recruitment of Eosinophils to the Lung

The pathobiology of eosinophils is highly relevant for eosinophilic lung diseases, as they represent the major culprit of tissue injury by these cells. Although the mechanisms by which eosinophils participate to disease pathogenesis are not fully

---

Box 1
Classification of the eosinophilic pneumonias in clinical practice

Eosinophilic pneumonias of unknown cause

Solitary idiopathic eosinophilic pneumonias

    Idiopathic chronic eosinophilic pneumonia

    Idiopathic acute eosinophilic pneumonia

Eosinophilic pneumonia in systemic syndromes

    Churg-Strauss syndrome

    Idiopathic hypereosinophilic syndromes (lymphocytic or myeloproliferative variant)

Eosinophilic pneumonias of known cause

Allergic bronchopulmonary aspergillosis and related syndromes (including bronchocentric granulomatosis)

Eosinophilic pneumonias of parasitic origin

Eosinophilic pneumonias of other infectious causes

Drug-induced eosinophilic pneumonias

Other pulmonary syndromes with possible usually mild eosinophilia

Organizing pneumonia, asthma, idiopathic pulmonary fibrosis, Langerhans cell histiocytosis, malignancies, and so forth

understood, blood and tissue eosinophilia have long been identified as major players in immunity against parasites and pathogenesis of allergic diseases.[3] Following differentiation of precursor cells in the bone marrow under the action of several cytokines, including interleukin (IL)-5, IL-3, and granulocyte macrophage colony-stimulating factor (GM-CSF),[4–6] eosinophils are recruited in the blood and tissue, including the lung in response mainly to circulating IL-5 and eotaxin and the C-C chemokine receptor-3, but tissue and blood eosinophilia are not necessarily associated. The importance of IL-5 in eosinophil biology has led to the development of anti–IL-5 antibodies, such as mepolizumab, to selectively target the eosinophil lineage in vivo with potential therapeutic approaches.[7–10]

Eosinophils and Innate Immunity

Eosinophils express cell membrane signaling molecules and receptors, including Toll-like receptors and receptors for cytokines, immunoglobulins, and complement,[4–6,11] resulting in interaction with basophils, endothelial cells, macrophages, platelets, fibroblasts, and mast cells that participate to innate immunity. Activated eosinophils release proinflammatory cytokines, arachidonic acid-derived mediators, enzymes, reactive oxygen species, complement proteins, chemokines, chemoattractants, metalloproteases, and other toxic granule proteins, especially cationic protein. Cationic proteins are released by degranulation of activated eosinophils and have a variety of proinflammatory properties, including direct cytotoxicity, up-regulation of chemoattraction, expression of adhesion molecules, regulation of vascular permeability, and contraction of smooth muscle cells.[4–6] Activated, degranulated (hypodense) eosinophils found in the BAL[12,13] and the lung[14] of patients with eosinophilic pneumonias denote the direct effect of eosinophilic cationic proteins. Cardiac damage in the hypereosinophilic syndrome or in tropical eosinophilia exemplifies tissue damage by eosinophils mediated by cationic proteins, which induce local thrombosis, necrosis, and eventually fibrosis.[11]

Eosinophils and Acquired Immunity

Eosinophils are involved in adaptive immunity against bacteria, viruses, and tumors through interaction with a variety of cell types and especially T lymphocytes.[4–6] Eosinophils present antigens to naive and antigen-primed T helper-2 cells in tissues and to T helper-0 cells in the draining lymph nodes in the context of major histocompatibility complex class II, thereby inducing T-cell development, activation, and migration to sites of inflammation. Eosinophils further secrete IL-4 and IL-13, thereby amplifying the T helper-2 response in the lung. In turn, the recruitment and activation of eosinophils is enhanced by T helper-2 cell–derived cytokines (IL-4, IL-5, and IL-13).

IDIOPATHIC CHRONIC EOSINOPHILIC PNEUMONIA

Individualized as an entity by Carrington and colleagues,[15] idiopathic chronic eosinophilic pneumonia (ICEP) is characterized by a progressive onset of symptoms leading within a few weeks to an infiltrative pulmonary disease with cough, increasing dyspnea, malaise, and weight loss.

Epidemiology and Risk Factors

ICEP is the commonest form of eosinophilic pneumonias in nontropical areas where the prevalence of parasitic infection is low. It is, however, a rare disease, representing less than 3% of cases of various interstitial lung diseases.[16] ICEP predominates in women (2:1 female/male ratio)[17,18] and may affect every age group, with a mean age of 45 years at diagnosis,[17] and no genetic predisposition.

Prior asthma is present in up to two-thirds of the patients.[17,18] About half the patients have a prior history of atopy, consisting in drug allergy, nasal polyposis, urticaria, and/or eczema.[17,18] As opposed to idiopathic acute eosinophilic pneumonia (IAEP), most patients with ICEP are nonsmokers.[17–19] These observations have led to the hypothesis that ICEP may occur predominantly in patients who are prone to develop a T helper-2 instead of T helper-1 response.[20]

Clinical Description

The onset of ICEP is progressive or subacute, with several weeks or months between the onset of symptoms and the diagnosis.[17,18] Dyspnea present in 60% to 90% of patients is usually moderate and associated with cough (90%), rhinitis or sinusitis (20%), and rarely chest pain or hemoptysis (10% or less).[17,18] In contrast with IAEP, respiratory failure requiring mechanical ventilation is exceptional.[21,22] Wheezes or crackles are found in one-third of patients at auscultation.

Respiratory manifestations are often accompanied by prominent systemic symptoms, with fatigue, malaise, fever, anorexia, night sweats, and weight loss (occasionally severe).[17,18] Although the disease is typically limited to the lungs and airways, mild extrathoracic manifestations (nonabundant pericardial effusion, arthralgia, nonspecific skin manifestations, and altered liver biology tests) are possible[15,17,23] and should systematically prompt further evaluation for CSS.

About 75% of the patients with ICEP experience asthma at some time throughout the course of disease. Asthma frequently precedes the onset of ICEP but occasionally occurs concomitantly with the diagnosis of ICEP (15%).[24] Asthma in ICEP is often severe and can progress to long-term persistent airflow obstruction in approximately 10% of patients despite oral and inhaled corticosteroid therapy.[24] Clinical and functional follow-up of patients is thus necessary even in the absence of recurrence of eosinophilic pneumonia.

Chest Imaging

The characteristic imaging features of ICEP consist of bilateral alveolar infiltrates with ill-defined margins present on the chest radiograph in almost all cases before initiation of treatment.[15,17,18,25–31] Spontaneous migration of the opacities in approximately a quarter of the cases suggests the diagnosis of either ICEP or cryptogenic organizing pneumonia.[17] A peripheral predominance of the lesions seen in approximately 25% of patients is also evocative of ICEP.[18,27,32,33]

On high-resolution CT (HRCT), confluent consolidations coexist with ground-glass opacities (**Figs. 1** and **2**).[17,26,30] Abnormalities are almost always bilateral[17] and predominate in the upper lobes and subpleural areas.[26] This pattern is sufficiently typical to suggest the diagnosis of ICEP in about 75% of cases in the appropriate setting.[29] Consolidation and ground-glass opacities rapidly decrease in extent and density with corticosteroid therapy.[26] Septal line thickening, band-like opacities parallel to the chest, or mediastinal lymph node enlargement are less characteristic.[17,25] Mild pleural effusions are present in only 10% of cases at HRCT, as opposed to IAEP. Cavitary lesions are exceedingly rare.[17,18,26]

Laboratory Findings

High-level peripheral blood eosinophilia present in most patients who have not yet received systemic corticosteroids[18] is the key to the diagnosis, with mean values of 5000 to 6000/mm^3 in large series (representing 20%–30% of blood leukocytes).[17]

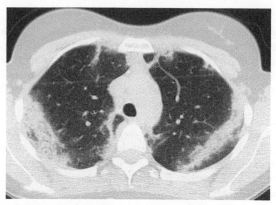

Fig. 1. Chest CT scan of a patient with ICEP, demonstrating peripheral airspace consolidation predominating in the upper lobes.

BAL eosinophilia (25% eosinophils or more at BAL differential cell count) is a major diagnostic feature in ICEP and is found in all patients evaluated before any corticosteroid intake. It is commonly greater than 40%, with a mean of 50% in large series. Sputum eosinophilia may be present.[18] Increase in blood C-reactive protein and total immunoglobulin E level lack specificity.

Pathogenesis

The release in urine of eosinophil-derived neurotoxin[34] and leukotriene E4[35] reflects eosinophilic activation and degranulation in vivo. Similarly, several studies have demonstrated the release of proinflammatory molecules or an increased expression of activation markers by eosinophils from patients with ICEP.[36,37]

Interestingly, clonality of the T-cell receptor-Vβ was reported in the BAL fluid of one patient with ICEP,[38] as well as clonality in the T-cell receptor-γ of peripheral blood lymphocytes,[39] similar to that seen in the lymphocytic variant of the idiopathic hypereosinophilic syndrome. Further investigation is warranted on the possible role of blood and lung tissue lymphocytes in the pathogenesis of ICEP.

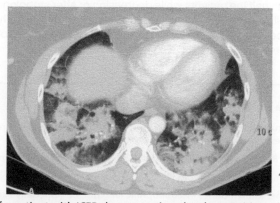

Fig. 2. Chest CT of a patient with ICEP, demonstrating alveolar opacities, with dense airspace consolidation and ground-glass opacities.

Lung Function

Approximately half the patients have an obstructive ventilatory defect, whereas the other half has a restrictive ventilatory defect associated to multiple consolidations at imaging.[17,18] Lung function tests rapidly normalize with treatment in most cases.[18] Mild hypoxemia is present in most patients.[17,18] Carbon monoxide transfer factor is frequently reduced[17,18] and transfer coefficient is reduced in about 25% of cases.[17]

Pathology

The diagnosis of ICEP only exceptionally requires a lung biopsy, which would not always be contributory especially in patients who already have taken systemic corticosteroids. It is characterized by prominent infiltration of the lung interstitium and the alveolar spaces by eosinophils[15,18] accompanied by a fibrinous exudate, with preservation of the lung architecture. Eosinophilic microabscesses, a nonnecrotizing nongranulomatous vasculitis, and occasional multinucleated giant cells (but no granuloma) can also be found. Some histologic overlap is common with organizing pneumonia.[1] Immunohistochemical and electron microscopic studies have demonstrated eosinophil degranulation within the site of eosinophilic pneumonia.[13,40]

Diagnosis

The diagnosis of ICEP relies on both characteristic clinical-imaging features and alveolar eosinophilia with or without peripheral blood eosinophilia, with no possible cause identified (**Box 2**). Before the disease can be considered idiopathic, potential causes of eosinophilia must be thoroughly investigated, especially drug intake, exposure to toxics, illicit drugs, and infections with parasites and fungi.

The presence of marked eosinophilia at BAL obviates lung biopsy, especially when exceeding 40% and when BAL eosinophils are more numerous than neutrophils and lymphocytes.[1] Markedly elevated peripheral blood eosinophilia, together with typical clinical radiologic features, also strongly suggests the diagnosis of ICEP. The main pitfall is the lack of blood or BAL eosinophilia in patients already receiving corticosteroid treatment.

Treatment and Outcome

Although spontaneous resolution can occur, management of ICEP is based on oral corticosteroids, with the goals of inducing remission of disease, reducing the risk of relapse, and minimizing the side effects of corticosteroids. Because relapses (which occur in more than half the patients while decreasing or after stopping corticosteroids) respond very well to resumed corticosteroid treatment, it is the authors' practice to progressively taper with tight control and then to stop corticosteroids to minimize side effects, while informing the patient of the possibility of relapse.

Box 2
Diagnostic criteria for ICEP

1. Diffuse pulmonary alveolar consolidation with air bronchogram and/or ground-glass opacities at chest imaging, especially with peripheral predominance

2. Eosinophilia at BAL differential cell count $\geq$40% (or peripheral blood eosinophils $\geq$1000/mm^3)

3. Respiratory symptoms present for at least 2 to 4 weeks

4. Absence of other known causes of eosinophilic lung disease (especially exposure to drug susceptible to induce pulmonary eosinophilia).

Although there are no established dose and duration of systemic corticosteroids in ICEP,[17,19,32,41,42] we usually use an initial dose of 0.5 mg/kg/d of oral prednisone for 2 weeks, followed by 0.25 mg/kg/d for 2 weeks, then corticosteroids are progressively reduced over a total duration of about 6 months and stopped.[1] ICEP responds dramatically to corticosteroids, with clinical improvement within 2 days,[18,19,43] and clearing of chest opacities within 1 week.[17,18] Relapses are usually treated with a dose of 20 mg/d of prednisone. Most patients need corticosteroids for 6 to 12 months.[17] Whether inhaled corticosteroids may be useful in nonasthmatic patients with ICEP is unknown.

At last follow-up, almost all patients are asymptomatic with a normal chest radiograph.[17] Death from ICEP is exceedingly rare. The main potential morbidity is related to adverse events of oral corticosteroids. Persistent airflow obstruction may develop in some patients despite bronchodilators and inhaled corticosteroids and often oral low-dose corticosteroids.[42] Therefore, long-term clinical and functional follow-up of patients is necessary.

IDIOPATHIC ACUTE EOSINOPHILIC PNEUMONIA

IAEP, the most dramatic of eosinophilic pneumonias, mimics infectious pneumonia or acute respiratory distress syndrome in previously healthy individuals. It differs from ICEP by its acute onset, the severity of hypoxemia, the usual lack of increased blood eosinophils at the onset of disease in contrast with a frank eosinophilia in BAL fluid, and the absence of relapse after recovery. It was first described by Badesch and colleagues[44] and later individualized by Allen and colleagues,[45] with characteristics confirmed in later series.[43,46–56]

Epidemiology and Risk Factors

IAEP occurs acutely in previously healthy young adults (without a history of asthma), with a mean age of about 30 years, and with male predominance.[44,45,48,55,56] Two-thirds of patients are smokers. The triggering role of various respiratory exposures has been well established, with the responsibility of a recent initiation of tobacco smoking (in a case-control study in militaries deployed in or near Iraq[56]), a recent change in smoking habits,[57] and restarting to smoke (rechallenge).[37,55,57–64] IAEP can occur within days after the initiation of smoking large quantities of cigarettes (or cigars). Patients should be informed about the responsibility of tobacco in the disease process and should be strongly encouraged to quit. Less frequently, short-term passive (massive) smoking may be sufficient to induce IAEP.[57,65] In addition, IAEP can develop a few days after environmental exposures to various inhaled contaminants,[1] suggesting triggering by nonspecific injurious agents. Whether this condition should be termed idiopathic in cases clearly related to tobacco smoking or other exposures is debatable.

Clinical Description

IAEP is very frequently misdiagnosed as community-acquired pneumonia, with acute onset of dyspnea (100% of patients), fever usually moderate (100%), cough (80%–100%), and thoracic pain (50%–70%) mostly pleuritic, sometimes with myalgias (30%–50%) or abdominal complaints (25%).[48,55–57,66] The delay between the first symptoms and hospital admission is typically less than 7 days,[48,55] but a duration of up to 1 month is possible.[55] Tachypnea, tachycardia, and crackles are present in most patients. Acute respiratory failure is frequent and admission to the intensive care unit and mechanical ventilation is often required.[55,56]

Chest Imaging

The chest radiograph shows bilateral infiltrates, with mixed alveolar and interstitial opacities, especially Kerley lines.[48,49,54] The coexistence on the chest radiograph areas of airspace consolidation, interlobular thickening, and pleural effusion can suggest the diagnosis.[54,55] These are better identified at chest HRCT, demonstrating the typical combination of poorly defined nodules of ground-glass attenuation (100%), interlobular septal thickening (90%), bilateral pleural effusion (76%), and airspace consolidation (55%) (**Fig. 3**).[67] Thickening of bronchovascular bundles, lymph node enlargement, and centrilobular nodules may also be seen.

Laboratory Findings

Blood eosinophil count is normal at presentation in most cases of IAEP.[48,56] This feature differs from all other eosinophilic lung diseases and can contribute to misdiagnosing IAEP as infectious pneumonia. The eosinophil count may rise to high values within days after presentation.[43,48,55,56] This finding is very evocative of IAEP. Given the usual lack of initial blood eosinophilia, BAL eosinophilia is the key to the diagnosis of IAEP, with 37% to 54% of eosinophils on average.[48,55,56] BAL bacterial cultures are sterile. BAL eosinophilia usually resolves with corticosteroid therapy but may persist for several weeks.[68] When performed, thoracentesis may show nonspecific pleural eosinophilia.

Several biomarkers have been found elevated in serum, urine, and BAL of patients with IAEP, especially IL-5, IL-18, and vascular endothelial growth factor; however, these are have no diagnostic value. The measurement of the serum levels of CCL17/TARC and KL6 (Krebs von den Lungen-6) might be useful in discriminating IAEP from other causes of acute lung injury.[69]

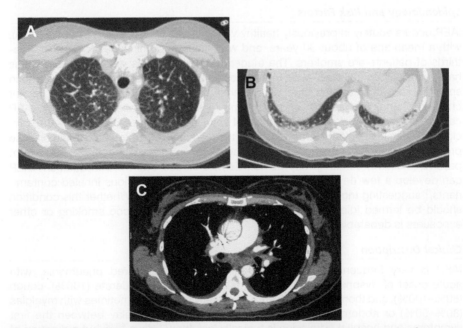

Fig. 3. Chest CT scan of a patient with acute eosinophilic pneumonia due to nitrofurantoin intake, showing (*A*) interlobular thickening in the upper areas of the lungs, (*B*) mild airspace consolidation in the lung bases, and (*C*) nonabundant bilateral pleural effusion and mediastinal lymphadenopathy. (*A, B*) Lung parenchymal windows. (*C*) Mediastinal window.

Lung Function

Because most patients fulfill diagnostic criteria for acute lung injury (including a Pao_2/fraction of inspired oxygen [Fio_2] ≤ 300 mmHg) or for acute respiratory distress syndrome ($Pao_2/Fio_2 \leq 200$ mmHg), arterial blood gas is warranted to evaluate hypoxemia, which is often severe owing to right-to-left shunting. Performed only in the less severe cases, lung function tests may show a mild restrictive ventilatory defect, reduced carbon monoxide transfer capacity, and increased alveolar-arterial oxygen gradient of Po_2.

Pathology

The lung biopsy shows acute and organizing diffuse alveolar damage together with interstitial alveolar and bronchiolar infiltration by eosinophils, intra-alveolar eosinophils, and interstitial edema.[66] Damage to the basal lamina is more pronounced than in ICEP.

Diagnosis

The lung biopsy is seldom necessary to ascertain the diagnosis of IAEP, which is established on clinical, radiological, and BAL findings (**Box 3**).[1] Alveolar eosinophilia at BAL and negative BAL cultures virtually exclude infectious pneumonia. Some patients with moderate disease severity may not fit established criteria.[70] The main characteristics that differ between IAEP and ICEP are listed in **Table 1**.

As in all eosinophilic lung diseases, a careful search for a potential cause of eosinophilia is mandatory. Potential causes include infectious agents, parasites, red spiders,[71] and illicit[72,73] and over-the-counter drugs, especially in the most severe cases or in cases of poor response to therapy. The etiologic enquiry is particularly important in IAEP because a similar presentation can be caused by drugs and infections, especially fungi[74–78] or viruses.[79] IAEP must be distinguished from AEP occurring after allogeneic hematopoietic stem cell transplantation[80] or in the context of acquired immunodeficiency virus infection.[81]

Treatment and Outcome

Most patients receive systemic corticosteroids for 2 to 4 weeks, with a starting dose of oral prednisone or intravenous methylprednisolone of 1 to 2 mg/kg/d. Extrapulmonary organ failure or shock is the exception; only a couple of lethal cases have been reported.[56,82] Extracorporeal membrane oxygenation has been used occasionally.[72]

Box 3
Diagnostic criteria for IAEP

1. Acute onset with febrile respiratory manifestations (≤ 1 month, and especially ≤ 7 days duration before medical examination)

2. Bilateral diffuse infiltrates on imaging

3. Pao_2 on room air ≤ 60 mmHg (8 kPa), or $Pao_2/Fio_2 \leq 300$ mmHg (40 kPa), or oxygen saturation on room air <90%

4. Lung eosinophilia, with $\geq 25\%$ eosinophils at BAL differential cell count (or eosinophilic pneumonia at lung biopsy when done)

5. Absence of determined cause of acute eosinophilic pneumonia (including infection or exposure to drugs known to induce pulmonary eosinophilia). Recent onset of tobacco smoking or exposure to inhaled dusts may be present.

Table 1
Distinctive features between ICEP and IAEP

	ICEP	IAEP
Onset	>2–4 wk	<1 mo
History of asthma	Yes	No
Smoking history	10% of smokers	2/3 of smokers, often recent initiation
Respiratory failure	No	Usual
Initial blood eosinophilia	Yes	No (delayed)
BAL eosinophilia	>25%	>25%
Chest imaging	Homogeneous peripheral airspace consolidation	Bilateral patchy areas of ground glass attenuation, airspace consolidation, interlobular septal thickening, bilateral pleural effusion
Relapse	Yes	No

Complete clinical recovery occurs rapidly on corticosteroid treatment. Parenchymal infiltrates and pleural effusions resolve within less than 1 month[48,54,55] and pulmonary function normalizes.[48,55] In contrast with ICEP, IAEP does not relapse.

CSS
Definition

CSS is a small-vessel vasculitis defined as an eosinophil-rich and granulomatous inflammation involving the respiratory tract and associated with asthma and eosinophilia. This eponymous syndrome was described by J. Churg and L. Strauss, in 1951, mainly from autopsied cases.[6] In the Chapel Hill Consensus Conference on the Nomenclature of Systemic Vasculitis,[66] CSS was included in the group of small vessel vasculitides and defined as an eosinophil-rich and granulomatous inflammation involving the respiratory tract, as a necrotizing vasculitis affecting small to medium-sized vessels, and as associated with asthma and eosinophilia. However, the coexistence of all three lesions on a biopsy is rare and the diagnosis is now more frequently made on the clinical presentation. In about 40% of cases, CSS is associated with antineutrophil cytoplasmic antibodies (ANCAs). The terminology of eosinophilic granulomatosis with polyangiitis has been recently proposed to replace the eponymous terminology.

Epidemiology and Risk Factors

CSS occurs at a mean age from 38 to 49 years at the onset of vasculitis, with no gender predominance.[83–86] The incidence has been estimated to 0.5 to 6.8 cases per million inhabitants per year, and the prevalence to 10.7 to 13 cases per million inhabitants.[87]

Allergy can be evidenced by specific serum IgE with corresponding clinical history in less than one-third of patients.[88] When present, allergy in CSS mainly consists of perennial allergies especially to *Dermatophagoides*, with seasonal allergies less frequent than in control asthmatics.[88] Familial CSS is an exception,[89] and genetic predisposition has been linked to the major histopathology complex DRB4 allele.[90]

The pathogenesis of CSS is largely unknown.[87] Several triggering or adjuvant factors have been suspected to play a role in CSS, which would result from an excessive inflammatory response to antigens,[1,87,91] including infectious agents (*Aspergillus*, *Candida*, *Ascaris*, *Actinomyces*), bird exposure, cocaine, drugs (sulfonamides used together with antiserum, diflunisal, macrolides, diphenylhydantoin, and recently omalizumab[92–97]), as well as allergic hyposensitizations and vaccinations.[98]

The possible link between leukotriene-receptor antagonists (montelukast, zafirlukast, and pranlukast) and the development of CSS is controversial.[99–103] There is increasing consideration that CSS may be mostly due to the flare of smoldering preexisting disease because of reducing oral or inhaled corticosteroids instead of to a direct effect of these drugs on the vasculitis pathogenesis.[87,102] However, in individual cases, CSS may occur following montelukast treatment in the absence of preexisting disease, may recur on rechallenge with leukotriene receptor antagonists, or may remit on withdrawal of this treatment without modifying other treatments.[99,101,103] The authors avoid leukotriene-receptor antagonists in asthmatics with eosinophilia and/or extrapulmonary manifestations compatible with smoldering CSS.

Clinical Description

The natural course of CSS has been described to follow three phases[84]: rhinosinusitis and asthma, blood and tissue eosinophilia, and eventually systemic vasculitis. These can significantly overlap in time.

Asthma is present in all patients with CSS. It is generally severe and becomes rapidly corticodependent, occurring at a mean age of about 35 to 50 years,[84,86,104–107] preceding the onset of the vasculitis by 3 to 6 years (ranging from 0–9 years).[83–86,107,108] Often severe, asthma may attenuate after the onset of the vasculitis[84,108]; however, this likely reflects the effect of systemic corticosteroids.[109,110] Other pulmonary manifestations of CSS consist in eosinophilic pneumonia, often similar to ICEP in presentation.[1]

Chronic rhinitis, present in about 75% of cases, is the most frequent extrathoracic manifestation. However, nasal and sinus manifestations lack specificity, consisting in chronic paraseptal sinusitis, crusty rhinitis, nasal obstruction, and nasal polyposis, often with eosinophilic infiltration at histopathology.[84,86,111–114] Septal nasal perforation does not occur as it does with granulomatosis with polyangiitis (Wegener syndrome).

General symptoms present in two-thirds of patients (eg, asthenia, weight loss, fever, arthralgias, and/or myalgias) often herald the onset of the vasculitis or its relapse. Any organ system can be affected by the systemic disease through eosinophilic infiltration and/or granulomatous vasculitis.[87,115] Heart and kidney involvement are frequently insidious and must be systematically investigated because of potential morbidity and mortality. Skin and gastrointestinal manifestations are also frequent.[87,115]

Cardiac involvement, although often asymptomatic, can lead to chronic cardiac failure requiring heart transplantation or sudden death.[84–86,107,108,116,117] It results from eosinophilic myocarditis or, much less commonly, from coronary arteritis.[118] Therefore, any patient with suspected CSS should undergo a strict cardiac evaluation with ECG, echocardiography, N-terminal pro-brain natriuretic peptide, and serum level of troponin I. MRI of the heart is currently the investigation preferred by most investigators to detect cardiac involvement.[117,119,120] MRI[117,120,121] and echocardiography[120,122] frequently detect cardiac abnormalities in asymptomatic patients, the clinical significance of which is unknown. Patients with CSS are at greater risk of venous thromboembolic events.[92]

Chest Imaging

Chest imaging abnormalities in patients with CSS are twofold:

- Pulmonary infiltrates (50%–70%) corresponding to eosinophilic pneumonia consist of ill-defined opacities, sometimes migratory, with peripheral predominance or random distribution, and density varying from ground-glass opacities to airspace consolidation (**Fig. 4**).[84,86,108,123–127] These abnormalities rapidly disappear with corticosteroid therapy.

- Airways abnormalities include centrilobular nodules, bronchial wall thickening, and bronchiectasis.[1,29,31,125]

Interlobular septal thickening, hilar or mediastinal lymphadenopathy, pleural effusion, or pericardial effusion may also be seen.[31,124,125,127,128] When present, pleural effusion should lead to consider cardiomyopathy as a possible cause.

Laboratory Findings

Peripheral blood eosinophilia is a major feature of CSS, with mean values generally between 5 and 20,000/mm^3 at diagnosis.[84,86,108] Blood eosinophilia usually parallels the vasculitis activity. BAL eosinophilia (sometimes >60%) is found in most cases.[129] Serum IgE levels and C-reactive protein levels are increased. High levels of urinary eosinophil-derived neurotoxin representing eosinophil degranulation in vivo reflect disease activity.[130] Serum IgG4 levels[131] and CCL17/TARC[132] may correlate with disease activity.

ANCAs, reported in about 40% of patients, are mainly perinuclear-ANCAs with myeloperoxidase (MPO) specificity.[85,133,134] Thus, absence of ANCAs does not exclude the diagnosis of CSS. No correlation was found in most studies between the titer of ANCA and the activity of disease. However, the clinical presentation and especially extrathoracic manifestations differ between ANCA-positive and ANCA-negative patients,[133,134] suggesting two clinical and pathophysiogic subtypes of CSS (**Table 2**).[135] Interestingly, the disease subtypes of CSS may have a genetic predisposition.[90,136]

Lung Function

Airflow obstruction is present in 70% of patients at diagnosis despite inhaled bronchodilator and corticosteroid therapy prescribed for asthma.[109] Improvement in lung function is obtained with oral corticosteroid therapy given for the systemic disease; however, mild airflow obstruction may persist.[109,110] Long-term oral corticosteroids are required for asthma in most patients despite inhaled therapy.[84,86,109] In patients with long-term follow-up, persistent airflow obstruction may be present in about

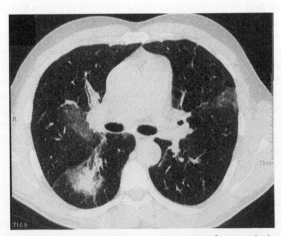

Fig. 4. Chest CT scan of a patient with CSS, showing areas of ground glass attenuation and of airspace consolidation.

Table 2
Distinct subtypes of Churg-Strauss syndrome

	Vasculitic Phenotype	Eosinophilic Tissular Disease Phenotype
Respective frequency	~40%	~60%
ANCA	Present (mostly perinuclear-ANCA with anti-MPO specificity)	Absent
Predominant manifestations	Glomerular renal disease Peripheral neuropathy Purpura Biopsy-proven vasculitis	Cardiac involvement (eosinophilic myocarditis) Eosinophilic pneumonia Fever

Data from Sablé-Fourtassou R, Cohen P, Mahr A, et al. Antineutrophil cytoplasmic antibodies and the Churg-Strauss syndrome. Ann Intern Med 2005;143:632–8; and Sinico RA, Di Toma L, Maggiore U, et al. Prevalence and clinical significance of antineutrophil cytoplasmic antibodies in Churg-Strauss syndrome. Arthritis Rheum 2005;52:2926–35.

40% of patients, in whom a transient sustained increase in the daily dose of oral corticosteroids may partially improve the lung function and restore some response to beta-2-agonists.[109]

Pathology

Because the diagnosis is now made earlier in the course of disease and based on clinical features, a lung biopsy is seldom necessary to confirm CSS. When a biopsy is performed (of skin, nerve, or muscle, in most cases[86]), the pathologic lesions[137,138] rarely comprise all the characteristic features on a single biopsy, including a vasculitis (necrotizing or not, involving mainly the medium-sized pulmonary arteries) and a granulomatous eosinophilic tissular infiltration (with palisading histiocytes and giant cells).

Diagnosis

In most patients, the diagnosis of CSS is currently based on clinical features. A pathologic diagnosis of CSS is not mandatory in patients with characteristic clinical features and marked eosinophilia; however, histology of vasculitis and presence of ANCAs further corroborate the diagnosis. Although the diagnosis is straightforward in patients with sub acute or chronic eosinophilic pneumonia and true vasculitis with positive ANCA, it may be more difficult in those with asthma, blood eosinophilia, and mild extrathoracic manifestations. Smoldering CSS may be suppressed by corticosteroid treatment of asthma, with disease flare on treatment tapering. Patients may present the so-called forms frustes of CSS[106,139,140] without overt vasculitis involving several organs. Diagnostic difficulties thus largely depend on the stage of disease, yet it is crucial that this diagnosis be established before severe organ involvement (especially renal or cardiac) is present.

The diagnostic criteria proposed by Lanham and colleagues[84] include (1) asthma, (2) eosinophilia exceeding 1.5×10^9/L, and (3) systemic vasculitis of two or more extrapulmonary organs (**Box 4**). Classification criteria have been established by the American College of Rheumatology.[141] The presence of ANCA deserves to be considered a major diagnostic criterion when present.

Treatment and Outcome

Corticosteroids remain the mainstay of treatment of CSS, with oral prednisone initiated at a dose of 1 mg/kg/d for 3 to 4 weeks, than tapered progressively to reach

---

Box 4
Diagnostic and classification criteria of CSS

Lanham and colleagues[84]

- Asthma
- Eosinophilia
- Evidence of vasculitis (clinical) involving at least two organs

American College of Rheumatology[139]

- Asthma
- Eosinophilia greater than 10%
- Mononeuropathy or polyneuropathy
- Pulmonary infiltrates, nonfixed
- Paranasal sinus abnormality
- Extravascular eosinophil infiltration on biopsy findings

Diagnosis is probable when four of the six criteria are present (sensitivity 85%, specificity 99.7%). These are classification criteria that may be used when the diagnosis of systemic vasculitis has been established by histopathology.

Chapel Hill Consensus conference[142]

- Eosinophil-rich and granulomatous inflammation involving the respiratory tract
- Necrotizing vasculitis affecting small-to-medium-size vessels
- Asthma
- Eosinophilia

Diagnostic criteria used by the authors

1. Asthma
2. Peripheral blood eosinophilia greater than 1500/mm^3 and/or alveolar eosinophilia greater than 25%
3. Extrapulmonary clinical manifestations of disease (other than rhinosinusitis), with at least one of the following:
   - Systemic manifestation typical of the disease: mononeuritis multiplex, cardiomyopathy confidently attributed to the eosinophilic disorder, or palpable purpura;
   - Any extrapulmonary manifestation with histopathological evidence of vasculitis as demonstrated especially by skin, muscle, or nerve biopsy
   - Any extrapulmonary manifestation with evidence of ANCAs with anti-MPO or antiproteinase 3 specificity.

When a single extrarespiratory manifestation attributable to the systemic disease is present, disease may be called forme fruste of CSS.

---

5 to 10 mg/d at 12 months of therapy.[87] An initial methylprednisolone bolus (15 mg/kg/d for 1–3 days) is useful in the most severe cases. Cyclophosphamide therapy (0.6–0.7 g/m^2 intravenously at days 1, 15, and 30; then every 3 weeks) should be added to corticosteroids to induce remission in patients with manifestations that could result in mortality or severe morbidity,[143] including one or more of the following criteria: age over 65 years; cardiac symptoms; gastrointestinal involvement; renal insufficiency with serum creatinine greater than 150 µg/L; and absence of ear, nose and throat

manifestation.[143] Subcutaneous interferon alpha, high-dose dose intravenous immunoglobulins, plasma exchange, and cyclosporine have been used successfully in a few cases refractory to corticosteroids.[2]

Once remission has been achieved, prolonged maintenance therapy is necessary to prevent relapses. Patients without poor prognosis criteria are generally treated by corticosteroids alone; the possible benefit of azathioprine to maintain remission in this setting (especially in patients who relapse despite 20 mg/d of prednisone or more) is currently evaluated. In patients with poor prognosis criteria, maintenance therapy for 18 to 24 months (after remission has been obtained using cyclophosphamide) is generally based on azathioprine, which has a favorable risk-to-benefit ratio.[87] Of note, rituximab, which is increasingly used in ANCA-associated vasculitis, can induce bronchospasm in this setting,[144] and should not be used routinely in patients with CSS.[87]

Interesting preliminary results have been obtained using the anti-IL5 antibody mepolizumab.[10,145,146] It is likely that strategies aiming at controlling the eosinophil cell line may become part of the treatment strategy in eosinophilic lung diseases and, especially, CSS in coming years.[147]

Despite strict management, about a quarter of CSS patients experience at least one relapse (generally with peripheral eosinophilia), which should be distinguished from severe asthma exacerbations. The 5-year overall survival in CSS is currently between 95% and 100%.[143,148,149] Most deaths during the first year of treatment are due to cardiac involvement,[150] whereas treatment-related side effects, difficult asthma, and persistent airflow obstruction later cause significant morbidity.[109,149]

ALLERGIC BRONCHOPULMONARY ASPERGILLOSIS
Epidemiology and Pathogenesis

Allergic bronchopulmonary aspergillosis (ABPA) occurs in 1% to 2% of asthmatic adults and in up to 7% to 10% of patients with cystic fibrosis,[151,152] but is exceptional in other contexts. However, isolated cases have been discussed in patients with chronic obstructive pulmonary disease and in peculiar occupational situations (eg, in workers in the bagasse-containing sites in sugar-cane mills[153]). ABPA may be associated with allergic Aspergillus sinusitis,[154] a sinusal equivalent of ABPA, resulting in a syndrome called sinobronchial allergic aspergillosis.[155]

ABPA is secondary to a complex chronic immune and inflammatory reaction in the bronchi and the surrounding parenchyma in response to the presence of Aspergillus growing in mucous plugs in the airways of asthmatics, progressively resulting in damage to bronchial and pulmonary tissue and impairment of the mucociliary clearance.[156] Both viscid mucus and exposure to fungus spores are necessary for this condition to develop. The immunologic response of the host includes, but is not restricted to, type I hypersensitivity mediated by IgE antibodies and type III hypersensitivity with the participation of IgG and IgA antibodies and of exaggerated Th2 CD4+ T-cell–mediated immune response. Excessive B-cell response and immunoglobulin production in response to circulating IL-4 seem to play a central role.[156]

Genetic predisposition has been demonstrated, especially with an increased prevalence of heterozygotic cystic fibrosis transmembrane conductance regulator gene mutations in non–cystic fibrosis patients with ABPA[157]; polymorphism within the IL-4 receptor alpha-chain gene, the IL-10 promoter, and surfactant protein A genes[158–160]; and association with HLA DR2/5 subtypes[161–163]; and familial cases have rarely been reported.[164] ABPA may, therefore, result from an abnormal host immune response to Aspergillus antigens in the setting of predisposing genetic factors.[156]

Clinical Description

Most patients with ABPA experience chronic cough, dyspnea, expectoration of brown or tan sputum plugs, low-grade fever, and chronic rhinitis with chronic evolution and repeated flares (exacerbations).[156,165] Sputum production may be abundant in patients with bronchiectasis, with sputum cultures often positive for *Pseudomonas aeruginosa*, *Staphylococcus aureus*, *Aspergillus fumigatus*, and/or non–tuberculous mycobacteria.[166]

Five stages of ABPA have been described: acute, remission, recurrent exacerbations, corticosteroid dependent asthma, and fibrotic end stage. ABPA may progress to chronic respiratory failure. However, patients do not necessarily progress from one stage to another. Pulmonary infiltrates or peripheral blood eosinophilia may only be present during the acute phase or recurrent exacerbations of the disease.

Chest Imaging

The imaging findings comprise prominent bronchial features with central bronchiectasis (including in the upper lobes), bronchial wall thickening, mucous plugging (mucoid impaction) with finger-in-glove pattern in about a quarter of patients,[167,168] ground-glass attenuation, and airspace consolidation.[29,169–171] The finger-in-glove sign corresponds to bronchial mucous impaction radiating from the hilum to the periphery.[170] Bronchiectases are most commonly cylindrical and suggest ABPA in asthmatics. HRCT direct signs of bronchiolitis resulting from extensive bronchiolar mucous impaction are also common in ABPA, with centrilobular nodules and tree-in-bud pattern (**Fig. 5**).[169,171] Overall, imaging abnormalities are evocative enough to suggest the diagnosis of ABPA in the appropriate context.[29]

Eosinophilic pneumonia is rare in ABPA, occurring especially during the early course of the disease. Consolidation should be differentiated from segmental or lobar atelectasis caused by mucous plugging.[165]

Laboratory Findings

Elevated blood eosinophils especially greater than 1000/mm^3 or elevated serum levels of total IgE levels should raise the suspicion of ABPA in asthmatics, as well as recurring infiltrates and central bronchiectasis.[156]

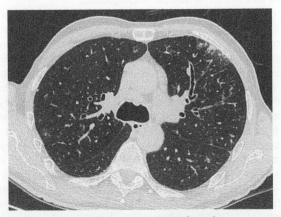

Fig. 5. Chest CT scan of a patient with allergic bronchopulmonary aspergillosis, showing proximal cylindrical bronchiectasis, bronchial wall thickening, centrilobular nodules, tree-in-bud pattern, and mild airspace subpleural consolidation.

Skin prick testing, and serum IgE and IgG (precipitin) reactions to *Aspergillus fumigatus* corroborate the diagnosis. In addition, total and *Aspergillus*-specific IgE levels generally increase during exacerbations of ABPA although they are not reliable markers of disease activity.[172] Fungal mycelia can be found at direct examination of sputum plugs. Whether antibodies specific for recombinant *Aspergillus* allergens (especially *Asp f4* and *Asp f6*) may contribute to diagnosis and help to differentiate ABPA from *Aspergillus*-sensitive asthma or eosinophilic asthma remains to be further investigated.

Pathology

A lung biopsy is not needed; however, limited resection is occasionally performed because of chronic pulmonary consolidation. Typical pathologic findings comprise bronchiectasis filled with mucous or mucopurulent plugs, granulomatous inflammation of the bronchiolar wall, peribronchiolar chronic eosinophilic infiltrates with areas of eosinophilic pneumonia, exudative bronchiolitis, and fungal hyphae or mucous impaction of bronchi.[173]

Diagnosis

The current primary diagnostic criteria are listed (**Box 5**). In patients with ABPA, typical proximal bronchiectasis may be absent; such cases are designated ABPA-seropositive.[174] The diagnosis of allergic bronchopulmonary syndromes associated with yeasts or fungi other than *Aspergillus fumigatus*[1] is particularly challenging.

Box 5
Minimal essential diagnostic criteria of ABPA

Patients with asthma and central bronchiectasis

1. Asthma

2. Central bronchiectasis (inner two-thirds of chest CT field)

3. Immediate cutaneous reactivity to *Aspergillus*

4. Total serum IgE concentration >417 kU/L (1000 ng/mL)

5. Elevated serum IgE-*A fumigatus* and/or IgG-*A fumigatus* (infiltrates on chest radiograph and serum precipitating antibodies to *A fumigatus* may be present but are not minimal essential diagnostic criteria)

Patients with asthma (ABPA-seropositive)

Patients with the above criteria 1, 3, 4, and 5 (infiltrates on chest radiograph may be present but are not a minimal essential diagnostic criteria)

Patients with cystic fibrosis

1. Clinical deterioration (increased cough, wheezing, exercise intolerance, increase sputum, and decrease in pulmonary function)

2. Immediate cutaneous reactivity to *Aspergillus* or presence of IgE-*A fumigatus*

3. Total serum IgE concentration ≥1000 kU/L

4. Precipitating antibodies to *A fumigatus* or serum IgG-*A fumigatus*

5. Abnormal chest radiograph (infiltrates, mucous plugging, or a change from earlier films)

Adapted from Greenberger PA. Allergic bronchopulmonary aspergillosis. J Allergy Clin Immunol 2002;110:685–92.

Treatment and Outcome

Management of patients with ABPA aims at treating asthma exacerbations and at preventing progression to bronchiectasis and severe fibrotic lung disease while minimizing corticosteroids side effects. The treatment mainly relies on corticosteroids during attacks, with long-term oral corticosteroids maintained only in patients with frequent symptomatic attacks or evidence of progressive lung damage. Treatment of episodes of pulmonary consolidation may prevent the progression of ABPA to the fibrotic end-stage.[175] Inhaled corticosteroids may reduce the need for long-term oral corticosteroids. However, persistent airflow obstruction may develop over the years.

Oral itraconazole reduces the burden of fungal colonization in the lung and has been demonstrated in two randomized trials to be a useful adjunct to corticosteroids.[176,177] Antifungal therapy leads to reduction of the doses of corticosteroids, reduction in sputum production, and frequency of exacerbations (with a trend for functional improvement) and decrease in biomarkers (sputum eosinophils, sputum eosinophil cationic protein levels, serum IgE levels, and serum IgG levels to A fumigatus).[176,177] Measuring total serum IgE level may be helpful for monitoring therapy.[156] Itraconazole is generally prescribed for 4 to 8 months. Itraconazole interacts with many medications and may further induce adrenal insufficiency. Experience with voriconazole in ABPA is limited. Treatment with the anti-IgE recombinant antibody omalizumab may be useful in cystic fibrosis patients[178–180] and in asthmatics.[181,182]

OTHER EOSINOPHILIC LUNG DISEASES
Idiopathic Hypereosinophilic Syndromes

The idiopathic hypereosinophilic syndrome, historically defined as a persistent eosinophilia greater than 1500/mm^3 for longer than 6 months, without a known cause of eosinophilia, and with presumptive signs and symptoms of organ involvement,[183] now encompasses two variants[184,185]:

- The myeloproliferative variant (about 20% of cases) shares common features with chronic myeloproliferative syndromes (including hepatomegaly, splenomegaly, anemia, thrombocythemia, increased serum vitamin B$_{12}$ and leukocyte alkaline phosphatase, and circulating leukocyte precursors) and is attributed to a constitutively activated tyrosine kinase fusion protein (Fip1L1-PDGFRα) because of an interstitial chromosomal deletion in 4q12.[186]
- The so called lymphocytic variant (about 30% of cases) is a T-cell disorder resulting from the production of chemokines (especially IL-5) by clonal Th2 lymphocytes bearing an aberrant antigenic surface phenotype (such as CD3$^-$CD4$^+$).[187]

At least half of the cases have neither fusion protein activity nor clonal proliferation of lymphocytes detected and thus they remain presently idiopathic.

Clinical manifestations of the idiopathic hypereosinophilic syndrome are dominated by fatigue, weight loss, and nonrespiratory involvement, especially targeting the skin, mucosa, heart, and nervous system.[185] In older series, respiratory manifestations present in up to 40% of patients were nonspecific and included cough, dyspnea, and patchy ground-glass attenuation, consolidation, and small nodules at chest imaging.[183] However, more recent studies in which the idiopathic hypereosinophilic syndromes were diagnosed according to current above standards indicate that respiratory manifestations may be generally of mild severity, rarely with eosinophilic pneumonia.[188]

Eosinophilic Pneumonias in Parasitic Diseases

Although it is the main cause of eosinophilic pneumonia in the world, parasitic infection is rare in Europe and North America. Clinical manifestations are nonspecific and presentation is rarely as typical as that of ICEP or IAEP.[1,189] Infection with the nematode *Ascaris lumbricoides* mainly causes Löffler syndrome (transient mild eosinophilic pneumonia) during the migration of the larvae through the lung, with transient cough, wheezing, fever, high blood eosinophilia, and pulmonary infiltrates. Visceral larva migrans syndrome caused by *Toxocara canis* occurs throughout the world. It causes fever, seizures, fatigue, blood eosinophilia, and transient pulmonary manifestations (cough, dyspnea, wheezes or crackles at pulmonary auscultation, and pulmonary infiltrates on chest radiograph). Infection with *Strongyloides stercoralis* may cause severe disease, affecting all organs (hyperinfection syndrome), especially in immunocompromised patients. Tropical pulmonary eosinophilia is caused by the filarial parasites *Wuchereria bancrofti* and *Brugia malayi*.[1]

Drug-Induced Eosinophilic Pneumonias

Drugs taken in the weeks or days before an eosinophilic disease must be thoroughly investigated. The possible association of pleural effusion and extrapulmonary manifestations, especially cutaneous rash, may be a clue for the diagnosis of drug-induced eosinophilic pneumonia.[1] Eosinophilic pneumonia has been reported in association with many drugs (www.pneumotox.com), but causality has been confidently established in fewer than 20.[91] Most drugs frequently causing eosinophilic pneumonias are antibiotics and nonsteroidal antiinflammatory drugs (**Box 6**).[91] Presentation may be similar to that of ICEP, or have an acute onset similar to IAEP, especially with minocycline[190] or nitrofurantoin (see **Fig. 3**).[191] Acute eosinophilic pneumonia may occur in the context of drug rash with eosinophilia and systemic symptoms (Dress syndrome).[192]

Toxics

The eosinophilia-myalgia syndrome that developed in 1989 in the United States was linked to impurities in L-tryptophan preparations in genetically-susceptible hosts.[193–195] One new case has been recently reported in a patient who had been taking L-tryptophan for 3 weeks as well as other dietary supplements.[196]

The toxic-oil syndrome, which affected about 20,000 people in Spain in 1981,[197] is a scleroderma-like disorder characterized in the acute phase by diffuse parenchymal lung disease and possibly respiratory failure with interstitial-alveolar pattern on chest imaging and blood eosinophilia.

Eosinophilic lung disease of varying presentation may be due to illicit drugs, especially cocaine or heroin but also cannabis.[72,73]

Box 6
Drugs commonly causing eosinophilic pneumonia

Antiinflammatory drugs and related drugs: acetylsalicylic acid, diclofenac, ibuprofen, naproxen, phenylbutazone, piroxicam, sulindac, and tolfenamic acid.

Antibiotics: ethambutol, fenbufen, minocycline, nitrofurantoin, penicillins, pyrimethamine, sulfamides, sulfonamides, and trimetoprim-sulfamethoxazole.

Other drugs: captopril, carbamazepine, and GM-CSF

A more extensive list of drugs reported to cause eosinophilic pneumonia may be found at www.pneumotox.com and Ref.[1]

Radiation Therapy

A condition similar to ICEP has been reported after radiation therapy for breast cancer in women (similar to the syndrome of radiation-induced organizing pneumonia), with a median delay of 3.5 months after completion of radiotherapy.[20,198,199] Relapse can occur after withdrawal of corticosteroid therapy.[20]

Miscellaneous

ICEP may overlap with, or mimic cryptogenic organizing pneumonia. Eosinophilia may be found in other bronchopulmonary disorders in which eosinophilic pneumonia is not prominent,[1] including the eosinophilic phenotype of asthma, asthma with marked blood eosinophilia (ie, >1500/mm^3) hypereosinophilic asthma, eosinophilic bronchitis (without asthma), bronchocentric granulomatosis, isolated cases of idiopathic interstitial pneumonias (idiopathic pulmonary fibrosis or usual interstitial pneumonia, nonspecific interstitial pneumonia, and desquamative interstitial pneumonia), pulmonary Langerhans cell histiocytosis, and sarcoidosis.

PRACTICAL APPROACH TO DIAGNOSIS AND TREATMENT

The diagnosis of eosinophilic lung diseases relies on characteristic clinical-imaging features and the demonstration of blood and/or alveolar eosinophilia. Lung biopsy is seldom necessary. Peripheral blood eosinophilia may be absent at presentation, especially in IAEP and in patients who have received corticosteroid treatment for even a few hours.

The etiologic diagnosis of eosinophilic lung diseases is of paramount importance because the identification of a potential cause may have practical consequences, especially when the disease is caused by medicinal drugs, illicit drugs, toxics, or infections with parasites or fungi.[1] Laboratory investigations for parasites must take into account the epidemiology of parasites. Biologic investigations for ABPA should be prompted by, but not restricted to, the presence of proximal bronchiectasis in patients with asthma or cystic fibrosis. When no cause is found, the eosinophilic lung disease is considered idiopathic. Systemic eosinophilic diseases such as CSS are suspected in the presence of extrathoracic manifestations. It is only once all known causes of eosinophilia and systemic manifestations have been excluded that idiopathic eosinophilic pneumonias (eg, ICEP and IAEP) may be considered.

Treatment of eosinophilic lung diseases involves oral corticosteroids in most cases, and withdrawal of the offending agent when identified. Cyclophosphamide is necessary in severe cases of CSS. The development of therapies that more specifically target the differentiation, activation, or recruitment of eosinophils to the lungs (with especially anti–IL-5 monoclonal antibodies) will likely complement available therapeutic approaches in the near future.

SUMMARY

The eosinophilic lung diseases are characterized by the prominent infiltration of the lungs by eosinophils. Eosinophilic pneumonia may present with chronic (with symptoms for more than 1 month before the patient seeks medical advice) or acute onset (less than 1 month), or as Löffler syndrome (which is of parasitic origin in most cases). The diagnosis of eosinophilic pneumonia relies on both characteristic clinical-imaging features and the demonstration of alveolar eosinophilia (greater than 25% eosinophils at BAL and, preferably, greater than 40%), with or without markedly elevated peripheral blood eosinophilia (greater than 1,000/mm^3 and preferably greater than 1,500/mm^3). Lung biopsy is generally not necessary for the diagnosis of eosinophilic pneumonia. Peripheral blood eosinophilia may be absent at presentation, especially in IAEP and in patients receiving corticosteroid treatment. IAEP may be misdiagnosed as severe infectious pneumonia. Particular attention should be paid to extrathoracic manifestations that may raise the suspicion of a systemic eosinophilic disease, especially CSS, thus necessitating specific diagnostic investigations. All possible causes of eosinophilia (especially fungus infection or drug or toxic exposure) must be thoroughly investigated before the diagnosis of idiopathic disease is made. Corticosteroids are the cornerstone of treatment of eosinophilic lung diseases.

REFERENCES

1. Cordier JF, Cottin V. Eosinophilic pneumonias. In: Schwarz MI, King TE Jr, editors. Interstitial lung disease. 5th edition. Shelton (CT): People's Medical Publishing House-USA; 2011. p. 833–93.
2. Cottin V, Cordier JF. Eosinophilic pneumonias. Allergy 2005;60:841–57.
3. Walsh ER, August A. Eosinophils and allergic airway disease: there is more to the story. Trends Immunol 2010;31:39–44.
4. Hogan SP, Rosenberg HF, Moqbel R, et al. Eosinophils: biological properties and role in health and disease. Clin Exp Allergy 2008;38:709–50.
5. Rothenberg ME, Hogan SP. The eosinophil. Annu Rev Immunol 2006;24:147–74.
6. Blanchard C, Rothenberg ME. Biology of the eosinophil. Adv Immunol 2009;101: 81–121.
7. Rothenberg ME, Klion AD, Roufosse FE, et al. Treatment of patients with the hypereosinophilic syndrome with mepolizumab. N Engl J Med 2008;358:1215–28.
8. Nair P, Pizzichini MM, Kjarsgaard M, et al. Mepolizumab for prednisone-dependent asthma with sputum eosinophilia. N Engl J Med 2009;360:985–93.
9. Haldar P, Brightling CE, Hargadon B, et al. Mepolizumab and exacerbations of refractory eosinophilic asthma. N Engl J Med 2009;360:973–84.
10. Kim S, Marigowda G, Oren E, et al. Mepolizumab as a steroid-sparing treatment option in patients with Churg-Strauss syndrome. J Allergy Clin Immunol 2010; 125:1336–43.
11. Akuthota P, Weller PF. Eosinophils and disease pathogenesis. Semin Hematol 2012;49:113–9.
12. Prin L, Capron M, Gosset P, et al. Eosinophil lung disease: immunological studies of blood and alveolar eosinophils. Clin Exp Immunol 1986;63:249–57.
13. Janin A, Torpier G, Courtin P, et al. Segregation of eosinophil proteins in alveolar macrophage compartments in chronic eosinophilic pneumonia. Thorax 1993;48: 57–62.
14. Fox B, Seed WA. Chronic eosinophilic pneumonia. Thorax 1980;35:570–80.
15. Carrington CB, Addington WW, Goff AM, et al. Chronic eosinophilic pneumonia. N Engl J Med 1969;280:787–98.
16. Thomeer MJ, Costabe U, Rizzato G, et al. Comparison of registries of interstitial lung diseases in three European countries. Eur Respir J Suppl 2001;32:114s–8s.
17. Marchand E, Reynaud-Gaubert M, Lauque D, et al. Idiopathic chronic eosinophilic pneumonia. A clinical and follow-up study of 62 cases. The Groupe d'Etudes et de Recherche sur les Maladies "Orphelines" Pulmonaires (GERM"O"P). Medicine (Baltimore) 1998;77:299–312.
18. Jederlinic PJ, Sicilian L, Gaensler EA. Chronic eosinophilic pneumonia. A report of 19 cases and a review of the literature. Medicine (Baltimore) 1988;67:154–62.
19. Naughton M, Fahy J, FitzGerald MX. Chronic eosinophilic pneumonia. A long-term follow-up of 12 patients. Chest 1993;103:162–5.

20. Cottin V, Frognier R, Monnot H, et al. Chronic eosinophilic pneumonia after radiation therapy for breast cancer. Eur Respir J 2004;23:9–13.
21. Libby DM, Murphy TF, Edwards A, et al. Chronic eosinophilic pneumonia: an unusual cause of acute respiratory failure. Am Rev Respir Dis 1980;122:497–500.
22. Ivanick MJ, Donohue JF. Chronic eosinophilic pneumonia: a cause of adult respiratory distress syndrome. South Med J 1986;79:686–90.
23. Weynants P, Riou R, Vergnon JM, et al. Pneumopathies chroniques à éosinophiles. Etude de 16 cases. Rev Mal Respir 1985;2:63–8 [in French].
24. Marchand E, Etienne-Mastroianni B, Chanez P, et al. Idiopathic chronic eosinophilic pneumonia and asthma: how do they influence each other? The Groupe d'Etudes et de Recherche sur les Maladies "Orphelines" Pulmonaires (GER-M"O"P). Eur Respir J 2003;22:8–13.
25. Mayo JR, Muller NL, Road J, et al. Chronic eosinophilic pneumonia: CT findings in six cases. AJR Am J Roentgenol 1989;153:727–30.
26. Ebara H, Ikezoe J, Johkoh T, et al. Chronic eosinophilic pneumonia: evolution of chest radiograms and CT features. J Comput Assist Tomogr 1994;18:737–44.
27. Gaensler E, Carrington C. Peripheral opacities in chronic eosinophilic pneumonia: the photographic negative of pulmonary edema. AJR Am J Roentgenol 1977;128:1–13.
28. Robertson CL, Shackelford GD, Armstrong JD. Chronic eosinophilic pneumonia. Radiology 1971;101:57–61.
29. Johkoh T, Muller NL, Akira M, et al. Eosinophilic lung diseases: diagnostic accuracy of thin-section CT in 111 patients. Radiology 2000;216:773–80.
30. Arakawa H, Kurihara Y, Niimi H, et al. Bronchiolitis obliterans with organizing pneumonia versus chronic eosinophilic pneumonia: high-resolution CT findings in 81 patients. AJR Am J Roentgenol 2001;176:1053–8.
31. Furuiye M, Yoshimura N, Kobayashi A, et al. Churg-Strauss syndrome versus chronic eosinophilic pneumonia on high-resolution computed tomographic findings. J Comput Assist Tomogr 2010;34:19–22.
32. Bancal C, Sadoun D, Valeyre D, et al. Chronic idiopathic eosinophilic pneumopathy. Carrington's disease. Presse Med 1989;18:1695–8 [in French].
33. Zimhony O. Photographic negative shadow of pulmonary oedema. Lancet 2002; 360:33.
34. Cottin V, Deviller P, Tardy F, et al. Urinary eosinophil-derived neurotoxin/protein X: a simple method for assessing eosinophil degranulation in vivo. J Allergy Clin Immunol 1998;101:116–23.
35. Ono E, Taniguchi M, Mita H, et al. Increased urinary leukotriene E4 concentration in patients with eosinophilic pneumonia. Eur Respir J 2008;32:437–42.
36. Cottin V, Cordier JF. Idiopathic eosinophilic pneumonias. Eur Respir Mon 2012; 134:118–39.
37. Vahid B, Marik PE. An 18-year-old woman with fever, diffuse pulmonary opacities, and rapid onset of respiratory failure: idiopathic acute eosinophilic pneumonia. Chest 2006;130:1938–41.
38. Shimizudani N, Murata H, Kojo S, et al. Analysis of T cell receptor V(beta) gene expression and clonality in bronchoalveolar fluid lymphocytes from a patient with chronic eosinophilic pneumonitis. Lung 2001;179:31–41.
39. Freymond N, Kahn JE, Legrand F, et al. Clonal expansion of T cells in patients with eosinophilic lung disease. Allergy;11:1506–8.
40. Grantham JG, Meadows JA, Gleich GJ. Chronic eosinophilic pneumonia. Evidence for eosinophil degranulation and release of major basic protein. Am J Med 1986;80:89–94.

41. Pearson DL, Rosenow EC 3rd. Chronic eosinophilic pneumonia (Carrington's): a follow-up study. Mayo Clin Proc 1978;53:73–8.
42. Durieu J, Wallaert B, Tonnel AB. Long term follow-up of pulmonary function in chronic eosinophilic pneumonia. Eur Respir J 1997;10:286–91.
43. Hayakawa H, Sato A, Toyoshima M, et al. A clinical study of idiopathic eosinophilic pneumonia. Chest 1994;105:1462–6.
44. Badesch DB, King TE, Schwartz MI. Acute eosinophilic pneumonia: a hypersensitivity phenomenon? Am Rev Respir Dis 1989;139:249–52.
45. Allen JN, Pacht ER, Gadek JE, et al. Acute eosinophilic pneumonia as a reversible cause of noninfectious respiratory failure. N Engl J Med 1989;321:569–74.
46. Buchheit J, Eid N, Rodgers G Jr, et al. Acute eosinophilic pneumonia with respiratory failure: a new syndrome? Am Rev Respir Dis 1992;145:716–8.
47. Davis WB, Wilson HE, Wall RL. Eosinophilic alveolitis in acute respiratory failure. A clinical marker for a non-infectious etiology. Chest 1986;90:7–10.
48. Pope-Harman AL, Davis WB, Allen ED, et al. Acute eosinophilic pneumonia. A summary of 15 cases and review of the literature. Medicine (Baltimore) 1996; 75:334–42.
49. Cheon JE, Lee KS, Jung GS, et al. Acute eosinophilic pneumonia: radiographic and CT findings in six patients. AJR Am J Roentgenol 1996;167:1195–9.
50. Chiappini J, Arbib F, Heyraud JD, et al. Subacute idiopathic eosinophilic pneumopathy with favorable outcome without corticotherapy. Rev Mal Respir 1995; 12:25–8 [in French].
51. Elcadi T, Morcos E, Lancrenon C, et al. Abdominal pain syndrome disclosing acute eosinophilic pneumonia. Presse Med 1997;26:416 [in French].
52. Balbi B, Fabiano F. A young man with fever, dyspnoea and nonproductive cough. Eur Respir J 1996;9:619–21.
53. Ogawa H, Fujimura M, Matsuda T, et al. Transient wheeze. Eosinophilic bronchobronchiolitis in acute eosinophilic pneumonia. Chest 1993;104:493–6.
54. King MA, Pope-Harman AL, Allen JN, et al. Acute eosinophilic pneumonia: radiologic and clinical features. Radiology 1997;203:715–9.
55. Philit F, Etienne-Mastroianni B, Parrot A, et al. Idiopathic acute eosinophilic pneumonia: a study of 22 patients. The Groupe d'Etudes et de Recherche sur les Maladies "Orphelines" Pulmonaires (GERM"O"P). Am J Respir Crit Care Med 2002;166:1235–9.
56. Shorr AF, Scoville SL, Cersovsky SB, et al. Acute eosinophilic pneumonia among US military personnel deployed in or near Iraq. JAMA 2004;292:2997–3005.
57. Uchiyama H, Suda T, Nakamura Y, et al. Alterations in smoking habits are associated with acute eosinophilic pneumonia. Chest 2008;133:1174–80.
58. Nakajima M, Manabe T, Niki Y, et al. A case of cigarette smoking-induced acute eosinophilic pneumonia showing tolerance. Chest 2000;118:1517–8.
59. Nakajima M, Manabe T, Niki Y, et al. Cigarette smoke-induced acute eosinophilic pneumonia. Radiology 1998;207:829–31.
60. Shintani H, Fujimura M, Ishiura Y, et al. A case of cigarette smoking-induced acute eosinophilic pneumonia showing tolerance. Chest 2000;117:277–9.
61. Shintani H, Fujimura M, Yasui M, et al. Acute eosinophilic pneumonia caused by cigarette smoking. Intern Med 2000;39:66–8.
62. Bok GH, Kim YK, Lee YM, et al. Cigarette smoking-induced acute eosinophilic pneumonia: a case report including a provocation test. J Korean Med Sci 2008; 23:134–7.
63. Dujon C, Guillaud C, Azarian R, et al. Pneumopathie aiguë à éosinophiles: rôle d'un tabagisme récemment débuté. Rev Mal Respir 2004;21:825–7.

64. Al-Saieg N, Moammar O, Kartan R. Flavored cigar smoking induces acute eosinophilic pneumonia. Chest 2007;131:1234–7.
65. Komiya K, Teramoto S, Kawashima M, et al. A case of acute eosinophilic pneumonia following short-term passive smoking: an evidence of very high level of urinary cotinine. Allergol Int 2010;59:421–3.
66. Tazelaar HD, Linz LJ, Colby TV, et al. Acute eosinophilic pneumonia: histopathologic findings in nine patients. Am J Respir Crit Care Med 1997;155:296–302.
67. Daimon T, Johkoh T, Sumikawa H, et al. Acute eosinophilic pneumonia: thin-section CT findings in 29 patients. Eur J Radiol 2008;65:462–7.
68. Taniguchi H, Kadota J, Fujii T, et al. Activation of lymphocytes and increased interleukin-5 levels in bronchoalveolar lavage fluid in acute eosinophilic pneumonia. Eur Respir J 1999;13:217–20.
69. Miyazaki E, Nureki S, Ono E, et al. Circulating thymus- and activation-regulated chemokine/CCL17 is a useful biomarker for discriminating acute eosinophilic pneumonia from other causes of acute lung injury. Chest 2007;131:1726–34.
70. Perng DW, Su HT, Tseng CW, et al. Pulmonary infiltrates with eosinophilia induced by nimesulide in an asthmatic patient. Respiration 2005;72:651–3.
71. Godeau B, Brochard L, Theodorou I, et al. A case of acute eosinophilic pneumonia with hypersensitivity to "red spider" allergens. J Allergy Clin Immunol 1995;95:1056–8.
72. Sauvaget E, Dellamonica J, Arlaud K, et al. Idiopathic acute eosinophilic pneumonia requiring ECMO in a teenager smoking tobacco and cannabis. Pediatr Pulmonol 2010;45:1246–9.
73. Brander PE, Tukiainen P. Acute eosinophilic pneumonia in a heroin smoker. Eur Respir J 1993;6:750–2.
74. Matsuno O, Ueno T, Takenaka R, et al. Acute eosinophilic pneumonia caused by Candida albicans. Respir Med 2007;101:1609–12.
75. Miyazaki E, Sugisaki K, Shigenaga T, et al. A case of acute eosinophilic pneumonia caused by inhalation of Trichosporon terrestre. Am J Respir Crit Care Med 1995;151:541–3.
76. Swartz J, Stoller JK. Acute eosinophilic pneumonia complicating Coccidioides immitis pneumonia: a case report and literature review. Respiration 2009;77:102–6.
77. Ricker DH, Taylor SR, Gartner JC Jr, et al. Fatal pulmonary aspergillosis presenting as acute eosinophilic pneumonia in a previously healthy child. Chest 1991; 100:875–7.
78. Trawick D, Kotch A, Matthay R, et al. Eosinophilic pneumonia as a presentation of occult chronic granulomatous disease. Eur Respir J 1997;10:2166–70.
79. Jeon EJ, Kim KH, Min KH. Acute eosinophilic pneumonia associated with 2009 influenza A (H1N1). Thorax 2010;65:268–70.
80. Wagner T, Dhedin N, Philippe B, et al. Acute eosinophilic pneumonia after allogeneic hematopoietic stem cell transplantation. Ann Hematol 2006;85:202–3.
81. Glazer CS, Cohen LB, Schwarz MI. Acute eosinophilic pneumonia in AIDS. Chest 2001;120:1732–5.
82. Kawayama T, Fujiki R, Morimitsu Y, et al. Fatal idiopathic acute eosinophilic pneumonia with acute lung injury. Respirology 2002;7:373–5.
83. Mouthon L, le Toumelin P, Andre MH, et al. Polyarteritis nodosa and Churg-Strauss angiitis: characteristics and outcome in 38 patients over 65 years. Medicine (Baltimore) 2002;81:27–40.
84. Lanham JG, Elkon KB, Pusey CD, et al. Systemic vasculitis with asthma and eosinophilia: a clinical approach to the Churg-Strauss syndrome. Medicine (Baltimore) 1984;63:65–81.

85. Keogh KA, Specks U. Churg-Strauss syndrome: clinical presentation, antineutrophil cytoplasmic antibodies, and leukotriene receptor antagonists. Am J Med 2003;115:284–90.
86. Guillevin L, Cohen P, Gayraud M, et al. Churg-Strauss syndrome. Clinical study and long-term follow-up of 96 patients. Medicine (Baltimore) 1999;78:26–37.
87. Dunogué B, Pagnoux C, Guillevin L. Churg-Strauss syndrome: clinical symptoms, complementary investigations, prognosis and outcome, and treatment. Semin Respir Crit Care Med 2011;32:298–309.
88. Bottero P, Bonini M, Vecchio F, et al. The common allergens in the Churg-Strauss syndrome. Allergy 2007;62:1288–94.
89. Tsurikisawa N, Morita S, Tsuburai T, et al. Familial Churg-Strauss syndrome in two sisters. Chest 2007;131:592–4.
90. Vaglio A, Martorana D, Maggiore U, et al. HLA-DRB4 as a genetic risk factor for Churg-Strauss syndrome. Arthritis Rheum 2007;56:3159–66.
91. Cottin V, Bonniaud P. Drug-induced infiltrative lung disease. Eur Respir Mon 2009;46:287–318.
92. Ruppert AM, Averous G, Stanciu D, et al. Development of Churg-Strauss syndrome with controlled asthma during omalizumab treatment. J Allergy Clin Immunol 2008;121:253–4.
93. Winchester DE, Jacob A, Murphy T. Omalizumab for asthma. N Engl J Med 2006;355:1281–2.
94. Puechal X, Rivereau P, Vinchon F. Churg-Strauss syndrome associated with omalizumab. Eur J Intern Med 2008;19:364–6.
95. Bargagli E, Madioni C, Olivieri C, et al. Churg-Strauss vasculitis in a patient treated with omalizumab. J Asthma 2008;45:115–6.
96. Wechsler ME, Wong DA, Miller MK, et al. Churg-Strauss syndrome in patients treated with omalizumab. Chest 2009;136:507–18.
97. Hamilos DL, Christensen J. Treatment of Churg-Strauss syndrome with high-dose intravenous immunoglobulin. J Allergy Clin Immunol 1991;88:823–4.
98. Guillevin L, Guittard T, Bletry O, et al. Systemic necrotizing angiitis with asthma: causes and precipitating factors in 43 cases. Lung 1987;165:165–72.
99. Nathani N, Little MA, Kunst H, et al. Churg-Strauss syndrome and leukotriene antagonist use: a respiratory perspective. Thorax 2008;63:883–8.
100. Harrold LR, Patterson MK, Andrade SE, et al. Asthma drug use and the development of Churg-Strauss syndrome (CSS). Pharmacoepidemiol Drug Saf 2007;16:620–6.
101. Beasley R, Bibby S, Weatherall M. Leukotriene receptor antagonist therapy and Churg-Strauss syndrome: culprit or innocent bystander? Thorax 2008;63:847–9.
102. Hauser T, Mahr A, Metzler C, et al. The leukotriene-receptor antagonist montelukast and the risk of Churg-Strauss syndrome: a case-crossover study. Thorax 2008;63(8):677–82.
103. Bibby S, Healy B, Steele R, et al. Association between leukotriene receptor antagonist therapy and Churg-Strauss syndrome: an analysis of the FDA AERS database. Thorax 2010;65:132–8.
104. Della Rossa A, Baldini C, Tavoni A, et al. Churg-Strauss syndrome: clinical and serological features of 19 patients from a single Italian centre. Rheumatology (Oxford) 2002;41:1286–94.
105. Solans R, Bosch JA, Perez-Bocanegra C, et al. Churg-Strauss syndrome: outcome and long-term follow-up of 32 patients. Rheumatology (Oxford) 2001;40:763–71.

106. Churg A, Brallas M, Cronin SR, et al. Formes frustes of Churg-Strauss syndrome. Chest 1995;108:320–3.

107. Reid AJ, Harrison BD, Watts RA, et al. Churg-Strauss syndrome in a district hospital. QJM 1998;91:219–29.

108. Chumbley LC, Harrison EG Jr, DeRemee RA. Allergic granulomatosis and angiitis (Churg-Strauss syndrome). Report and analysis of 30 cases. Mayo Clin Proc 1977;52:477–84.

109. Cottin V, Khouatra C, Dubost R, et al. Persistent airflow obstruction in asthma of patients with Churg-Strauss syndrome and long-term follow-up. Allergy 2009; 64:589–95.

110. Szczeklik W, Sokolowska BM, Zuk J, et al. The course of asthma in Churg-Strauss syndrome. J Asthma 2011;48:183–7.

111. Bacciu A, Bacciu S, Mercante G, et al. Ear, nose and throat manifestations of Churg-Strauss syndrome. Acta Otolaryngol 2006;126:503–9.

112. Bacciu A, Buzio C, Giordano D, et al. Nasal polyposis in Churg-Strauss syndrome. Laryngoscope 2008;118:325–9.

113. Olsen KD, Neel HB, De Remee RA, et al. Nasal manifestations of allergic granulomatosis and angiitis (Churg-Strauss syndrome). Otolaryngol Head Neck Surg 1995;88:85–9.

114. Srouji I, Lund V, Andrews P, et al. Rhinologic symptoms and quality-of-life in patients with Churg-Strauss syndrome vasculitis. Am J Rhinol 2008;22:406–9.

115. Cottin V, Cordier JF. Churg-Strauss syndrome. Allergy 1999;54:535–51.

116. Vinit J, Bielefeld P, Muller G, et al. Heart involvement in Churg-Strauss syndrome: retrospective study in French Burgundy population in past 10 years. Eur J Intern Med 2010;21:341–6.

117. Neumann T, Manger B, Schmid M, et al. Cardiac involvement in Churg-Strauss syndrome: impact of endomyocarditis. Medicine (Baltimore) 2009;88:236–43.

118. Ginsberg F, Parrillo JE. Eosinophilic myocarditis. Heart Fail Clin 2005;1:419–29.

119. Courand PY, Croisille P, Khouatra C, et al. Churg-Strauss syndrome presenting with acute myocarditis and cardiogenic shock. Heart Lung Circ 2012;21:178–81.

120. Dennert RM, van Paassen P, Schalla S, et al. Cardiac involvement in Churg-Strauss syndrome. Arthritis Rheum 2010;62:627–34.

121. Marmursztejn J, Vignaux O, Cohen P, et al. Impact of cardiac magnetic resonance imaging for assessment of Churg-Strauss syndrome: a cross-sectional study in 20 patients. Clin Exp Rheumatol 2009;27:S70–6.

122. Pela G, Tirabassi G, Pattoneri P, et al. Cardiac involvement in the Churg-Strauss syndrome. Am J Cardiol 2006;97:1519–24.

123. Degesys GE, Mintzer RA, Vrla RF. Allergic granulomatosis: Churg-Strauss syndrome. AJR Am J Roentgenol 1980;135:1281–2.

124. Choi YH, Im JG, Han BK, et al. Thoracic manifestation of Churg-Strauss syndrome: radiologic and clinical findings. Chest 2000;117:117–24.

125. Kim YK, Lee KS, Chung MP, et al. Pulmonary involvement in Churg-Strauss syndrome: an analysis of CT, clinical, and pathologic findings. Eur Radiol 2007;17:3157–65.

126. Chung MP, Yi CA, Lee HY, et al. Imaging of pulmonary vasculitis. Radiology 2010;255:322–41.

127. Johkoh T. Imaging of idiopathic interstitial pneumonias. Clin Chest Med 2008;29: 133–47, vi.

128. Worthy SA, Muller NL, Hansell DM, et al. Churg-Strauss syndrome: the spectrum of pulmonary CT findings in 17 patients. AJR Am J Roentgenol 1998;170: 297–300.

129. Wallaert B, Gosset P, Prin L, et al. Bronchoalveolar lavage in allergic granulomatosis and angiitis. Eur Respir J 1993;6:413–7.
130. Cottin V, Tardy F, Gindre D, et al. Urinary eosinophil-derived neurotoxin in Churg-Strauss syndrome. J Allergy Clin Immunol 1995;96:261–4.
131. Vaglio A, Strehl JD, Manger B, et al. IgG4 immune response in Churg-Strauss syndrome. Ann Rheum Dis 2012;71:390–3.
132. Dallos T, Heiland GR, Strehl J, et al. CCL17/thymus and activation-related chemokine in Churg-Strauss syndrome. Arthritis Rheum 2010;62:3496–503.
133. Sable-Fourtassou R, Cohen P, Mahr A, et al. Antineutrophil cytoplasmic antibodies and the Churg-Strauss syndrome. Ann Intern Med 2005;143:632–8.
134. Sinico RA, Di Toma L, Maggiore U, et al. Prevalence and clinical significance of antineutrophil cytoplasmic antibodies in Churg-Strauss syndrome. Arthritis Rheum 2005;52:2926–35.
135. Kallenberg CG. Churg-Strauss syndrome: just one disease entity? Arthritis Rheum 2005;52:2589–93.
136. Wieczorek S, Hellmich B, Arning L, et al. Functionally relevant variations of the interleukin-10 gene associated with antineutrophil cytoplasmic antibody-negative Churg-Strauss syndrome, but not with Wegener's granulomatosis. Arthritis Rheum 2008;58:1839–48.
137. Katzenstein AL. Diagnostic features and differential diagnosis of Churg-Strauss syndrome in the lung. A review. Am J Clin Pathol 2000;114:767–72.
138. Churg A. Recent advances in the diagnosis of Churg-Strauss syndrome. Mod Pathol 2001;14:1284–93.
139. Lie JT. Limited forms of Churg-Strauss syndrome. Pathol Annu 1993;28:199–220.
140. Wechsler ME, Garpestad E, Flier SR, et al. Pulmonary infiltrates, eosinophilia, and cardiomyopathy following corticosteroid withdrawal in patients with asthma receiving zarfirlukast. JAMA 1998;279:455–7.
141. Masi AT, Hunder GG, Lie JT, et al. The American College of Rheumatology 1990 criteria for the classification of Churg-Strauss syndrome (allergic granulomatosis and angiitis). Arthritis Rheum 1990;33:1094–100.
142. Jennette JC, Falk RJ, Andrassy K, et al. Nomenclature of systemic vasculitides. Proposal of an international consensus conference. Arthritis Rheum 1994;37:187–92.
143. Guillevin L, Pagnoux C, Seror R, et al. The Five-Factor Score revisited: assessment of prognoses of systemic necrotizing vasculitides based on the French Vasculitis Study Group (FVSG) cohort. Medicine (Baltimore) 2011;90:19–27.
144. Bouldouyre MA, Cohen P, Guillevin L. Severe bronchospasm associated with rituximab for refractory Churg-Strauss syndrome. Ann Rheum Dis 2009;68:606.
145. Kahn JE, Grandpeix-Guyodo C, Marroun I, et al. Sustained response to mepolizumab in refractory Churg-Strauss syndrome. J Allergy Clin Immunol 2010;125:267–70.
146. Moosig F, Gross WL, Herrmann K, et al. Targeting interleukin-5 in refractory and relapsing Churg-Strauss syndrome. Ann Intern Med 2011;155:341–3.
147. Rosenwasser LJ, Rothenberg ME. IL-5 pathway inhibition in the treatment of asthma and Churg-Strauss syndrome. J Allergy Clin Immunol 2010;125:1245–6.
148. Cohen P, Pagnoux C, Mahr A, et al. Treatment of Churg-Strauss syndrome (CSS) without poor prognosis factor at baseline with corticosteroids (CS) alone. Preliminary results of a prospective multicenter trial. Arthritis Rheum 2003;48:S209.

149. Ribi C, Cohen P, Pagnoux C, et al. Treatment of Churg-Strauss syndrome without poor-prognosis factors: a multicenter, prospective, randomized, open-label study of seventy-two patients. Arthritis Rheum 2008;58:586–94.
150. Bourgarit A, Le Toumelin P, Pagnoux C, et al. Deaths occurring during the first year after treatment onset for polyarteritis nodosa, microscopic polyangiitis, and Churg-Strauss syndrome: a retrospective analysis of causes and factors predictive of mortality based on 595 patients. Medicine (Baltimore) 2005;84:323–30.
151. Geller DE, Kaplowitz H, Light MJ, et al. Allergic bronchopulmonary aspergillosis in cystic fibrosis: reported prevalence, regional distribution, and patient characteristics. Chest 1999;116:639–46.
152. Mastella G, Rainisio M, Harms HK, et al. Allergic bronchopulmonary aspergillosis in cystic fibrosis. A European epidemiological study. Epidemiologic Registry of Cystic Fibrosis. Eur Respir J 2000;16:464–71.
153. Mehta SK, Sandhu RS. Immunological significance of *Aspergillus fumigatus* in cane-sugar mills. Arch Environ Health 1983;38:41–6.
154. Leonard CT, Berry GJ, Ruoss SJ. Nasal-pulmonary relations in allergic fungal sinusitis and allergic bronchopulmonary aspergillosis. Clin Rev Allergy Immunol 2001;21:5–15.
155. Venarske DL, deShazo RD. Sinobronchial allergic mycosis: the SAM syndrome. Chest 2002;121:1670–6.
156. Bains SN, Judson MA. Allergic bronchopulmonary aspergillosis. Clin Chest Med 2012;33:265–81.
157. Marchand E, Verellen-Dumoulin C, Mairesse M, et al. Frequency of cystic fibrosis transmembrane conductance regulator gene mutations and 5T allele in patients with allergic bronchopulmonary aspergillosis. Chest 2001;119:762–7.
158. Knutsen AP, Kariuki B, Consolino JD, et al. IL-4 alpha chain receptor (IL-4Ralpha) polymorphisms in allergic bronchopulmonary aspergillosis. Clin Mol Allergy 2006;4:3.
159. Brouard J, Knauer N, Boelle PY, et al. Influence of interleukin-10 on *Aspergillus fumigatus* infection in patients with cystic fibrosis. J Infect Dis 2005;191: 1988–91.
160. Saxena S, Madan T, Shah A, et al. Association of polymorphisms in the collagen region of SP-A2 with increased levels of total IgE antibodies and eosinophilia in patients with allergic bronchopulmonary aspergillosis. J Allergy Clin Immunol 2003;111:1001–7.
161. Chauhan B, Santiago L, Kirschmann DA, et al. The association of HLA-DR alleles and T cell activation with allergic bronchopulmonary aspergillosis. J Immunol 1997;159:4072–6.
162. Chauhan B, Santiago L, Hutcheson PS, et al. Evidence for the involvement of two different MHC class II regions in susceptibility or protection in allergic bronchopulmonary aspergillosis. J Allergy Clin Immunol 2000;106:723–9.
163. Chauhan B, Knutsen A, Hutcheson PS, et al. T cell subsets, epitope mapping, and HLA-restriction in patients with allergic bronchopulmonary aspergillosis. J Clin Invest 1996;97:2324–31.
164. Shah A, Khan ZU, Chaturvedi S, et al. Concomitant allergic *Aspergillus* sinusitis and allergic bronchopulmonary aspergillosis associated with familial occurrence of allergic bronchopulmonary aspergillosis. Ann Allergy 1990;64:507–12.
165. Agarwal R. Allergic bronchopulmonary aspergillosis. Chest 2009;135:805–26.
166. Mussaffi H, Rivlin J, Shalit I, et al. Nontuberculous mycobacteria in cystic fibrosis associated with allergic bronchopulmonary aspergillosis and steroid therapy. Eur Respir J 2005;25:324–8.

167. Agarwal R, Gupta D, Aggarwal AN, et al. Clinical significance of hyperattenuating mucoid impaction in allergic bronchopulmonary aspergillosis: an analysis of 155 patients. Chest 2007;132:1183–90.

168. Logan PM, Muller NL. High-attenuation mucous plugging in allergic bronchopulmonary aspergillosis. Can Assoc Radiol J 1996;47:374–7.

169. Agarwal R, Gupta D, Aggarwal AN, et al. Allergic bronchopulmonary aspergillosis: lessons from 126 patients attending a chest clinic in north India. Chest 2006;130:442–8.

170. Martinez S, Heyneman LE, McAdams HP, et al. Mucoid impactions: finger-in-glove sign and other CT and radiographic features. Radiographics 2008;28:1369–82.

171. Ward S, Heyneman L, Lee MJ, et al. Accuracy of CT in the diagnosis of allergic bronchopulmonary aspergillosis in asthmatic patients. AJR Am J Roentgenol 1999;173:937–42.

172. Rosenberg M, Patterson R, Roberts M, et al. The assessment of immunologic and clinical changes occurring during corticosteroid therapy for allergic bronchopulmonary aspergillosis. Am J Med 1978;64:599–606.

173. Bosken C, Myers J, Greenberger P, et al. Pathologic features of allergic bronchopulmonary aspergillosis. Am J Surg Pathol 1988;12:216–22.

174. Greenberger PA. Allergic bronchopulmonary aspergillosis. J Allergy Clin Immunol 2002;110:685–92.

175. Patterson R, Greenberger PA, Lee TM, et al. Prolonged evaluation of patients with corticosteroid-dependent asthma stage of allergic bronchopulmonary aspergillosis. J Allergy Clin Immunol 1987;80:663–8.

176. Salez F, Brichet A, Desurmont S, et al. Effects of itraconazole therapy in allergic bronchopulmonary aspergillosis. Chest 1999;116:1665–8.

177. Wark P. Pathogenesis of allergic bronchopulmonary aspergillosis and an evidence-based review of azoles in treatment. Respir Med 2004;98:915–23.

178. van der Ent CK, Hoekstra H, Rijkers GT. Successful treatment of allergic bronchopulmonary aspergillosis with recombinant anti-IgE antibody. Thorax 2007;62:276–7.

179. Zirbes JM, Milla CE. Steroid-sparing effect of omalizumab for allergic bronchopulmonary aspergillosis and cystic fibrosis. Pediatr Pulmonol 2008;43:607–10.

180. Kanu A, Patel K. Treatment of allergic bronchopulmonary aspergillosis (ABPA) in CF with anti-IgE antibody (omalizumab). Pediatr Pulmonol 2008;43:1249–51.

181. Tillie-Leblond I, Germaud P, Leroyer C, et al. Allergic bronchopulmonary aspergillosis and omalizumab. Allergy 2011;66:1254–6.

182. Perez-de-Llano LA, Vennera MC, Parra A, et al. Effects of omalizumab in Aspergillus-associated airway disease. Thorax 2011;66:539–40.

183. Chusid MJ, Dale DC, West BC, et al. The hypereosinophilic syndrome: analysis of fourteen cases with review of the literature. Medicine (Baltimore) 1975;54:1–27.

184. Klion A. Hypereosinophilic syndrome: current approach to diagnosis and treatment. Annu Rev Med 2009;60:293–306.

185. Ogbogu PU, Bochner BS, Butterfield JH, et al. Hypereosinophilic syndrome: a multicenter, retrospective analysis of clinical characteristics and response to therapy. J Allergy Clin Immunol 2009;124:1319–25.e3.

186. Cools J, DeAngelo DJ, Gotlib J, et al. A tyrosine kinase created by fusion of the PDGFRA and FIP1L1 genes as a therapeutic target of imatinib in idiopathic hypereosinophilic syndrome. N Engl J Med 2003;348:1201–14.

187. Simon HU, Plotz SG, Dummer R, et al. Abnormal clones of T cells producing interleukin-5 in idiopathic eosinophilia. N Engl J Med 1999;341:1112–20.

188. Dulohery MM, Patel RR, Schneider F, et al. Lung involvement in hypereosinophilic syndromes. Respir Med 2011;105:114–21.
189. Kunst H, Mack D, Kon OM, et al. Parasitic infections of the lung: a guide for the respiratory physician. Thorax 2011;66:528–36.
190. Sitbon O, Bidel N, Dussopt C, et al. Minocycline pneumonitis and eosinophilia. A report on eight patients. Arch Intern Med 1994;154:1633–40.
191. Sovijarvi AR, Lemola M, Stenius B, et al. Nitrofurantoin-induced acute, subacute and chronic pulmonary reactions. Scand J Respir Dis 1977;58:41–50.
192. Favrolt N, Bonniaud P, Collet E, et al. Severe drug rash with eosinophilia and systemic symptoms after treatment with minocycline. Rev Mal Respir 2007;24: 892–5 [in French].
193. Belongia EA, Hedberg CW, Gleich GJ, et al. An investigation of the cause of the eosinophilia-myalgia syndrome associated with tryptophan use. N Engl J Med 1990;323:357–65.
194. Hertzman PA, Blevins WL, Mayer J, et al. Association of the eosinophilia-myalgia syndrome with the ingestion of tryptophan. N Engl J Med 1990;322:869–73.
195. Silver RM, Heyes MP, Maize JC, et al. Scleroderma, fasciitis, and eosinophilia associated with the ingestion of tryptophan. N Engl J Med 1990;322:874–81.
196. Allen JA, Peterson A, Sufit R, et al. Post-epidemic eosinophilia myalgia syndrome associated with L-Tryptophan. Blood 2011. http://dx.doi.org/ 10.1002/art.30514.
197. Alonso-Ruiz A, Calabozo M, Perez-Ruiz F, et al. Toxic oil syndrome. A long-term follow-up of a cohort of 332 patients. Medicine (Baltimore) 1993;72:285–95.
198. Miranowski AC, Ditto AM. A 59-year-old woman with fever, cough, and eosinophilia. Ann Allergy Asthma Immunol 2006;96:483–8.
199. Cottin V, Cordier JF. Eosinophilic pneumonia in a patient with breast cancer: idiopathic or not? Ann Allergy Asthma Immunol 2006;97:557–8.

Update on Diffuse Alveolar Hemorrhage and Pulmonary Vasculitis

Megan L. Krause, MD[a], Rodrigo Cartin-Ceba, MD[b],
Ulrich Specks, MD[b], Tobias Peikert, MD[b,c,*]

KEYWORDS

- Pulmonary vasculitis • Diffuse alveolar hemorrhage • ANCA-associated vasculitis
- Granulomatosis with polyangiitis • Microscopic polyangiitis
- Eosinophilic granulomatosis with polyangiitis

KEY POINTS

- Diffuse alveolar hemorrhage (DAH) represents the most common and potentially life-threatening manifestation of pulmonary vasculitis.
- Identification and treatment of the underlying cause of DAH are crucial for therapeutic success.
- Pulmonary vasculitis, including antineutrophil cytoplasmic antibody–associated vasculitis (AAV), represents the most common immune-mediated cause of DAH.
- Rituximab has an increasing role in the treatment of AAV, particularly in patients with severe relapsing or refractory disease.

Pulmonary vasculitis is characterized by inflammation and necrosis of the pulmonary blood vessels. Even though it can involve all parts of the pulmonary vasculature, pulmonary arteries, capillaries, and pulmonary veins, it most commonly affects the pulmonary capillaries. Diffuse alveolar hemorrhage (DAH), characterized by the widespread extravasation of red blood cells into the pulmonary alveolar spaces, is the most common clinical manifestation of pulmonary vasculitis (**Fig. 1**). DAH is typically attributable to disseminated injury of the pulmonary capillaries. It is associated with a disruption of the alveolar and capillary basement membranes facilitating the entry of red blood cells into the alveoli. Independent of the underlying cause, pulmonary capillaritis represents the most common histologic finding if lung-tissue biopsies are

Funding sources/Conflicts of interest: Ulrich Specks: Research grant from Genentech/BiogenIDEC.
[a] Department of Internal Medicine, Mayo Clinic, 200 First Street Southwest, Rochester, MN 55905, USA; [b] Division of Pulmonary and Critical Care, Department of Internal Medicine, Mayo Clinic, 200 First Street Southwest, Rochester, MN 55905, USA; [c] Department of Immunology, Mayo Clinic, 200 First Street Southwest, Rochester, MN 55905, USA
* Corresponding author. Mayo Clinic, 200 First Street Southwest, Rochester, MN 55905.
E-mail address: Peikert.Tobias@mayo.edu

Immunol Allergy Clin N Am 32 (2012) 587–600
http://dx.doi.org/10.1016/j.iac.2012.08.001
0889-8561/12/$ – see front matter © 2012 Elsevier Inc. All rights reserved.

immunology.theclinics.com

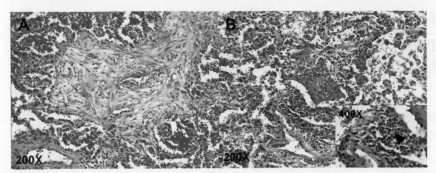

Fig. 1. Pathologic findings of diffuse alveolar hemorrhage. (A) Organizing diffuse alveolar hemorrhage with hemosiderin-laden macrophages with surrounding fibrosis. (B) Pulmonary capillaritis. Arrowhead indicates leukocytoclastic inflammation. (Courtesy of Dr MC. Aubry, MD, Mayo Clinic, Rochester, MN.)

obtained in these patients (see **Fig. 1**).[1] DAH can occur in the context of various systemic disorders or present in isolation. The etiology of DAH can be broadly divided into immune-mediated and non–immune-mediated causes.

As a group, antineutrophil cytoplasmic antibody (ANCA)-associated vasculitis (AAV) represents the most common cause of pulmonary vasculitis. Even though all these diseases remain idiopathic, over the last few decades our understanding of their pathogenesis has improved significantly. In a recent effort to eliminate eponyms and establish more descriptive disease names reflective of the associated pathology and disease associations, a new nomenclature for AAV was proposed by an international expert panel.[2] Wegener's granulomatosis was renamed as granulomatosis with polyangiitis (Wegener's) GPA, highlighting the granulomatous nature and vascular inflammation associated with the disease as well as its similarities to microscopic polyangiitis (MPA). To emphasize the contribution of eosinophilic inflammation and the resemblance to GPA, Churg-Strauss was renamed as eosinophilic granulomatosis with polyangiitis (Churg-Strauss) EGPA.[2]

CLINICAL PRESENTATION AND DIAGNOSIS OF DAH

The clinical presentation of DAH is highly variable. Patients can present within a spectrum ranging from asymptomatic radiographic abnormalities to severe life-threatening respiratory failure. Even though the majority of patients experience a variable degree of hemoptysis, approximately one-third of all patients with DAH are lacking this symptom.[3] Other common symptoms include dyspnea, cough, fever, and chest pain. Laboratory studies frequently demonstrate anemia and/or decreasing hemoglobin values as a marker of intrapulmonary blood loss.[4,5] In addition, patients presenting with DAH frequently report signs and symptoms related to an etiologically related systemic disorder. Such abnormalities may include rashes, ocular, sinus, nasal, or ear symptoms, airway obstruction, renal dysfunction owing to glomerular inflammation characterized by an active urinary sediment, neurologic symptoms such as mononeuritis multiplex, inflammatory arthritis, muscle weakness, and many other symptoms. Patients presenting with DAH and concurrent glomerulonephritis are typically classified as pulmonary-renal syndrome. The vast majority of these cases are attributable to immune-mediated causes, most frequently AAV, systemic lupus erythematosus (SLE), or anti–glomerular basement membrane antibody (anti-GBM) syndrome. A careful history including review of systems, review of exposures, and medical history, as well as a comprehensive physical examination are critically important for the characterization of any underlying systemic disease causing DAH.

Imaging studies, specifically high-resolution computed tomography, provide additional information to support a diagnosis of DAH (**Fig. 2**). However, radiologic findings are frequently nonspecific and subject to change throughout the course of the disease. Typical patterns include focal or diffuse areas of ground-glass opacification and/or consolidation as a consequence of alveolar filling. On cessation of the alveolar bleeding, most of the associated radiologic abnormalities resolve within a few days to weeks. The resolution of this process is slower than that of the infiltrates related to pulmonary edema but faster than the disappearance of the inflammatory/infectious radiologic changes observed in pneumonias. During the resolution of the acute hemorrhage, "crazy paving" with associated interlobular septal thickening may become more prominent.[6,7] Additional radiologic abnormalities may be attributable to many of the underlying systemic disorders or represent infectious complications related to systemic immunosuppression. Some of these findings include cavitating pulmonary nodules and masses and large-airway inflammation and stenosis caused by granulomatous inflammation in GPA, fibrosis and bronchiectasis in MPA, airway inflammation and inflammatory infiltrates in EGPA, and pleural effusions in SLE (see **Fig. 2**).

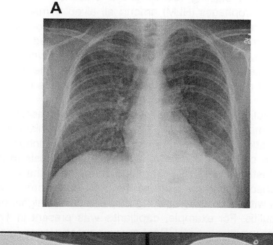

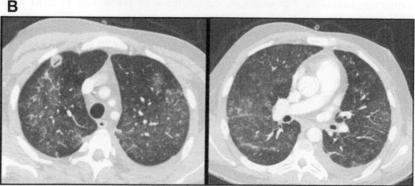

Fig. 2. Radiographic findings of diffuse alveolar hemorrhage. (*A*) Chest radiograph shows bilateral patchy infiltrate. (*B*) Computed tomography images show bilateral ground-glass infiltrates with associated necrotizing nodule in right upper lobe.

Because of the relatively nonspecific nature of the clinical-radiologic signs and symptoms of pulmonary vasculitis, additional laboratory tests and bronchoscopy with bronchoalveolar lavage (BAL) are frequently required to accurately diagnose and optimally manage patients with DAH. Laboratory studies typically include: complete blood count with differential, coagulation studies, serum creatinine and blood urea nitrogen, ANCA testing (by indirect immunofluorescence [cytoplasmic ANCA and perinuclear ANCA] and antigen-specific enzyme-linked immunosorbent assay [PR3-ANCA and MPO-ANCA]), anti-GBM antibodies, antinuclear antibodies (ANA), anticyclic citrullinated peptide antibodies (anti-CCP), rheumatoid factor (RF), antiphospholipid antibodies, creatine kinase, urinalysis with urinary sediment, and urine drug screen.

A transient, reversible increase in the diffusing capacity for carbon monoxide (DLCO) has been previously reported in patients with DAH.[8] This increase is attributed to the enhanced uptake of carbon monoxide by extravascular blood. However, because of the acute onset, the often severe clinical manifestations of DAH, and a lack of comparison baseline DLCO values, DLCO measurements are not routinely used to evaluate patients with suspected DAH.

The purpose of bronchoscopy with BAL is primarily to confirm the presence of intra-alveolar blood, exclude the large airways as a source of bleeding, and rule out infection. Alveolar blood results in an increasingly hemorrhagic appearance of consecutive BAL aliquots.[4] BAL iron staining revealing the presence of greater than 20% hemosiderin-laden macrophages (HLM) among all alveolar macrophages provides additional support for a diagnosis of DAH.[9] However, it is important that in cases of acute hemorrhage, increasingly bloody BAL returns may precede the appearance of HLM. By contrast, HLM may be detectable in the BAL fluid weeks to months after the intra-alveolar red cells have disappeared. Unfortunately, the presence of HLM is not restricted to DAH and is also commonly seen in patients with diffuse alveolar damage.[10]

Because most established diagnostic criteria for pulmonary vasculitis (eg, the American College of Rheumatology criteria for GPA) do require the histologic confirmation of vascular inflammation by tissue biopsy, tissue transbronchoscopic (TBBx) or surgical biopsies are often considered to establish a diagnosis in these patients. However, the diagnostic yield of TBBx remains suboptimal, the histologic findings are frequently nonspecific, and the risks of the procedure commonly outweigh its benefits. Compared with TBBx, surgical lung biopsies have a higher diagnostic yield for pulmonary vasculitis. For example, capillaritis was present in 17% to 43% of surgical lung biopsies in patients with GPA; however, these procedures are also associated with a substantial risk for these patients.[11,12] Consequently, recent efforts have focused on the development of diagnostic criteria that use clinical, radiologic, and serologic information (eg, ANCA for AAV) to establish a diagnosis.[13]

DIFFERENTIAL DIAGNOSIS OF DAH

The etiology of DAH can be broadly divided into immune-mediated and non–immune-mediated causes (**Table 1**). The list of diagnostic considerations is long, and a careful history and physical examination represents a key component in the evaluation of these patients.

In a 28-year retrospective cohort of patients presenting with DAH, immune-mediated causes including vasculitis, anti-GBM disease, and other connective tissue disease were identified in 36% of patients (35 of 97). Twenty-five patients had a diagnosis of vasculitis. Among the non–immune-mediated causes, systolic or diastolic

Table 1	
Differential diagnosis of diffuse alveolar hemorrhage	
Immune Mediated	**Non–Immune Mediated**
ANCA-Associated Vasculitis	Cardiac disease
Granulomatosis with polyangiitis (GPA)	Left ventricular dysfunction
Microscopic polyangiitis (MPA)	Valvular disease
Eosinophilic granulomatosis with polyangiitis	Infection
(EGPA)	Medications
Isolated pulmonary capillaritis	Acute respiratory distress syndrome
Anti–glomerular basement membrane antibody	Idiopathic pulmonary hemosiderosis
syndrome	Coagulopathy
Connective tissue disease	Radiation exposure
Systemic lupus erythematosus	Occupational exposure
Rheumatoid arthritis	Crack cocaine inhalation
Inflammatory myopathies	Bone marrow transplant[a]
Antiphospholipid antibody syndrome	
Henoch-Schönlein purpura/IgA vasculitis	
Cryoglobulinemic vasculitis	
Behçet disease	
Lung transplant rejection	
Hypocomplementemic urticarial vasculitis (anti-C1q vasculitis)	
Drug-induced vasculitis	
Bone marrow transplant[a]	

[a] In autopsy series of patients with bone marrow transplant with diffuse alveolar hemorrhage, there were complications of diffuse alveolar damage, rather than capillaritis, suggesting a non–immune-mediated mechanism of diffuse alveolar hemorrhage.

cardiac dysfunction of the left ventricle and valvular heart disease accounted for 27% (26 of 97) of the cases.[3] Similarly, among critically ill patients with DAH, vasculitis accounted for 19% (7 of 37) of all cases.[14] Because capillaritis, independent of the underlying etiology, represents the most common histologic finding in DAH, it is certainly possible that pulmonary vasculitis is responsible for up to 88% of these cases.[1]

Among DAH patients with pulmonary vasculitis, AAV including GPA, MPA, and more rarely, EGPA and isolated pulmonary capillaritis account for the majority of cases.[15] Although all AAV have been associated with pulmonary capillaritis and DAH, their frequency differs between the syndromes. The incidence of DAH ranges from 12% to 29% for MPA, 8% to 18% for GPA, and 0% to 4% for EGPA.[16–20] Other less frequent causes of immune-mediated pulmonary small-vessel vasculitis include Henoch-Schönlein purpura, capillaritis including connective tissue disease (SLE, inflammatory myopathies, and rheumatoid arthritis), antiphospholipid syndrome, and anti-GBM-disease. DAH is also increasingly recognized as a pulmonary complication of bone marrow transplantation. However, whether this represents an immune-mediated or non–immune-mediated phenomenon remains controversial.

ACUTE MANAGEMENT OF DAH

Acute management of DAH involves supportive care, including ventilatory support ranging from oxygen supplementation to mechanical ventilation.[21] The coagulation cascade should be evaluated, and identified coagulation abnormalities should be corrected accordingly. Commonly accepted targets include a platelet count greater than

50,000/μL and an international normalized ratio of less than 1.5. Depending on the cause of the coagulopathy, platelet transfusions, vitamin K and fresh frozen plasma are used for correction.

It is crucial to identify and treat the underlying etiology of the DAH. Non–immune-mediated causes are treated by addressing the cause (eg, heart-failure management or discontinuation of any causative drugs). To quickly control the inflammatory activity in immune-mediated DAH, prompt initiation of high-dose methylprednisolone therapy is critical. Because of the high mortality associated with DAH, glucocorticoids are frequently started while diagnostic test results are pending.

If a non–immune-mediated cause is not effectively controlled by supportive care or addressing the underlying etiology or when all other options are exhausted in immune-mediated cases that are refractory to aggressive initial immunosuppressive therapy, consideration can be given to recombinant factor VIIa (rVIIa). Several recent case reports and small case series suggest that rVIIa may represent a treatment option for refractory cases. rVIIa is approved by the Food and Drug Administration (FDA) for the prevention and management of hemorrhagic complications in patients with hemophilia A or B. However, it has also been used for hemostasis in patients without hemophilia. Activated factor VIIa is thought to bind to activated platelets and activate factor X, resulting in the generation of thrombin in a tissue factor–independent fashion. In refractory cases of immune-mediated and non–immune-mediated DAH, including cases attributable to pulmonary vasculitis, rVIIa has been successfully administered both systemically (intravenously) or bronchoscopically. The optimal dose and dosing intervals remain to be determined. Systemic administration usually involves the intravenous administration of 90 to 180 μg/kg as either a single dose or, if needed, repeated doses every 2 to 4 hours. Endobronchial therapy typically includes the bronchoscopic delivery of a total dose of 50 μg/kg of activated factor VIIa diluted in 50 mL of normal saline. During the procedure 25 mL are instilled into each of the mainstem bronchi.[22–25] It must be noted that this represents an off-label use of rVIIa. Thrombotic complications involving both arterial and venous events have been reported in some patients treated with rVIIa, and patients should be monitored carefully. This risk is further increased in the known prothrombotic state of AAV. Therefore, this agent should be used with great caution when treating AAV.[26]

Another option includes the inhibition of fibrinolysis with the plasminogen inhibitor aminocaproic acid. The addition of aminocaproic acid to corticosteroids in patients with post–bone marrow transplant DAH was demonstrated to result in a lower 100-day disease-related mortality rate in comparison with corticosteroids alone.[27]

ADVANCES IN THE TREATMENT OF AAV

The treatment of AAV is typically stratified based on disease extent/severity and disease activity. The disease extent is classified as either nonsevere (limited) or severe disease. Severe disease is defined as the presence of life-threatening and/or organ-threatening disease manifestations, which includes all cases of pulmonary vasculitis and DAH. Active disease typically requires the initiation of remission induction therapy. Once remission has been achieved (after 3–6 months of therapy) patients are transitioned to remission maintenance therapy. At present, a minimum of 18 months is the accepted duration of remission maintenance therapy. The optimal length is not yet known. However, it is being evaluated in a randomized clinical trial comparing 24 months with 48 months.

In patients with severe disease, the selection of the appropriate remission induction and maintenance regimens appears to be independent of a clinical diagnosis of GPA or MPA. Recent clinical trials have stratified patients based on their ANCA type rather than the specific underlying diagnosis. ANCA are classified based on their target antigens (either PR3 or MPO) and their staining pattern by indirect immunofluorescence on ethanol-fixed neutrophils (cytoplasmic [c] or perinuclear [p]). The most common pattern is c-ANCA/PR3-ANCA (GPA), p-ANCA/MPO-ANCA (MPA and EGPA).

Remission Induction Therapy for Severe AAV

Historically AAV was almost universally fatal; however, over the past decades new treatment strategies resulted in a dramatic decrease in AAV morbidity and mortality. Disease severity typically dictates the aggressiveness of the treatment strategy used. Traditionally combination therapy with high-dose corticosteroids (intravenous high-dose methylprednisolone, 1000 mg/d for 3–5 days followed by oral prednisone, 1 mg/kg/d [maximum 80 mg/d] tapered over approximately 6 months) and oral cyclophosphamide (CYC), 2 mg/kg/d was used for almost all cases of severe GPA and MPA, including cases of DAH. Approximately 75% of patients treated with prednisone/CYC will achieve remission, but disease relapse rates are as high as 50%.[28] Unfortunately, this regimen carries a substantial risk of severe treatment-related toxicity. Treatment-related complications include leukopenia and neutropenia owing to bone marrow suppression, opportunistic infections, hemorrhagic cystitis, female and male infertility, bladder cancer, and hematologic malignancies.[29,30] To decrease the occurrence of these side effects, intermittent intravenous pulse-dose CYC has been compared with the daily oral administration of the drug. Despite a significant decrease in the cumulative CYC dose in patients treated intravenously, differences in the side-effect profile were limited to fewer non–life-threatening leukopenias in patients receiving intravenous CYC. There were no differences in remission induction.[31] However, the relapse rate was higher in the intravenous-pulse CYC group, a finding that was recently confirmed during the long-term follow up of the study.[31,32] Even though methotrexate (MTX) is effective for remission induction therapy in patients with nonsevere (limited) GPA, this should not be used in the setting of DAH.[33]

Despite major advances in AAV remission induction, morbidity and mortality of patients with pulmonary vasculitis/DAH remains high and disease relapses occur frequently. Although the precise role of ANCA in the pathogenesis of AAV remains unclear, increasing clinical and experimental data suggest that these antibodies are at least modifying the autoimmune response. The presence of ANCA varies with the phenotype and the extent of disease. Whereas ANCA is absent in up to 30% to 40% of patients with nonsevere (limited) AAV, they are almost universally detectable in patients with pulmonary vasculitis/DAH. Consequently, several new therapeutic approaches have recently focused on the elimination of ANCA by depletion of B lymphocytes as the precursors of antibody-producing plasma cells or the direct removal of circulating antibodies.

Plasma Exchange for AAV

In an uncontrolled retrospective cohort study, 20 patients with AAV and DAH underwent plasma exchange (PLEX) in addition to standard immunosuppressive therapy. This approach resulted in excellent patient outcomes; DAH resolved in all cases and only 1 of 20 patients (5%) died, compared with historical controls.[34] However, earlier other investigators had reported a high mortality (50%) among 14 patients with pulmonary-renal syndrome despite the use of PLEX in 12 of 14 patients.[34,35] Furthermore, in the MEPEX trial the addition of PLEX to immunosuppressive therapy was found to improve 12-month renal outcomes in AAV patients presenting with severe renal dysfunction (serum creatinine >5.8 mg/dL).[36] Nevertheless, according to the recently reported long-term follow-up data, these benefits were not sustained. In accordance with the evidence-based guidelines of the American Society for Apheresis, the authors are currently using PLEX in AAV patients with DAH presenting with hypoxemic respiratory failure requiring either high-flow supplemental oxygen or mechanical ventilation.[37] PLEX is typically performed daily or on alternating days for 14 days. Each exchange involves 1 to 1.5 times the total plasma volume. The volume is replaced with albumin but fresh frozen plasma is used at the end of each treatment. Nevertheless, the therapeutic indications of PLEX in AAV specifically for patients with DAH and glomerulonephritis remains controversial and is currently being investigated in an international randomized controlled clinical trial, the Plasma Exchange and Glucocorticoids for Treatment of AAV (PEXIVAS; NCT00987389).[38]

Rituximab in AAV

Rituximab (RTX) is a monoclonal chimeric antibody targeting CD20, a cell-surface protein expressed on B lymphocytes. These cells are the precursors for ANCA producing short-lived plasma cells. Antibody-mediated modification and/or depletion of B lymphocytes represents the proposed mechanism for this approach to decrease autoantibody production and control disease activity. Based on this rationale, RTX was evaluated on a compassionate-use basis for patients with refractory AAV. RTX is highly effective in patients with refractory AAV.[39–42] Successful treatment has been reported in more than 200 patients in at least 19 uncontrolled studies.[43] Therapeutic failures are uncommon and usually occur in patients with otherwise specific disease manifestations that are difficult to treat, such as retro-orbital pseudotumor. These very encouraging results led to 2 randomized controlled trials evaluating the use of RTX for remission induction therapy in patients with severe AAV.

The RTX in AAV (RAVE) trial compared combination therapy of glucocorticoids plus RTX or glucocorticoids plus CYC. After remission was achieved, patients in the CYC group were transitioned (after 3–6 months) to azathioprine (AZA) to complete 18 months of remission maintenance therapy, whereas RTX-treated patients were observed in the absence of further therapy. The RAVE trial was a double-blind, double-dummy controlled trial with a primary end point of noninferiority. All patients received either 4 weekly infusions of 375 mg/m^2 RTX or 2 mg/kg/d oral CYC. Based on the primary outcome measure (complete remission at 6 months: a Birmingham Vasculitis Assessment Score = 0 in the absence of corticosteroid therapy), RTX was found to be noninferior to CYC for remission induction therapy for severe AAV, including patients with pulmonary vasculitis and DAH. However, it must be noted that patients with severe DAH causing respiratory failure requiring mechanical ventilation were excluded from participation in this study. Both medications demonstrated similar efficacy in the subgroup of patients with DAH. Rituximab was superior to CYC for remission induction in patients who had a severe disease flare at the time of enrollment.[44] Somewhat surprisingly, relapse rates were similar between the 2 treatment groups at 18 months despite the absence of any active remission maintenance therapy in the RTX group.[45] Patients treated with RTX had fewer protocol-defined adverse events. This difference was mainly due to an increased frequency of leukopenia in the CYC-treated patients. Based on these data, RTX became the first FDA-approved drug for remission induction therapy in AAV.

Another study, the RTX versus CYC in ANCA-associated renal vasculitis study (RITUXVAS), enrolled 44 patients with newly diagnosed AAV (GPA and MPA) with renal involvement. Remission induction therapy included corticosteroids in combination with either RTX (4 weekly doses of 375 mg/m^2) and 2 pulses of intravenous CYC (15 mg/kg with the first and the third RTX infusion) or monthly intravenous CYC pulses for 3 to 6 months (control patients received 15 mg/kg intravenous CYC every 2 weeks × 3, followed by every 3 weeks thereafter until stable remission, minimum 6, maximum 10 doses). Patients were randomized at a 3:1 ratio to experimental treatment (RTX plus 2 intravenous pulses of CYC) versus control treatment (intravenous pulse treatment with CYC for 6 months, followed by oral AZA for remission maintenance). Low-dose corticosteroids (5 mg/d) were continued in both treatment arms through 18 months. Similar to the RAVE study, there was no difference in remission induction and relapse rates between RTX and CYC.[46] Long-term data regarding the efficacy and safety of RTX is beginning to become available.[42]

Remission Maintenance Therapy for AAV

Remission induction therapy alone regardless of regimen is insufficient to prevent relapses, and prolonged CYC treatment has been associated with unacceptable toxicities. Consequently, several different remission maintenance regimens have been investigated. In a landmark randomized controlled trial, maintenance therapy with AZA (2 mg/kg for 18 months) was demonstrated to be as effective as long-term CYC treatment.[47] MTX (25 mg weekly) has also been demonstrated to be effective as remission maintenance therapy for AAV, and a recent randomized trial showed its equal efficiency in comparison with AZA.[48,49]

Mycophenolate mofetil is another safe alternative for remission maintenance therapy. However, in a recent randomized controlled trial it was found to be inferior to AZA. Consequently it is mainly used as a second-line option for patients who have contraindications to AZA or MTX or who have failed the first-line remission maintenance options.[50,51]

The intermittent administration of RTX without corticosteroids may represent another option for remission maintenance treatment of AAV. RTX will be investigated as such in an upcoming randomized controlled trial. Meanwhile, recent data regarding the long-term use of RTX in patients with refractory AAV is very promising.[42]

MONITORING AND PROPHYLAXIS

To minimize treatment-related morbidity, preemptive monitoring of the appropriate laboratory parameters should be conducted at regular intervals. Pneumocystis pneumonia prophylaxis should be prescribed to all patients on high doses of glucocorticoids, CYC, AZA, MTX, mycophenolate mofetil, or RTX. All patients on long-term glucocorticoid therapy should be offered prophylactic therapy for osteoporosis. Furthermore, patients exposed to CYC should be monitored for the development of bladder cancer, and reproductive issues should be addressed in patients of child-bearing age. All patients treated with MTX should receive folic acid supplementation.

SELECTED OTHER DISEASES ASSOCIATED WITH PULMONARY VASCULITIS AND DAH
Primary Antiphospholipid Syndrome

DAH represents a rare, frequently fatal nonthrombotic pulmonary complication of primary antiphospholipid syndrome (APLS). Pulmonary capillaritis without thrombosis has been demonstrated in lung biopsies from APLS patients presenting with DAH.[52] A proposed mechanism for the pathogenesis includes binding of antiphospholipid antibodies to endothelial cells, promoting the increased expression of endothelial cell adhesion molecules, neutrophil binding, and ultimately injury of alveolar capillaries and alveolar basement membrane.[52]

DAH in APLS is very difficult to treat. Historically, combination therapy of glucocorticoids and other immunosuppressants (CYC, AZA, or mycophenolate mofetil) is combined with the intravenous administration of immunoglobulin G (IVIG) and/or PLEX.[52,53] However, a recent review of 17 consecutive cases of DAH in APLS demonstrated the limited success of aggressive standard immunosuppressive therapy in these patients. None of the patients treated with AZA or mycophenolate mofetil achieved remission, and remission was only seen in a subgroup of patients treated with CYC, IVIG, PLEX, or RTX.[54] A recent case report also demonstrated a potential role for RTX for patients with primary APLS and DAH.[55] In addition to these challenging decisions regarding the appropriate immunosuppressive therapy, the clinical management of these cases is typically complicated by the fact that many of these individuals are on therapeutic anticoagulation to treat previous thrombotic complications. Because the DAH almost universally requires at least the temporary discontinuation of the anticoagulation, these patients are at high risk for recurrent venous and/or arterial thrombosis.

Hematopoietic Stem Cell Transplant

DAH can complicate both allogeneic and autologous hematopoietic stem cell transplantation. It typically occurs early after stem cell transplantation.[56] The incidence of DAH is approximately 2%.[57,58] The mortality is commonly greater than 50% in these patients. Outcomes are worse in allogeneic transplants and in patients presenting with DAH more than 30 days after their transplant.[59] While risk factors for DAH (older age and treatment regimens including intensive pretransplant chemotherapy and total body irradiation) have been identified, the underlying pathogenesis remains poorly understood. Based on data from selected retrospective case series, the current standard therapy frequently includes high-dose corticosteroids, implying that the nature of this disease is immune mediated.[56] A diagnosis of DAH in these typically immunocompromised patients is characteristically established based on clinical, radiologic, and bronchoscopic data (respiratory decompensation in a patient with pulmonary infiltrates and BAL findings suggestive of DAH). Similar findings are also typically present in patients with diffuse alveolar damage with or without associated coagulopathy, both of which are frequently present after bone marrow transplant. Because of the associated risks, lung biopsies are usually not obtained in these patients. It is interesting that in a large autopsy series most of these cases demonstrated a histologic pattern of diffuse alveolar damage, and capillaritis was notably absent in all cases. This information argues against the immune-mediated nature of DAH in the context of bone marrow transplantation, and caution is warranted against the indiscriminate use of glucocorticoid therapy. This caution is especially important in a patient population with a high incidence of invasive fungal infections, in whom further immunosuppressive therapy may result in worse clinical outcomes.

SUMMARY

Pulmonary vasculitis most frequently manifests with DAH and represents its most common immune-mediated cause. The acute management of these patients primarily focuses on respiratory support and the correction of abnormalities in the coagulation cascade. A careful history taking and physical examination in conjunction with a focused laboratory investigation (including serologic testing for autoantibodies) frequently facilitates targeted therapy by identifying the underlying systemic disease. AAV, specifically GPA and MPA, represents the most common cause of pulmonary vasculitis and immune-mediated DAH. Because of their life-threatening nature, these cases are typically categorized as severe disease and treated accordingly. Based on the data from recent randomized controlled trials, RTX represents an equally effective and likely less toxic alternative to CYC for remission induction therapy in these patients. The role of PLEX remains unclear, and appropriate patients should be considered for participation in clinical trials.

Patients with pulmonary vasculitis benefit from a multidisciplinary team approach, and expedited referral to an appropriate center with these resources should be considered for these patients. Further research is needed to continue to optimize the care of these challenging patients.

REFERENCES

1. Travis WD, Colby TV, Lombard C, et al. A clinicopathologic study of 34 cases of diffuse pulmonary hemorrhage with lung biopsy confirmation. Am J Surg Pathol 1990;14(12):1112–25.
2. Falk RJ, Gross WL, Guillevin L, et al. Granulomatosis with polyangiitis (Wegener's): an alternative name for Wegener's granulomatosis. Arthritis Rheum 2011;63(4): 863–4.
3. de Prost N, Parrot A, Picard C, et al. Diffuse alveolar haemorrhage: factors associated with in-hospital and long-term mortality. Eur Respir J 2010;35(6):1303–11.
4. Cordier JF, Cottin V. Alveolar hemorrhage in vasculitis: primary and secondary. Semin Respir Crit Care Med 2011;32(3):310–21.
5. Lara AR, Schwarz MI. Diffuse alveolar hemorrhage. Chest 2010;137(5):1164–71.
6. Castaner E, Alguersuari A, Gallardo X, et al. When to suspect pulmonary vasculitis: radiologic and clinical clues. Radiographics 2010;30(1):33–53.
7. Hansell DM. Small-vessel diseases of the lung: CT-pathologic correlates. Radiology 2002;225(3):639–53.
8. Ewan PW, Jones HA, Rhodes CG, et al. Detection of intrapulmonary hemorrhage with carbon monoxide uptake. Application in Goodpasture's syndrome. N Engl J Med 1976;295(25):1391–6.
9. De Lassence A, Fleury-Feith J, Escudier E, et al. Alveolar hemorrhage. Diagnostic criteria and results in 194 immunocompromised hosts. Am J Respir Crit Care Med 1995;151(1):157–63.
10. Maldonado F, Parambil JG, Yi ES, et al. Haemosiderin-laden macrophages in the bronchoalveolar lavage fluid of patients with diffuse alveolar damage. Eur Respir J 2009;33(6):1361–6.
11. Mark EJ, Matsubara O, Tan-Liu NS, et al. The pulmonary biopsy in the early diagnosis of Wegener's (pathergic) granulomatosis: a study based on 35 open lung biopsies. Hum Pathol 1988;19(9):1065–71.
12. Travis WD, Hoffman GS, Leavitt RY, et al. Surgical pathology of the lung in Wegener's granulomatosis. Review of 87 open lung biopsies from 67 patients. Am J Surg Pathol 1991;15(4):315–33.
13. Watts R, Lane S, Hanslik T, et al. Development and validation of a consensus methodology for the classification of the ANCA-associated vasculitides and polyarteritis nodosa for epidemiological studies. Ann Rheum Dis 2007;66(2): 222–7.
14. Rabe C, Appenrodt B, Hoff C, et al. Severe respiratory failure due to diffuse alveolar hemorrhage: clinical characteristics and outcome of intensive care. J Crit Care 2010;25(2):230–5.
15. Papiris SA, Manali ED, Kalomenidis I, et al. Bench-to-bedside review: pulmonary-renal syndromes—an update for the intensivist. Crit Care 2007;11(3):213.
16. Savage CO, Winearls CG, Evans DJ, et al. Microscopic polyarteritis: presentation, pathology and prognosis. Q J Med 1985;56(220):467–83.

17. Serra A, Cameron JS, Turner DR, et al. Vasculitis affecting the kidney: presentation, histopathology and long-term outcome. Q J Med 1984;53(210):181–207.
18. Guillevin L, Durand-Gasselin B, Cevallos R, et al. Microscopic polyangiitis: clinical and laboratory findings in eighty-five patients. Arthritis Rheum 1999;42(3): 421–30.
19. Guillevin L, Cohen P, Gayraud M, et al. Churg-Strauss syndrome. Clinical study and long-term follow-up of 96 patients. Medicine (Baltimore) 1999;78(1):26–37.
20. Keogh KA, Specks U. Churg-Strauss syndrome: clinical presentation, antineutrophil cytoplasmic antibodies, and leukotriene receptor antagonists. Am J Med 2003;115(4):284–90.
21. Khan SA, Subla MR, Behl D, et al. Outcome of patients with small-vessel vasculitis admitted to a medical ICU. Chest 2007;131(4):972–6.
22. Henke D, Falk RJ, Gabriel DA. Successful treatment of diffuse alveolar hemorrhage with activated factor VII. Ann Intern Med 2004;140(6):493–4.
23. Heslet L, Nielsen JD, Levi M, et al. Successful pulmonary administration of activated recombinant factor VII in diffuse alveolar hemorrhage. Crit Care 2006;10(6): R177.
24. Pastores SM, Papadopoulos E, Voigt L, et al. Diffuse alveolar hemorrhage after allogeneic hematopoietic stem-cell transplantation: treatment with recombinant factor VIIa. Chest 2003;124(6):2400–3.
25. Hicks K, Peng D, Gajewski JL. Treatment of diffuse alveolar hemorrhage after allogeneic bone marrow transplant with recombinant factor VIIa. Bone Marrow Transplant 2002;30(12):975–8.
26. Merkel PA, Lo GH, Holbrook JT, et al. Brief communication: high incidence of venous thrombotic events among patients with Wegener granulomatosis: the Wegener's Clinical Occurrence of Thrombosis (WeCLOT) study. Ann Intern Med 2005;142(8):620–6.
27. Wanko SO, Broadwater G, Folz RJ, et al. Diffuse alveolar hemorrhage: retrospective review of clinical outcome in allogeneic transplant recipients treated with aminocaproic acid. Biol Blood Marrow Transplant 2006;12(9):949–53.
28. Hoffman GS, Kerr GS, Leavitt RY, et al. Wegener granulomatosis: an analysis of 158 patients. Ann Intern Med 1992;116(6):488–98.
29. Talar-Williams C, Hijazi YM, Walther MM, et al. Cyclophosphamide-induced cystitis and bladder cancer in patients with Wegener granulomatosis. Ann Intern Med 1996;124(5):477–84.
30. Clowse ME, Copland SC, Hsieh TC, et al. Ovarian reserve diminished by oral cyclophosphamide therapy for granulomatosis with polyangiitis (Wegener's). Arthritis Care Res 2011;63(12):1777–81.
31. de Groot K, Harper L, Jayne DR, et al. Pulse versus daily oral cyclophosphamide for induction of remission in antineutrophil cytoplasmic antibody-associated vasculitis: a randomized trial. Ann Intern Med 2009;150(10):670–80.
32. Harper L, Morgan MD, Walsh M, et al. Pulse versus daily oral cyclophosphamide for induction of remission in ANCA-associated vasculitis: long-term follow-up. Ann Rheum Dis 2012;71(6):955–60.
33. De Groot K, Rasmussen N, Bacon PA, et al. Randomized trial of cyclophosphamide versus methotrexate for induction of remission in early systemic antineutrophil cytoplasmic antibody-associated vasculitis. Arthritis Rheum 2005;52(8): 2461–9.
34. Klemmer PJ, Chalermskulrat W, Reif MS, et al. Plasmapheresis therapy for diffuse alveolar hemorrhage in patients with small-vessel vasculitis. Am J Kidney Dis 2003;42(6):1149–53.

35. Gallagher H, Kwan JT, Jayne DR. Pulmonary renal syndrome: a 4-year, single-center experience. Am J Kidney Dis 2002;39(1):42–7.

36. Jayne DR, Gaskin G, Rasmussen N, et al. Randomized trial of plasma exchange or high-dosage methylprednisolone as adjunctive therapy for severe renal vasculitis. J Am Soc Nephrol 2007;18(7):2180–8.

37. Szczepiorkowski ZM, Winters JL, Bandarenko N, et al. Guidelines on the use of therapeutic apheresis in clinical practice–evidence-based approach from the Apheresis Applications Committee of the American Society for Apheresis. J Clin Apheresis 2010;25(3):83–177.

38. Plasma exchange and glucocorticoids for treatment of anti-neutrophil cytoplasm antibody (ANCA)-associated vasculitis. Available at: http://clinicaltrials.gov/ct2/results?term=pexivas. Accessed May 26, 2012.

39. Specks U, Fervenza FC, McDonald TJ, et al. Response of Wegener's granulomatosis to anti-CD20 chimeric monoclonal antibody therapy. Arthritis Rheum 2001; 44(12):2836–40.

40. Keogh KA, Wylam ME, Stone JH, et al. Induction of remission by B lymphocyte depletion in eleven patients with refractory antineutrophil cytoplasmic antibody-associated vasculitis. Arthritis Rheum 2005;52(1):262–8.

41. Keogh KA, Ytterberg SR, Fervenza FC, et al. Rituximab for refractory Wegener's granulomatosis: report of a prospective, open-label pilot trial. Am J Respir Crit Care Med 2006;173(2):180–7.

42. Cartin-Ceba R, Golbin JM, Keogh KA, et al. Rituximab for remission induction and maintenance in refractory granulomatosis with polyangiitis (Wegener's): a single-center ten-year experience. Arthritis Rheum 2012. http://dx.doi.org/10.1002/art.34584.

43. Cartin-Ceba R, Fervenza FC, Specks U. Treatment of antineutrophil cytoplasmic antibody-associated vasculitis with rituximab. Curr Opin Rheumatol 2012;24(1):15–23.

44. Stone JH, Merkel PA, Spiera R, et al. Rituximab versus cyclophosphamide for ANCA-associated vasculitis. N Engl J Med 2010;363(3):221–32.

45. Specks U, Stone JH, Group RR. Long-term efficacy and safety results of the rave trial [abstract]. Clin Exp Immunol 2011;164(Suppl 1):65.

46. Jones RB, Tervaert JW, Hauser T, et al. Rituximab versus cyclophosphamide in ANCA-associated renal vasculitis. N Engl J Med 2010;363(3):211–20.

47. Jayne D, Rasmussen N, Andrassy K, et al. A randomized trial of maintenance therapy for vasculitis associated with antineutrophil cytoplasmic autoantibodies. N Engl J Med 2003;349(1):36–44.

48. Pagnoux C, Mahr A, Hamidou MA, et al. Azathioprine or methotrexate maintenance for ANCA-associated vasculitis. N Engl J Med 2008;359(26):2790–803.

49. Langford CA, Talar-Williams C, Barron KS, et al. A staged approach to the treatment of Wegener's granulomatosis: induction of remission with glucocorticoids and daily cyclophosphamide switching to methotrexate for remission maintenance. Arthritis Rheum 1999;42(12):2666–73.

50. Hiemstra TF, Walsh M, Mahr A, et al. Mycophenolate mofetil vs azathioprine for remission maintenance in antineutrophil cytoplasmic antibody-associated vasculitis: a randomized controlled trial. JAMA 2010;304(21):2381–8.

51. Langford CA, Talar-Williams C, Sneller MC. Mycophenolate mofetil for remission maintenance in the treatment of Wegener's granulomatosis. Arthritis Rheum 2004;51(2):278–83.

52. Deane KD, West SG. Antiphospholipid antibodies as a cause of pulmonary capillaritis and diffuse alveolar hemorrhage: a case series and literature review. Semin Arthritis Rheum 2005;35(3):154–65.

53. Waterer GW, Latham B, Waring JA, et al. Pulmonary capillaritis associated with the antiphospholipid antibody syndrome and rapid response to plasmapheresis. Respirology 1999;4(4):405–8.

54. Cartin-Ceba R, Peikert T, Ashrani A, et al. Diffuse alveolar hemorrhage caused by primary antiphospholipid syndrome [abstract]. Vienna (Austria): European Respiratory Society Annual Congress; 2012.

55. Scheiman Elazary A, Klahr PP, Hershko AY, et al. Rituximab induces resolution of recurrent diffuse alveolar hemorrhage in a patient with primary antiphospholipid antibody syndrome. Lupus 2012;21(4):438–40.

56. Afessa B, Tefferi A, Litzow MR, et al. Diffuse alveolar hemorrhage in hematopoietic stem cell transplant recipients. Am J Respir Crit Care Med 2002;166(5): 641–5.

57. Majhail NS, Parks K, Defor TE, et al. Diffuse alveolar hemorrhage and infection-associated alveolar hemorrhage following hematopoietic stem cell transplantation: related and high-risk clinical syndromes. Biol Blood Marrow Transplant 2006;12(10):1038–46.

58. Afessa B, Abdulai RM, Kremers WK, et al. Risk factors and outcome of pulmonary complications after autologous hematopoietic stem cell transplant. Chest 2012; 141(2):442–50.

59. Afessa B, Tefferi A, Litzow MR, et al. Outcome of diffuse alveolar hemorrhage in hematopoietic stem cell transplant recipients. Am J Respir Crit Care Med 2002; 166(10):1364–8.

Bronchiolitis

Brian T. Garibaldi, MD[a], Peter Illei, MD[b],
Sonye K. Danoff, MD, PhD[c],*

KEYWORDS

- Bronchiolitis • Constrictive bronchiolitis • Bronchiolitis obliterans
- Small airways obstruction

KEY POINTS

- Bronchiolitis is a disease of the small airways accompanied by progressive and often irreversible airflow obstruction.
- Bronchiolitis can be caused by several different processes including infectious, toxic exposure, collagen vascular disease, post lung and stem cell transplant, and idiopathic.
- Symptoms of chronic cough and sputum production are often mistaken for chronic obstructive pulmonary disease or asthma, leading to a delay in diagnosis.
- Mosaic perfusion and expiratory air trapping on high-resolution computed tomography are the hallmarks of bronchiolitis.
- Treatment of bronchiolitis depends in part on etiology, but is often ineffective.

INTRODUCTION

Bronchiolitis refers to inflammation occurring in the smaller conducting airways of the lung, typically in segments that are less than 2 mm in diameter.[1] Bronchiolitis was first reported in the literature by Wilhelm Lange in 1901 when he used the term "bronchiolitis obliterans" in an autopsy report of 2 patients who likely had what would now be described as cryptogenic organizing pneumonia (COP) (an entity formerly known as bronchiolitis obliterans organizing pneumonia [BOOP]).[2,3] Soon thereafter Fraenkel described the pathology of bronchiolitis obliterans caused by inhalation of nitrogen oxide.[3,4] Bronchiolitis is often a confusing entity because it may develop in isolation

Funding sources: Dr Garibaldi: None. Dr Illei: None. Dr Danoff: American College of Rheumatology Within Our Reach, Lisa Sandler Spaeth and Robert M. Fisher Funds for Pulmonary Fibrosis.
Conflicts of interest: None.
[a] Division of Pulmonary and Critical Care Medicine, Johns Hopkins University School of Medicine, 5501 Hopkins Bayview Circle, Baltimore, MD 21224, USA; [b] Department of Pathology, Johns Hopkins University School of Medicine, 600 North Wolfe Street, Baltimore, MD 21287, USA; [c] Division of Pulmonary and Critical Care Medicine, Johns Hopkins Interstitial Lung Disease Clinic, Johns Hopkins University School of Medicine, 1830 East Monument Street, Baltimore, MD 21205, USA
* Corresponding author.
E-mail address: sdanoff@jhmi.edu

Immunol Allergy Clin N Am 32 (2012) 601–619
http://dx.doi.org/10.1016/j.iac.2012.08.002
immunology.theclinics.com

or as a secondary feature of a diffuse lung disease. The number of potential causes of bronchiolitis, ranging from infectious etiology to environmental insults to autoimmune disease, further complicates the clinician's approach to bronchiolitis.

Anatomy of Bronchioles

Bronchioles, in contrast to larger bronchi, do not have cartilage, glands, or goblet cells. Bronchioles are arranged in parallel, which maximizes cross-sectional area while minimizing their contribution to overall airflow resistance in the healthy lung.[5] However, because of their relatively thin walls, bronchioles become narrowed at low lung volumes and their resistance increases as the lung approaches residual volume.[6] In the context of inflammation or obstruction, their contribution to overall airflow resistance can become substantial and can lead to significant respiratory impairment.

Causes of Bronchiolitis

Bronchiolitis can be classified based on histopathologic or radiologic criteria, but it is perhaps most useful to think about bronchiolitis in terms of the likely clinical etiology (**Box 1**). In children younger than 2 years, bronchiolitis is the most frequently diagnosed respiratory disorder,[7] with the vast majority of cases attributable to viral infection, particular respiratory syncytial virus (RSV), enteroviruses, and rhinoviruses.[8] While less common in adults, infectious bronchiolitis can be the result of viral infections (adenovirus, influenza and parainfluenza, and so forth) as well as *Legionella pneumophila* and *Mycoplasma pneumonia*.[9,10] Mycobacterial infections can also cause subacute and chronic bronchiolitis.[11] Common noninfectious causes of adult bronchiolitis include inhalational injury (including tobacco smoke), drug-induced, collagen vascular disease, post lung transplant, post bone marrow transplant, and idiopathic.[12] The term bronchiolitis obliterans (BO) is often used to describe these seemingly unrelated conditions in which the common finding is functional obstruction of bronchioles.[13]

CLINICAL PRESENTATION

The clinical presentation of bronchiolitis depends in part on the etiology. In children, infectious bronchiolitis is typically acute in onset and is associated with fever, cough, rhinorrhea, expiratory wheezing and, occasionally, frank respiratory distress.[14] In older children and adults, isolated infectious bronchiolitis in the absence of bronchopneumonia is extremely rare, but may occur with *Mycoplasma pneumonia*. Such patients present with acute onset cough, dyspnea, fever, and even pleuritic chest pain.[15]

Box 1
Potential causes of bronchiolitis

Infectious

Postinfectious

Inhalational injury

Diffuse panbronchiolitis

Toxic ingestion

Collagen vascular disease associated

Post lung transplant

Post stem cell transplant

Idiopathic

In most cases of infectious bronchiolitis, the disease is self-limited and rarely lasts longer than 7 to 10 days.[14]

In the case of inhalational exposures, patients may present with acute symptoms related to airway injury or chemical pneumonitis, or they may have a delayed onset of cough and breathlessness weeks after the initial insult.[16] In most other forms of adult bronchiolitis, patients present with a more subacute and slowly progressive course. Patients may complain of several weeks to months of worsening dyspnea and cough, often accompanied by signs and symptoms of air trapping and irreversible airflow obstruction. Patients may also have intermittent episodes of acute bronchiolitis accompanied by symptom worsening.[1] These symptoms are often attributed to underlying chronic obstructive pulmonary disease (COPD) or asthma, leading to a substantial delay in diagnosis.[17]

The presence of an underlying disease known to be associated with small airways disease (ie, post bone marrow transplant, post lung transplant, collagen vascular disease, and so forth) should prompt a search for bronchiolitis in patients with unexplained breathlessness, cough, or airflow obstruction. Patients with bronchiolitis may be asymptomatic in the early stages of disease, so screening with pulmonary function testing, imaging, and even bronchoscopy can identify high-risk patients before overt pulmonary symptoms develop.[18]

PHYSICAL EXAMINATION

The physical examination in patients with bronchiolitis is often nonspecific, but may suggest the presence of small airways disease including diffuse expiratory wheezing.[19] Mid-inspiratory squeaks are present in 40% to 60% of patients.[20] Patients with advanced BO may have inspiratory crackles on auscultation.[19] In patients with systemic disorders such as a collagen vascular disease, there may be findings associated with the systemic disorder on physical examination.

RADIOGRAPHIC FINDINGS

Radiographic findings in patients with bronchiolitis are often nonspecific but may provide clues to the presence of an underlying bronchiolar disorder. Bronchioles are not visible on standard chest radiographs, but obstruction of small airways may result in air trapping or hyperinflation. Sequential radiographs may show worsening hyperinflation in the absence of parenchymal disease.[19] High-resolution computed tomography (HRCT) has revolutionized the contribution of imaging to the diagnostic workup of suspected bronchiolitis. Even though normal bronchioles are too small to be effectively imaged by HRCT, both direct and indirect signs of diseased bronchioles can be seen (**Table 1**).[21]

Direct Signs of Bronchiolitis

Thickening of bronchiolar walls by an inflammatory infiltrate or filling of the lumen or surrounding interstitium with an exudate will make the bronchial wall directly visible

Table 1 Radiographic signs of bronchiolitis	
Direct Signs of Bronchiolitis	**Indirect Signs of Bronchiolitis**
Centrilobular thickening and peripheral nodules	Mosaic attenuation
Tree-in-bud opacities	Air trapping (accentuated on expiratory CT)
Bronchiolectasis	

on computed tomography (CT). Centrilobular thickening is the earliest sign of inflammation and may be seen as small peripheral nodules. Worsening bronchiolar inflammation associated with early mucoid impaction will create a "tree-in-bud" appearance visible as centrilobular branching structures that terminate in a nodule (**Fig. 1A**). The presence of tree-in-bud-opacities most often indicates an infectious bronchiolitis.[22] Progressive inflammation and obstruction may lead to bronchiolar dilation (bronchiolectiasis) identified as a cystic or tubular structure in the secondary pulmonary lobule (**Fig. 1B**).[11]

Indirect Signs of Bronchiolitis

Indirect signs of bronchiolitis may be seen on standard HRCT performed at end-inspiration. Luminal obstruction of bronchioles will result in a segment of underventilated, and subsequently underperfused lung from compensatory hypoxic-pulmonary vasoconstriction. This process results in a patchy "mosaic attenuation pattern" whereby areas of bronchiolitis appear darker secondary to decreased perfusion (**Fig. 2**). The mosaic pattern is enhanced by obtaining images at end-expiration. Areas with luminal obstruction will not empty on expiration and will appear darker in comparison with unobstructed areas (**Fig. 3**).[21,23,24] This "air trapping" is essentially the radiographic correlate to airflow obstruction seen on pulmonary function testing in patients with bronchiolitis. Findings of unilateral hypoattenuation and air trapping are suggestive of the Swyer-James and Macleod syndrome, which is likely the consequence of a postinfectious bronchiolitis.[25,26] However, the isolated finding of air trapping on expiratory CT must be interpreted in the clinical context because healthy subjects, particularly smokers, can have expiratory air trapping on HRCT in the absence of overt clinical disease.[27]

PULMONARY FUNCTION TESTING

Bronchiolitis is a disease of the small airways. As a result, the classic finding on pulmonary function testing is airflow obstruction on spirometry with or without evidence of air trapping or hyperinflation on lung volumes.[12,28] In general, this airflow obstruction is less responsive to bronchodilators than are asthma or COPD, although the degree of reversibility varies depending on the underlying etiology. Diffusing capacity may be normal or reduced depending on the specific etiology and the presence or absence of associated bronchopneumonia or interstitial disease.[19]

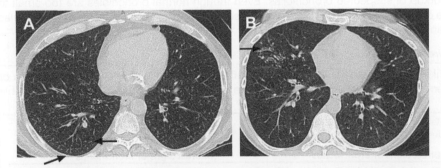

Fig. 1. (A) Computed tomography (CT) showing multiple small centrilobular nodules as well as tree-in-bud opacities (*arrows*) in an immunocompromised patient with disseminated aspergillosis. (B) CT showing bronchiolectasis (*arrow*) and bronchiectasis in a patient with common variable immune deficiency.

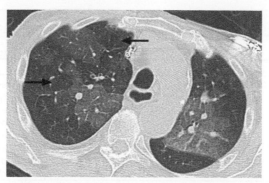

Fig. 2. CT showing mosaic perfusion in a patient with bronchiolitis associated with collagen vascular disease (*arrows*).

PATHOLOGIC FINDINGS

The pathologic findings in bronchiolitis depend in part on the underlying cause of the disorder. Several histopathologic classification systems have been developed, which has led to some degree of confusion regarding terminology. This section reviews the most commonly described types of bronchiolitis (**Table 2**).

Cellular Bronchiolitis

Cellular bronchiolitis refers to the presence of any inflammatory cells in the bronchiolar wall or lumen. It is commonly observed in infectious bronchiolitis as well as in association with asthma, chronic bronchitis, bronchiectasis, and hypersensitivity pneumonitis. There are 4 types of cellular bronchiolitis that deserve particular attention: follicular bronchiolitis, diffuse panbronchiolitis (DPB), lymphocytic bronchiolitis, and respiratory bronchiolitis.[23]

Follicular bronchiolitis refers to the presence of lymphoid hyperplasia with secondary germinal centers along the bronchioles (**Fig. 4**).[22] Centrilobular and peribronchial nodules are the radiographic correlate of this lymphoid hyperplasia.[29] Follicular bronchiolitis may result from immunodeficiency, hypersensitivity reactions, and collagen vascular disease (especially rheumatoid arthritis and Sjögren syndrome), and as a distal reaction in the setting of bronchiectasis of any cause.[23]

DPB is a type of bronchiolitis most commonly seen in East Asian men. It is characterized histopathologically by chronic inflammation and the accumulation of foamy macrophages in the walls of respiratory bronchioles.[30]

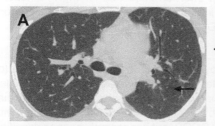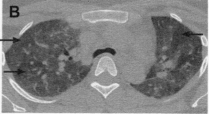

Fig. 3. (*A*) Inspiratory CT showing subtle areas of mosaic perfusion (*arrow*) in a patient with bronchiolitis. (*B*) Expiratory CT in same patient showing multiple areas of hypoattenuation consistent with air trapping (*arrows*). The bowing forward of the cartilaginous component of the trachea confirms that this is an expiratory CT. (*Courtesy of* David Feigin, MD, Department of Radiology, Johns Hopkins University School of Medicine.)

Table 2
Pathologic classification of bronchiolitis

Classification	Pathologic Features	Clinical Associations
Cellular bronchiolitis		
Follicular bronchiolitis	Lymphoid hyperplasia with secondary germinal centers	Collagen vascular disease (especially rheumatoid arthritis and Sjögren), immunodeficiency, hypersensitivity, lymphoproliferative disease, diffuse panbronchiolitis
Diffuse panbronchiolitis	Chronic inflammation with foamy macrophages in bronchiole walls	Clinical syndrome in East Asia, often associated with chronic sinusitis
Lymphocytic bronchiolitis	Lymphocyte infiltration in bronchiole walls	Rejection post lung transplant, infection, in association with lymphocytic interstitial pneumonia
Respiratory bronchiolitis	Pigmented macrophages in bronchiole lumen	Tobacco smoking in isolation or with associated interstitial lung disease
Proliferative bronchiolitis	Intraluminal buds of fibrotic tissue	Commonly occurs with organizing pneumonia (ie, cryptogenic organizing pneumonia)
Constrictive bronchiolitis	Concentric narrowing or obliteration of bronchiole lumen by submucosal and peribronchiolar fibrosis	Idiopathic, postinfectious, collagen vascular disease, inhalational or toxic exposure, post lung transplant, post stem cell transplant

Lymphocytic bronchiolitis is characterized by the presence of lymphocyte infiltration in the walls of the respiratory bronchioles. It can be seen in several infectious and inflammatory states, but is most commonly associated with acute allograft rejection in lung transplantation (**Fig. 5**).[31]

Respiratory bronchiolitis is characterized by the presence of pigmented macrophages in the bronchiolar lumen. It is most often an incidental finding in smokers, but may be associated with a mild form of interstitial lung disease called respiratory bronchiolitis–interstitial lung disease (RB-ILD) (**Fig. 6**).[32]

Proliferative Bronchiolitis

Proliferative bronchiolitis is characterized by intraluminal buds of fibrotic tissue (or Masson bodies) in the respiratory bronchioles (**Fig. 7**). Proliferative bronchiolitis may occur in isolation, but is most often associated with an organizing pneumonia that extends into the alveolar ducts and alveoli.[13,33,34] This bronchiolitis obliterans with organizing pneumonia was historically called BOOP, but has recently been reclassified as cryptogenic organizing pneumonia (COP). This change in nomenclature underscores the fact that the features of organizing pneumonia, and not airflow obstruction, dominate the clinical picture.[23] A more detailed description of COP is provided elsewhere in this issue.

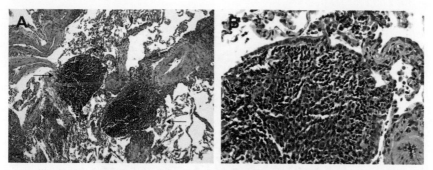

Fig. 4. Follicular bronchiolitis in a patient with bronchiectasis secondary to chronic *Mycobacterium avium-intracellulare* infection. (*A*) Low-power view demonstrates the presence of lymphoid hyperplasia with secondary germinal centers (*arrows*) (hematoxylin and eosin, original magnification ×100). (*B*) Higher-power view of germinal center showing dense lymphoid aggregates (hematoxylin and eosin, original magnification ×400).

Constrictive Bronchiolitis

Constrictive bronchiolitis is characterized by narrowing and eventual obliteration of respiratory bronchioles by peribronchiolal and submucosal fibrosis (**Fig. 8**).[23] The term BO used to describe the clinical syndrome of irreversible airflow obstruction most often refers to constrictive bronchiolitis. Constrictive bronchiolitis can be the consequence of several different insults including inhalational injury, infection, collagen vascular disease, and post lung transplant and stem cell transplant.[14] Several of these causes are discussed in more detail in the following section.

BRONCHIOLITIS TREATMENT

Bronchiolitis is a challenging airway disorder to treat. The airflow obstruction in bronchiolitis is usually not responsive to bronchodilator therapy.[19] Corticosteroids and other immunomodulating therapies have been used in several bronchiolar diseases, often with little or no response, although they may be effective in certain subtypes

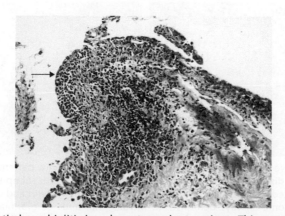

Fig. 5. Lymphocytic bronchiolitis in a lung transplant patient. This transbronchial biopsy shows a bronchiole with dense lymphocytic transmural infiltrate (*arrow*). The infiltrate is seen in all layers of the respiratory mucosa and in surrounding soft tissue, and includes scattered plasma cells and mononuclear cells (hematoxylin and eosin, magnification ×200).

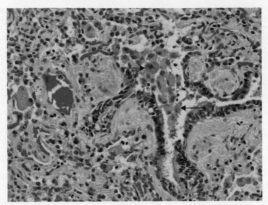

Fig. 6. Respiratory bronchiolitis in an active tobacco smoker. This high-magnification (×400) view of a bronchiole shows a cluster of dusky pigmented macrophages in the lumen (*arrows*) and thickening of the basement membrane. The surrounding alveoli are also filled with similar dusky pigmented macrophages. No significant interstitial fibrosis or remodeling is present (Hematoxylin and eosin).

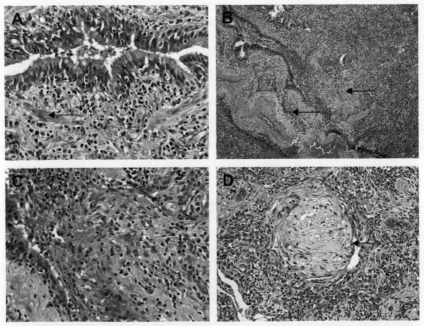

Fig. 7. Proliferative bronchiolitis with organizing pneumonia in a patient with suspected collagen vascular disease. (*A*) The bronchioles show variable chronic subepithelial inflammation with associated proliferation of fibroblasts (*arrow*) (Hematoxylin and eosin, magnification ×400). (*B*) Some airways demonstrate intraluminal buds of granulation tissue with associated inflammation (*arrows*) (Hematoxylin and eosin, magnification ×100). (*C*) Higher-power view of airway intraluminal buds (Hematoxylin and eosin, magnification ×400). (*D*) The surrounding parenchyma shows organization with numerous intra-alveolar fibroblast plugs filling the lumina (*arrow*) (Hematoxylin and eosin, magnification ×400).

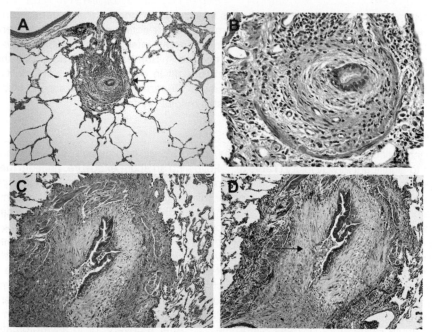

Fig. 8. Constrictive bronchiolitis. (*A*) Lung biopsy in a previously healthy 56-year-old woman showing scattered small airways with concentric subepithelial fibrosis and marked narrowing of the lumen (*arrow*) (Hematoxylin and eosin, magnification ×100). (*B*) Higher-power view demonstrating marked bronchiolar narrowing and fibrosis (Hematoxylin and eosin, magnification ×400). (*C*) Lung biopsy from a stem cell transplant patient showing marked subepithelial fibrosis (Hematoxylin and eosin, magnification ×400). (*D*) Movat stain from the same biopsy highlighting the subepithelial fibrosis (*arrow*).

of bronchiolitis. Specific therapies are discussed next, in the context of the bronchiolitis subtypes.

SPECIFIC CAUSES OF BRONCHIOLITIS

There are several conditions associated with the development of bronchiolitis. Although the pathologic presence of isolated bronchiolitis is by itself nonspecific, the finding of bronchiolitis should prompt an evaluation for an associated or known cause.[1] Some of the more commonly encountered causes of bronchiolitis are reviewed here.

Postinfectious

As already described, acute infection is an extremely common cause of bronchiolitis in children and can also occur in adults. Although this acute bronchiolitis is usually self-limited, a small number of both pediatric and adult patients will develop a progressive BO.[35,36] Postinfectious bronchiolitis in children is frequently caused by adenovirus infection.[37] Histopathology may reveal an initial proliferative bronchiolitis followed by a later constrictive pattern, depending on the timing of the biopsy.[12,38] Patients ultimately recover, although long-term sequelae such as the Swyer-James and Macleod syndrome may develop, characterized by regional airflow obstruction, often in a unilateral distribution.[12,25,26,35]

Treatment of postinfectious bronchiolitis includes both inhaled and systemic corticosteroids in an attempt to reduce inflammation, short-acting and long-acting bronchodilators for wheezing, antibiotics for recurrent infection from poor airway clearance, and supplemental oxygen as needed.[37] Some clinicians advocate the use of azithromycin based on its apparent benefit in other forms of bronchiolitis, although its efficacy in this context is unknown.[39] In rare cases, lung transplantation may be indicated in the setting of progressive respiratory failure.[12]

Inhalational Injury

The inhalation of a variety of different gases, fumes, dusts, or organic substances may lead to significant airway injury (**Table 3**).[23] Following an acute exposure, patients may experience severe symptoms including laryngospasm, bronchiolar spasm, reflex respiratory arrest, or asphyxia. Death may occur following a massive exposure. If patients inhale the substance deeply enough into the lungs, acute pulmonary edema can develop from a chemical pneumonitis. Following the initial exposure, patients will uncommonly develop 1 of 2 syndromes: (1) prolonged reactive airways disease, termed the reactive airway dysfunction syndrome (RADS); or (2) constrictive bronchiolitis.[12,33,40]

The most commonly recognized cause of bronchiolitis after inhalational exposure is nitrogen dioxide. Nitrogen dioxide can reach the periphery of the lung, where it forms both nitric and nitrous acids as well as nitrous oxide. If inhaled in high enough concentrations, patients may develop acute or delayed (3–30 hours later) pulmonary edema and Acute Respiratory Distress Syndrome.[12,41] After recovery, or in asymptomatic patients, symptoms of cough and progressive dyspnea may develop 2 to 6 weeks after the initial exposure, accompanied by progressive and usually irreversible airflow obstruction.[42,43] The airflow obstruction correlates with a progressive constrictive bronchiolitis seen on histopathology.[13,23]

The first death from acute inhalation of nitrogen dioxide was reported by Desgranges in 1804 when he described the case of a man who died of respiratory failure after a bottle of nitric acid broke and reacted with a woodpile.[41,44] Fraenkel was the first to report histopathologic BO in association with nitrogen gas exposure.[4] Today, inhalational injury from nitrogen dioxide is commonly referred to as silo filler's disease because nitrogen dioxide and dinitrogen tetroxide are found in the air on the surface of silage in agricultural silos.[12,43]

Table 3	
Exposures that may result in bronchiolitis	
Toxic Inhalation/Ingestion	**Potential Source**
Nitrogen dioxide	Grain silos
Sulfur	Chemical warfare (ie, mustard gas)
Diacetyl	Artificial butter flavoring in microwave popcorn
Chlorine	Household or industrial bleach; chemical warfare
Phosgene	Pesticides and plastics manufacturing; chemical warfare
Flock	Synthetic fabric manufacturing
Mineral dust	Asbestos, aluminum, silica, iron oxide, coal
Gastric contents	Acute large-volume aspiration; chronic aspiration
Penicillamine	Treatment of collagen vascular disease
Gold	Treatment of rheumatoid arthritis
Sauropus androgynus	Raw vegetable used in Asia for weight loss

Several other gases and volatile compounds have been reported in association with the development of BO. Perhaps the best known is the development of BO in several employees at a microwave popcorn factory, thought to be secondary to exposure to diacetyl, a ketone used as an artificial butter flavoring.[17,45] Constrictive bronchiolitis has recently been described in soldiers returning from Iraq and Afghanistan. In some of these cases, exposure to a sulfur-mine fire may have been the direct cause.[46] Survivors of the World Trade Center bombing on September 11, 2001, as well as other terrorist attacks, have been reported to have features of BO following massive dust particle exposure.[47]

A history of known exposure to a potentially toxic irritant should be sought in all patients with a suspected or confirmed diagnosis of bronchiolitis. Patients who present following an acute inhalational exposure should be observed for at least 48 hours in the hospital and then followed expectantly for the development of BO in the weeks to months following the index event.[12] If acute respiratory symptoms develop, clinical experience with nitrogen dioxide injury suggests that corticosteroids may improve symptoms and prevent disease progression.[16,42,48] Relapse of BO after removal of steroids has been described, prompting some clinicians to advocate at least a 2-month course of treatment.[12] Removal of the inciting toxic agent is critical and in some cases may result in complete recovery. For example, BO secondary to nylon fibers in synthetic fabrics (ie, flock worker's lung) may improve substantially after the exposure is removed.[49] BO from diacetyl inhalation does not appear to resolve after removal of the exposure, but lung function will generally not worsen.[17]

Drug-Induced

Whereas COP has been reported as a potential adverse reaction to several different medications, isolated BO associated with pharmacologic treatments is rare. Isolated BO has been reported after gold therapy and penicillamine treatment in patients with rheumatoid arthritis (RA). It is difficult to determine if the therapy or the disease process was the cause because BO has been described in RA patients in the absence of these therapies.[50,51] BO has also been reported after rituximab therapy in a patient with B-cell lymphoma.[52] Over-the-counter and herbal therapies have been associated with the development of BO. For example, ingestion of uncooked *Sauropus androgynus*, a vegetable with supposed weight-loss properties, led to an outbreak of BO in young women in both Taiwan and Japan.[53,54] Even though drug-induced BO is rare, a thorough exposure history, including over-the-counter and herbal remedies, should be obtained from any patient presenting with unexplained bronchiolitis. Corticosteroids may play some role in the treatment of drug-induced BO in the setting of collagen vascular disease, but were of limited benefit in BO caused by *S androgynus*.[53]

Diffuse Panbronchiolitis

DPB is a distinct form of bronchiolitis that is found almost exclusively in East Asia. It was first recognized in Japan in the 1960s[55] and has since been seen in both Korea and China. Rare cases have been reported outside of Asia.[56] This may in part be explained by a close association of DPB with HLA Bw54, which is predominantly found in Asian populations.[57] The incidence of DPB was as high as 11.1 per 100,000 in Japan in 1980, but may have decreased in recent years.[58] Mean age at presentation is 50 years, with a 2:1 male/female predominance. Most patients have a history of long-standing chronic sinusitis before they develop pulmonary manifestations. Symptoms include chronic cough and copious purulent sputum production, in some cases up to 50 mL per day.[58,59] Pulmonary function testing reveals marked obstruction that is not responsive to bronchodilators. Chest radiographs may reveal bilateral nodular infiltrates, particularly in a lower lobe distribution. HRCT will characteristically show centrilobular nodules and may also show a tree-in-bud pattern. Bronchiectasis is often present in advanced disease.[11,58] Patients with DPB often have marked elevation in serum cold agglutinins with negative *Mycoplasma pneumonia* antibody titers, suggesting that this is in response to chronic inflammation and not acute *Mycoplasma* infection.[12] The most distinctive feature on biopsy is chronic inflammation accompanied by the presence of foam cells in the walls of respiratory bronchioles.[1,30] If untreated, 50% of patients with DPB die within 5 years of diagnosis, in part because of secondary bacterial infections associated with bronchiectasis and poor airway clearance.

In the 1980s, physicians in Japan realized that patients with DPB who were treated with erythromycin appeared to do better over the long term. Subsequent studies revealed that survival in patients on low-dose erythromycin increased from 63% to 91%.[60] Since then, these observations have been extended to include other macrolides such as clarithromycin and azithromycin.[61] The effectiveness of macrolide therapy is not thought to be secondary to its antibacterial properties, because patients with *Pseudomonas* infection also improve with therapy. Several mechanisms have been postulated to play a role including decreased neutrophil recruitment, reduction in mucus production, decreased lymphocyte accumulation, and modulation of bacterial virulence.[58,61] These observations have led to the use of macrolides in other forms of bronchiolitis.

Collagen Vascular Disease–Associated Bronchiolitis

Bronchiolitis has been described in association with several connective tissue diseases. In fact, in nontransplant-related cases of BO, connective tissue disease has been estimated to account for 25% to 50% of reported cases.[20,62] The incidence of isolated bronchiolitis appears to be highest in patients with RA and Sjögren syndrome, although cases have been reported in patients with systemic lupus erythematosus, scleroderma, and even inflammatory bowel disease (**Table 4**).[20,63,64]

Rheumatoid arthritis

Perhaps the best-known association between collagen vascular disease and bronchiolar disorders occurs in patients with RA. Although several pulmonary complications can be seen in patients with RA, it has been estimated that up to 68% of asymptomatic patients with RA have evidence of bronchiolar disease on HRCT imaging.[20,65] Pulmonary function testing in RA patients with normal HRCT scans suggests that an additional 30% of asymptomatic patients have some degree of airflow obstruction.[66] In patients who develop severe, symptomatic airflow obstruction (defined as forced expiratory volume in 1 second/forced vital capacity less than 50% or residual volume/total lung capacity greater than 140% predicted), the predominant histologic

Table 4
Collagen vascular diseases commonly associated with bronchiolar involvement

Collagen Vascular Disease	Bronchiolar Complications
Rheumatoid arthritis	Follicular bronchiolitis, constrictive bronchiolitis, bronchiectasis, cryptogenic organizing pneumonia (COP)
Sjögren syndrome	Lymphocytic bronchiolitis, constrictive bronchiolitis (usually in secondary Sjögren syndrome), rare COP
Systemic lupus erythematosus	COP, rare constrictive bronchiolitis
Inflammatory bowel disease	Lymphocytic bronchiolitis

pattern is usually constrictive bronchiolitis, although some patients may also have features of follicular bronchiolitis.[67] Patients with constrictive bronchiolitis will have characteristic mosaic perfusion and expiratory air trapping on HRCT. Follicular bronchiolitis may produce centrilobular and peribronchial nodules.[68] Up to 40% of patients will also have evidence of coexisting bronchiectasis on HRCT. Patients with significant airflow obstruction will complain of dyspnea on exertion and almost half will have bronchorrhea. Almost all patients with symptomatic bronchiolar disease have a preexisting diagnosis of RA at the time of symptom onset.[67] Prognosis in these patients is poor, with progression to respiratory failure within 3 to 4 years of diagnosis.[33,67] RA patients with secondary Sjögren syndrome may be at increased risk for developing BO.[20,69] As mentioned previously, treatment of RA with both gold and penicillamine has been associated with a higher risk of developing BO, although the role of these drugs in such development is controversial.[50,51]

Several agents have been used to treat BO in RA patients, with limited success. Corticosteroids with the addition of either azathioprine or cyclophosphamide have been reported to cause a transient improvement but have not resulted in long-term remission.[20,70] Erythromycin has been used to treat both follicular bronchiolitis and BO in patients with RA. In one small case series, 11 of 15 patients symptomatically improved and none died over a 2-year follow-up period.[71]

Sjögren syndrome

Sjögren syndrome may occur as an isolated disease or as a secondary phenomenon in patients with another connective tissue disease, most commonly RA and SLE. The prevalence of symptomatic airflow obstruction in association with bronchiolitis is not well described. Air trapping is present on pulmonary function testing in as many as half of patients with primary Sjögren syndrome.[20,72] HRCT may reveal bronchial wall thickening, bronchiectasis, bronchiolectasis, tree-in-bud opacities, and air trapping. Sjögren patients can develop lymphocytic bronchiolitis with or without coexisting lymphocytic interstitial pneumonia (LIP). In both cases, lymphocytic infiltration into the walls of the small bronchioles leads to obstruction, which can present as small nodules and even cystic structures on HRCT.[68] Constrictive bronchiolitis has been described in patients with RA and secondary Sjögren syndrome, but is not commonly seen as an isolated lesion in primary Sjögren syndrome.[28]

The optimal treatment of bronchiolitis in patients with Sjögren syndrome is unknown. In cases of lymphocytic bronchiolitis associated with LIP, corticosteroids are generally used, as about half of patients with "idiopathic" LIP will improve on corticosteroids.[73] Similarly, if follicular bronchiolitis is seen in conjunction with either LIP or nonspecific interstitial pneumonia (NSIP), treatment is directed at the associated interstitial lung disease. Corticosteroids appear to be beneficial in follicular bronchiolitis, and progression to respiratory failure is rare.[74]

Post Lung Transplant

Post lung transplant bronchiolitis obliterans syndrome (BOS) is the most common cause of BO and continues to be one of the most important factors limiting survival in lung transplant recipients. BOS is the clinical manifestation of chronic allograft rejection and is defined by progressive airflow obstruction in the absence of acute rejection, infection, or other known cause.[75] In patients who survive to 5 years after transplant, more than 50% will develop BOS.[76] The onset of BOS confers a 5-year mortality of 50% to 70%.[18,77] Patients who present earlier after transplant or with severe disease have increased mortality.[78] On histopathology BOS usually manifests as a constrictive bronchiolitis, but may have features of a proliferative bronchiolitis.[19] Several mechanisms are thought to play a role in the development of BOS including T-cell activation, circulating antibodies, innate immune responses to environmental insults (ie, infection), and even autoimmunity directed against type 5 collagen.[79] BOS is closely associated with episodes of acute rejection (AR) and is seen at a higher frequency in patients who have had multiple episodes of AR.[80] Lymphocytic bronchiolitis, either in isolation or as part of AR, appears to be of particular importance in causing epithelial injury and downstream fibroproliferation, and has been shown to be highly associated with the development of BOS.[31,75] Few therapies improve outcomes in patients once BOS has developed, and despite advances in the early detection and treatment of acute rejection, the prevalence of BOS has not appreciably changed in recent years.[79]

Changing the primary immunosuppressive regimen (ie, converting cyclosporine to tacrolimus or azathioprine to mycophenolate mofetil) has been shown in small studies to stabilize the course of BOS.[81,82] Extracorporeal photopheresis (ECP) and total lymphoid irradiation (TLI) have been shown to slow the decline in lung function in patients with BOS, although the side effects of TLI may be poorly tolerated.[83–86] Several small studies have shown that low-dose azithromycin 3 times per week may slow or even reverse the decline in lung function from BOS.[85] Azithromycin may prevent the development of chronic rejection and BOS in some patients,[87] although recent data regarding the risk of sudden cardiac death after treatment of bacterial infections with azithromycin may temper its routine use in all transplant patients.[88]

Post Bone Marrow Transplant

Patients who undergo allogeneic stem cell transplantation (SCT) are at risk of developing a BOS that is similar in clinical presentation and pathology to post lung transplantation BOS. It is likely that both syndromes represent an alloimmune response: host versus graft in the case of lung transplant, and graft versus host in the case of SCT.[89] BOS was first reported as a complication of graft-versus-host disease (GVHD) in 1982.[90] It has since been recognized as the most common and significant pulmonary manifestation of GVHD, and is included in the National Institutes of Health consensus criteria for diagnosing chronic GVHD.[91] The prevalence of BOS after SCT has been reported to be as high as 5.5% in all SCT patients and up to 14% in patients with chronic GVHD.[92] It usually occurs within the first 2 years post transplant but has been reported up to 5 years after SCT. Patients usually lack respiratory symptoms during the initial phases of BOS but may manifest other signs of chronic GVHD such as liver, skin, and eye involvement.[93] As BOS progresses patients experience dyspnea on exertion and a persistent nonproductive cough, similar to other forms of BO.[94]

Despite effective therapies for other tissue complications of chronic GVHD, long-term outcomes for patients with SCT-related BOS are dismal; survival is 20% at 2 years and only 13% at 5 years.[93,95–97] Patients who present more than 1 year after SCT may have a slightly improved survival. Most centers monitor SCT patients with routine pulmonary function testing to detect the presence of asymptomatic small airways disease in the hope that identification of patients at risk for BOS will allow for earlier treatment that might halt airway obliteration.[93,98] Once BOS is recognized, several therapies have been used based on the lung transplant experience. No therapy has been rigorously studied in the SCT population.[89,93]

Corticosteroids remain the mainstay of treatment with or without the addition of calcineurin inhibitors, rapamycin, and mycophenolate mofetil. Azithromycin has been used with mixed results in small case series.[89,99] ECP and TLI have also been used, with limited success.[89] Recently, pulmonary rehabilitation has been shown to improve 6-minute walk distance, dyspnea, and exercise tolerance in SCT patients with BOS, and may be an important adjunctive therapy.[100]

SUMMARY

Bronchiolitis can result from several infectious, inflammatory, and environmental insults. It is often a confusing clinical entity because of overlapping terminology and the existence of several histopathologic, radiographic, and clinical classification systems. Patients may present with chronic cough and dyspnea and are often thought to have asthma or COPD, leading to a delay in diagnosis. Chest radiography may be unremarkable but high-resolution CT often reveals mosaic perfusion and expiratory air trapping. Treatment and long-term prognosis are determined in part by the underlying etiology, although many types of bronchiolitis are poorly responsive to therapy. Post lung transplant and stem cell transplant bronchiolitis are the most frequently encountered, and provide important insights into the immune pathogenesis and treatment of this diverse group of disorders.

REFERENCES

1. Visscher DW, Myers JL. Bronchiolitis. Proc Am Thorac Soc 2006;3:41–7.
2. Lange W. Ueber eine eigenthümliche Erkrankung der kleinen Bronchien und Bronchiolen. Dtsch Arch Klin Med 1901;70:342–64.
3. Poletti V, Costabel U. Bronchiolar disorders: classification and diagnostic approach. Semin Respir Crit Care Med 2003;24(5):457–64.
4. Fraenkel A. Ueber Bronchiolitis fibrosa obliterans, nebst Bemerkungen über Lungenhyperaemie und indurierende Pneumonie. Dtsch Arch Klin Med 1902; 73:484–510.
5. Albertine KH. Anatomy of the lungs. In: Mason RD, Broaddus VC, Martin TR, et al, editors. Murray and Nadel's textbook of respiratory medicine. 5th edition. Philadelphia: Elsevier; 2010. p. 3–25.
6. Hughes JM, Rosenzweig DY, Kivitz PB. Site of airway closure in excised dog lungs: histologic demonstration. J Appl Phys 1970;29:340–4.
7. Flaherman V, Ragins A, Li S, et al. Frequency, duration and predictors of bronchiolitis episodes of care among infants [greater than or equal to] 32 weeks gestation in a large integrated healthcare system: a retrospective cohort study. BMC Health Serv Res 2012;12:144.
8. Huguenin A, Moutte L, Renois F, et al. Broad respiratory virus detection in infants hospitalized for bronchiolitis by use of a multiplex RT-PCR DNA microarray system. J Med Virol 2012;84:979–85.
9. Cha SI, Shin KM, Kim M, et al. Mycoplasma pneumoniae bronchiolitis in adults: clinicoradiologic features and clinical course. Scand J Infect Dis 2009;41:515–9.
10. Andersen P. Pathogenesis of lower respiratory tract infections due to Chlamydia, Mycoplasma, Legionella and viruses. Thorax 1998;53:302–7.
11. Lynch DA. Imaging of small airways disease and chronic obstructive pulmonary disease. Clin Chest Med 2008;29(1):165–79.
12. King TE. Miscellaneous causes of bronchiolitis: inhalational, infectious, drug-induced, and idiopathic. Semin Respir Crit Care Med 2003;24(5):567–76.
13. Epler GR, Colby TV. The spectrum of bronchiolitis obliterans. Chest 1983;83(2): 161–2.
14. American Academy of Pediatrics Subcommittee on Diagnosis and Management of Bronchiolitis. Diagnosis and management of bronchiolitis. Pediatrics 2006; 118:1774–93.
15. Chan ED, Kalayanamit T, Lynch DA, et al. Mycoplasma pneumoniae-associated bronchiolitis causing severe restrictive lung disease in adults: report of three cases and literature review. Chest 1999;115:1188–94.

16. Milne JE. Nitrogen dioxide inhalation and bronchiolitis obliterans. A review of the literature and report of a case. J Occup Med 1969;11(10):538–47.
17. van Rooy FG, Rooyackers JM, Prokop M, et al. Bronchiolitis obliterans syndrome in chemical workers producing diacetyl for food flavorings. Am J Respir Crit Care Med 2007;176:498–504.
18. Belperrio JA, Lake K, Tazelaar H, et al. Bronchiolitis obliterans syndrome complicating lung or heart-lung transplantation. Semin Respir Crit Care Med 2003; 24(5):499–530.
19. Angel L, Homma A, Levine SM. Bronchiolitis obliterans. Semin Respir Crit Care Med 2000;21(2):123–34.
20. White E, Tazelaar HD, Lynch JP. Bronchiolar complications of connective tissue diseases. Semin Respir Crit Care Med 2003;24(5):543–66.
21. Hansell DM. HRCT of obliterative bronchiolitis and other small airways diseases. Semin Roentgenol 2001;36:51–65.
22. Devakonda A, Raoof S, Sung A, et al. bronchiolar disorders: a clinical-radiological diagnostic algorithm. Chest 2010;137:938–51.
23. Kang E, Woo OH, Shin BK, et al. Bronchiolitis: classification, computed tomographic and histopathologic features, and radiologic approach. J Comput Assist Tomogr 2009;33(1):32–41.
24. Jensen SP, Lynch DA, Brown KK, et al. High-resolution CT features of severe asthma and bronchiolitis obliterans. Clin Radiol 2002;57:1078–85.
25. Swyer P, James G. Case of unilateral pulmonary emphysema. Thorax 1953;8:133–6.
26. Macleod WM. Abnormal translucency of one lung. Thorax 1954;9:147–53.
27. Lee KW, Chung SY, Yang I, et al. Correlation of aging and smoking with air trapping at thin-section CT of the lung in asymptomatic subjects1. Radiology 2000; 214:831–6.
28. Turton CW, Williams G, Green M. Cryptogenic obliterative bronchiolitis in adults. Thorax 1981;36(11):805–10.
29. Howling SJ, Hansell DM, Wells AU, et al. Follicular bronchiolitis: thin-section CT and histologic findings. Radiology 1999;212:637–42.
30. Iwata M, Colby TV, Kitaichi M. Diffuse panbronchiolitis: diagnosis and distinction from various pulmonary diseases with centrilobular interstitial foam cell accumulations. Hum Pathol 1994;25:357–63.
31. Girgis RE, Berry GJ, Reichenspurner H, et al. Risk factors for the development of obliterative bronchiolitis after lung transplantation. J Heart Lung Transplant 1996;15:1200–8.
32. Wright JL, Tazelaar HD, Churg A. Fibrosis with emphysema. Histopathology 2011;58:517–24.
33. Epler GR. Bronchiolar disorders with airflow obstruction. Curr Opin Pulm Med 1996;2(2):134–40.
34. Epler GR, Colby TV, McLoud TC, et al. Bronchiolitis obliterans organizing pneumonia. N Engl J Med 1985;312:152–8.
35. Kurland G, Michelson P. Bronchiolitis obliterans in children. Pediatr Pulmonol 2005;39:193–208.
36. Wright JL. Diseases of the small airways. Lung 2002;176(6):375–96.
37. Fischer GB, Sarria EE, Mattiello R, et al. Post infectious bronchiolitis obliterans in children. Paediatr Respir Rev 2010;11:233–9.
38. Mauad T, Dolhnikoff M. Histology of childhood bronchiolitis obliterans. Pediatr Pulmonol 2002;33:466–74.
39. De Baets F. Bronchiolitis obliterans in children: a ghostly journey to the origin. Allergol Immunopathol 2011;39:251–2.

40. Brooks SM, Weiss MA, Bernstein IL. Reactive airways dysfunction syndrome (RADS). Persistent asthma syndrome after high level irritant exposures. Chest 1985;88:376–84.
41. Smith DL. Criteria for a recommended standard: occupational exposures to oxides of nitrogen (nitrogen dioxide and nitric oxide). Washington, DC: National Institute for Occupational Safety and Health; 1976. p. 76–149.
42. Fleming GM, Chester EH, Montenegro HD. Dysfunction of small airways following pulmonary injury due to nitrogen dioxide. Chest 1979;75(6):720–1.
43. Gurney JW, Unger JM, Dorby CA, et al. Agricultural disorders of the lung. Radiographics 1991;11:625–34.
44. Desgranges JB. Observation and comments on a sudden death caused by nitrous gas. J Med Chir Pharm 1804;8:487–505.
45. Kreiss K, Gomaa A, Kullman G, et al. Clinical bronchiolitis obliterans in workers at a microwave-popcorn plant. N Engl J Med 2002;347:330–8.
46. King MS, Eisenberg R, Newman JH, et al. Constrictive bronchiolitis in soldiers returning from Iraq and Afghanistan. N Engl J Med 2011;365:222–30.
47. Ghanei M, Harandi AA, Tazelaar HD. Isolated bronchiolitis obliterans: high incidence and diagnosis following terrorist attacks. Inhal Toxicol 2012;24:340–1.
48. Horvath EP, doPico GA, Barbee RA, et al. Nitrogen dioxide-induced pulmonary disease: five new cases and a review of the literature. J Occup Med 1978;20(2):103–10.
49. Kern DG, Kuhn C III, Ely EW, et al. Flock worker's lung—broadening the spectrum of clinicopathology, narrowing the spectrum of suspected etiologies. Chest 2000;117:251–9.
50. Tomioka R, King TE. Gold-induced pulmonary disease: clinical features, outcome, and differentiation from rheumatoid lung disease. Am J Respir Crit Care Med 1997;155:1011–20.
51. Turner-Warnick M. Adverse reactions affecting the lung: possible association with D-penicillamine. J Rheumatol Suppl 1981;7:166–8.
52. Shen T, Braude S. Obliterative bronchiolitis after rituximab administration: a new manifestation of rituximab-associated pulmonary toxicity. Intern Med J 2012;42:597–9.
53. Lai RS, Chiang AA, Wu MT, et al. Outbreak of bronchiolitis obliterans associated with consumption of Sauropus androgynus in Taiwan. Lancet 1996;348:83–5.
54. Oonakahara K, Matsuyama W, Higashimoto J, et al. Outbreak of bronchiolitis obliterans associated with consumption of Sauropus androgynus in Japan—alert of food-associated pulmonary disorders from Japan. Respiration 2005;72:221.
55. Homma H, Yamanaka A, Tanimoto S, et al. Diffuse panbronchiolitis. A disease of the transitional zone of the lung. Chest 1983;83:63–9.
56. Fitzgerald JE, King TE, Lynch DA, et al. Diffuse panbronchiolitis in the United States. Am J Respir Crit Care Med 1996;154:497–503.
57. Sugiyama Y, Kudoh S, Maeda H, et al. Analysis of HLA antigens in patients with diffuse panbronchiolitis. Am J Respir Crit Care Med 1990;141:1459–62.
58. Kudoh S, Keicho N. Diffuse panbronchiolitis. Clin Chest Med 2012;33:297–305.
59. Homma H. Diffuse panbronchiolitis. Jpn J Med 1986;25:329–34.
60. Kudoh S, Azuma A, Yamamoto M, et al. Improvement of survival in patients with diffuse panbronchiolitis treated with low-dose erythromycin. Am J Respir Crit Care Med 1998;157:1829–32.
61. Li H, Zhou Y, Fan F, et al. Effect of azithromycin on patients with diffuse panbronchiolitis: retrospective study of 51 cases. Intern Med 2011;50:1663–9.

62. Katzenstein AL, Myers JL, Prophet WD, et al. Bronchiolitis obliterans and usual interstitial pneumonia. A comparative clinicopathologic study. Am J Surg Pathol 1986;10(6):373–81.

63. Yousem SA. The pulmonary manifestations of the CREST syndrome. Hum Pathol 1990;21(5):467–74.

64. Camus P, Piard F, Ashcroft T, et al. The lung in inflammatory bowel disease. Baltimore (MD): Medicine; 1993. 151–183.

65. Demir R, Bodur H, Tokoglu F, et al. High resolution computed tomography of the lungs in patients with rheumatoid arthritis. Rheumatol Int 1999;19:19–22.

66. Mori S, Koga Y, Sugimoto M. Small airway obstruction in patients with rheumatoid arthritis. Mod Rheumatol 2011;21:164–73.

67. Devouassoux G, Cottin V, Lioté H, et al. Characterisation of severe obliterative bronchiolitis in rheumatoid arthritis. Eur Respir J 2009;33:1053–61.

68. Lynch DA. Lung disease related to collagen vascular disease. J Thorac Imaging 2009;24:299–309.

69. Bégin R, Massé S, Cantin A, et al. Airway disease in a subset of nonsmoking rheumatoid patients: characterization of the disease and evidence for an auto-immune pathogenesis. Am J Med 1982;72:743–50.

70. Wells AU, du Bois RM. Bronchiolitis in association with connective tissue disorders. Clin Chest Med 1993;14:655–66.

71. Hayakawa H, Sato A, Imokawa S, et al. Bronchiolar disease in rheumatoid arthritis. Am J Respir Crit Care Med 1996;154:1531–6.

72. Lahdensuo A, Korpela M. Pulmonary findings in patients with primary Sjögren's syndrome. Chest 1995;108:316–9.

73. Cha SI, Fessler MB, Cool CD, et al. Lymphoid interstitial pneumonia: clinical features, associations and prognosis. Eur Respir J 2006;28:364–9.

74. Aerni MR, Vassallo R, Myers JL, et al. Follicular bronchiolitis in surgical lung biopsies: clinical implications in 12 patients. Respir Med 2008;102:307–12.

75. Estenne M, Maurer JR, Boehler A, et al. Bronchiolitis obliterans syndrome 2001: an update of the diagnostic criteria. J Heart Lung Transplant 2002;21:297–310.

76. Christie JD, Edwards LB, Kucheryavaya AY, et al. The registry of the international society for heart and lung transplantation: twenty-seventh official adult lung and heart-lung transplant report—2010. J Heart Lung Transplant 2010; 29:1104–18.

77. Valentine VG, Robbins RC, Berry GJ, et al. Actuarial survival of heart-lung and bilateral sequential lung transplant recipients with obliterative bronchiolitis. J Heart Lung Transplant 1996;15:371–83.

78. Finlen Copeland CA, Snyder LD, Zaas DW, et al. Survival after bronchiolitis obliterans syndrome among bilateral lung transplant recipients. Am J Respir Crit Care Med 2010;182:784–9.

79. Todd JL, Palmer SM. Bronchiolitis obliterans syndrome in lung transplantation: the final frontier for lung transplantation. Chest 2011;140:502–8.

80. Husain AN, Siddiqui MT, Holmes EW, et al. Analysis of risk factors for the development of bronchiolitis obliterans syndrome. Am J Respir Crit Care Med 1999; 159:829–33.

81. Whyte RI, Rossi SJ, Mulligan MS, et al. Mycophenolate mofetil for obliterative bronchiolitis syndrome after lung transplantation. Ann Thorac Surg 1997;64: 945–8.

82. Cairn J, Yek T, Banner NR, et al. Time-related changes in pulmonary function after conversion to tacrolimus in bronchiolitis obliterans syndrome. J Heart Lung Transplant 2003;22:50–7.

83. Morrell MR, Despotis GJ, Lublin DM, et al. The efficacy of photopheresis for bronchiolitis obliterans syndrome after lung transplantation. J Heart Lung Transplant 2010;29:424–31.
84. Benden C, Speich R, Hofbauer GF, et al. Extracorporeal photopheresis after lung transplantation: a 10-year single-center experience. Transplantation 2008;86:1625–7.
85. Hayes D. A review of bronchiolitis obliterans syndrome and therapeutic strategies. J Cardiovasc Surg 2011;6:92.
86. Verleden GM, Lievens Y, Dupont LJ, et al. Efficacy of total lymphoid irradiation in azithromycin nonresponsive chronic allograft rejection after lung transplantation. Transplant Proc 2009;41:1816–20.
87. Vos R, Vanaudenaerde BM, Ottevaere A, et al. Long-term azithromycin therapy for bronchiolitis obliterans syndrome: divide and conquer? J Heart Lung Transplant 2010;29:1358–68.
88. Ray WA, Murray KT, Hall K, et al. Azithromycin and the risk of cardiovascular death. N Engl J Med 2012;366:1881–90.
89. Sengsayadeth SM, Srivastava S, Jagasia M, et al. Time to explore preventive and novel therapies for bronchiolitis obliterans syndrome after allogeneic hematopoietic stem cell transplantation. Biol Blood Marrow Transplant 2012. [Epub ahead of print].
90. Roca J, Granena A, Rodriguez-Roisin R, et al. Fatal airway disease in an adult with chronic graft-versus-host disease. Thorax 1982;37:77–8.
91. Filipovich AH, Weisdorf D, Pavletic S, et al. National Institutes of Health consensus development project on criteria for clinical trials in chronic graft-versus-host disease: I. Diagnosis and staging working group report. Biol Blood Marrow Transplant 2005;11:945–56.
92. Au BK, Au MA, Chien JW. Bronchiolitis obliterans syndrome epidemiology after allogeneic hematopoietic cell transplantation. Biol Blood Marrow Transplant 2011;17:1072–8.
93. Williams KM, Chien JW, Gladwin MT, et al. Bronchiolitis obliterans after allogeneic hematopoietic stem cell transplantation. JAMA 2009;302:306–14.
94. Clark JG, Crawford SW, Madtes DK, et al. Obstructive lung disease after allogenic marrow transplantation. Ann Intern Med 1989;111:368.
95. Chien JW, Martin PJ, Gooley TA, et al. Airflow obstruction after myeloablative allogeneic hematopoietic stem cell transplantation. Am J Respir Crit Care Med 2003;168:208–14.
96. Chan CK, Hyland RH, Hutcheon MA, et al. Small-airways disease in recipients of allogeneic bone marrow transplants. An analysis of 11 cases and a review of the literature. Medicine (Baltimore) 1987;66:327–40.
97. Dudek AZ, Mahaseth H, DeFor TE, et al. Bronchiolitis obliterans in chronic graft-versus-host disease: analysis of risk factors and treatment outcomes. Biol Blood Marrow Transplant 2003;9:657–66.
98. Forslöw U, Mattsson J, Gustafsson T, et al. Donor lymphocyte infusion may reduce the incidence of bronchiolitis obliterans after allogeneic stem cell transplantation. Biol Blood Marrow Transplant 2011;17:1214–21.
99. Lam DC, Lam B, Wong MK, et al. Effects of azithromycin in bronchiolitis obliterans syndrome after hematopoietic SCT—a randomized double-blinded placebo-controlled study. Bone Marrow Transplant 2011;46:1551–6.
100. Tran J, Norder EE, Diaz PT, et al. Pulmonary rehabilitation for bronchiolitis obliterans syndrome after hematopoietic stem cell transplantation. Biol Blood Marrow Transplant 2012;18(8):1250–4.

Granulomatous Lymphocytic Interstitial Lung Disease

Evans R. Fernández Pérez, MD, MS

KEYWORDS

- Common variable immunodeficiency • Interstitial lung diseases • Granuloma
- Sarcoidosis • Lymphoproliferative disorders

KEY POINTS

- GLILD is a distinctive manifestation of CVID and is characterized by a combination of granulomatous and lymphoproliferative interstitial features.
- Confident diagnosis of GLILD can be challenging and requires a multidisciplinary approach.
- Other causes of granulomatous and lymphoproliferative lung disorders must be definitively excluded before a GLILD diagnosis is rendered.
- On imaging, in contrast to sarcoidosis, GLILD findings commonly demonstrate a mid and lower lung zone predominance.
- In GLILD, pulmonary nodules are common and tend to wax and wane.
- Immunosuppressive treatment is generally reserved for patients with GLILD with persistent respiratory symptoms or evidence of radiographic or physiologic progressive lung disease.

INTRODUCTION

Common variable immunodeficiency (CVID) is a heterogeneous syndrome characterized immunologically by hypogammaglobulinemia and impaired antibody response. It is the most common of the primary immune deficiencies, and clinically characterized by a host of systemic manifestations, including recurrent sinopulmonary infections, autoimmune disorders, and lymphoproliferation. The pulmonary manifestations of CVID may be infectious or noninfectious (**Box 1**). The infectious complications are more common and must be excluded before a noninfectious, CVID-associated, pulmonary diagnosis is rendered. Examples of infectious complications include

Conflict of interests: None.
Autoimmune Lung Center and Interstitial Lung Disease Program, Division of Pulmonary and Critical Care Medicine, National Jewish Health, B'nai B'rith Building, Office #M322, 1400 Jackson Street, Denver, CO 80206, USA
E-mail address: fernandezevans@njhealth.org

Immunol Allergy Clin N Am 32 (2012) 621–632
http://dx.doi.org/10.1016/j.iac.2012.08.003
0889-8561/12/$ – see front matter © 2012 Elsevier Inc. All rights reserved.

Box 1
Pulmonary complications in CVID

Infectious disorders

- Primary infections

  - Bacterial, fungal, and viral pneumonias

  - Granulomatous lung disease (eg, nontuberculous mycobacteria)

- Recurrent or postinfectious

  - Bronchitis

  - Bronchiectasis

  - Bronchiolitis

  - Cavitary and bullous lung disease

Noninfectious disorders

- ILD

  - GLILD

  - Idiopathic concurrent disorders (eg, UIP)

- Neoplastic disorders

  - Primary malignancy (eg, primary pulmonary lymphoma)

  - Secondary malignancies (eg, secondary lymphomatous spread from neighboring sites, such as mediastinal lymph nodes)

- Primary airway-centered disorders[a] (eg, follicular bronchiolitis)

- Isolated benign local (eg, NLH) or diffuse lymphoproliferative disorders (eg, LIP)

Mixed infectious and noninfectious disorders

Abbreviations: CVID, common combined immunodeficiency disorder; ILD, interstitial lung disease; LIP, lymphocytic interstitial pneumonia; NLH, nodular lymphoid hyperplasia; UIP, usual interstitial pneumonia.
[a] Might be associated with hyperreactive airway disease.

---

bronchiectasis, cavities, and postinfection scarring. Noninfectious manifestations can be subdivided into primary (eg, pulmonary MALToma) or secondary malignancies (eg, pulmonary involvement from neighboring sites, such as mediastinal lymphoma); airway-limited entities (eg, follicular bronchiolitis); parenchymal or interstitial lung disease (ILD); and benign lymphoproliferative disorders (eg, nodular lymphoid hyperplasia [NLH]). Although patients with CVID have anecdotally been reported to develop ILD in a variety of pathologic patterns,[1–4] granulomatous-lymphocytic ILD (GLILD) is unique to CVID. The classic histopathologic pattern of GLILD is a cellular interstitial pneumonia with a combination of granulomatous and lymphoproliferative (a combination of lymphocytic interstitial pneumonia [LIP], follicular bronchiolitis, and lymphoid hyperplasia) features.[3] However, in some patients only lymphoproliferative changes are found, whereas in others granulomatous inflammation dominates. Thus, arriving at a confident diagnosis of GLILD can be challenging and requires a multidisciplinary approach with thoughtful integration of clinical, radiologic, and physiologic data. This article focuses on the diagnosis and management of GLILD.

PREVALENCE

The prevalence of ILD in one retrospective analysis of 69 patients with CVID was 26% (18 of 69), and more than two-thirds of these had GLILD.[3] However, larger-scale epidemiologic data for GLILD are unknown.[2]

DIAGNOSTIC EVALUATION
Clinical Evaluation

In patients with known CVID, the development of respiratory symptoms or signs should prompt a focused respiratory evaluation. The clinician embarks on a diagnostic evaluation that includes taking an in-depth medical history with the focus on the severity and course of respiratory symptoms, with special attention to identifying historical features that suggest recurrent respiratory tract infections, the most common presenting feature of patients with CVID. GLILD generally presents insidiously with cough and exertional dyspnea.

Comprehensive occupational and environmental histories, a full systems review, and a thorough physical examination are necessary for an accurate diagnosis. In a patient with recognized CVID without infection, significant environmental exposures or an established diagnosis of connective tissue disease, finding splenomegaly, oligoarticular or polyarticular arthritis, lymphadenopathy, and a nodular pattern on high-resolution chest computed tomography (CT) point strongly toward a diagnosis of GLILD. In contrast, "B" symptoms in a patient with CVID, especially when lung nodules or masses are also identified, raise suspicion for lymphoma.

Because the granulomatous/lymphocytic inflammatory process that leads to GLILD in the lung can affect other organs, screening for evidence of other organ dysfunction is important. Anemia, malabsortion, enteropathies (eg, intestinal NLH), liver disease (eg, secondary to granulomatous infiltration, autoimmune hepatitis, and nodular regenerative hyperplasia), and kidney involvement should all be considered.[5,6]

In some cases, GLILD is the initial manifestation of CVID. In cases in which CVID is yet to be recognized, there is often delay in making an accurate diagnosis of GLILD.[7] For example, a patient with nonnecrotizing granulomas in the liver or spleen and bilateral hilar adenopathy with interstitial changes on chest imaging may erroneously be diagnosed with sarcoidosis if CVID goes unappreciated. Thus, an exhaustive search for lymphoproliferative disorders, granulomatous infections (eg, mycobacterial and fungal), and other causes of granulomatous lung diseases, such as drug reactions, occupational exposures (ie, berylliosis), sarcoidosis, hypersensitivity pneumonitis, or vasculitis, must be undertaken before GLILD is diagnosed. The fact that patients with CVID are at risk for developing autoimmune phenomenon and infections further complicates matters: in these patients GLILD may occur before or after diagnosis of another systemic inflammatory disorder (eg, Sjögren syndrome) or granulomatous infection (eg, nontuberculous mycobacterial infection).

In patients with CVID, microbiologic testing should be pursued based on clinical suspicion. Components of the evaluation may include sputum, urine, sinus, stool, synovial fluid (eg, ureaplasma), or blood cultures. When chest imaging reveals parenchymal lung abnormalities, bronchoalveolar lavage (BAL) should be performed to exclude active pulmonary infection. Consultation with an infectious disease specialist is frequently beneficial in addressing potential infectious etiologies.

Pulmonary function testing is useful for quantifying pulmonary impairment and for monitoring response to therapy in GLILD. A mixed obstructive-restrictive defect, or more commonly an isolated restrictive ventilatory defect, with a low diffusing capacity for carbon monoxide is observed in patients with GLILD. However, some patients (even some with extensive radiologic abnormalities) have normal pulmonary function testing.[3] Maximal cardiopulmonary exercise testing can be a valuable tool in the early detection of subtle pulmonary gas exchange abnormalities and in predicting the degree of impairment in functional capacity in subjects with GLILD; however, its limited availability detracts from its usefulness.[8]

Invasive Testing and Histopathology

Besides ruling out infection, bronchoscopy with BAL can be a useful tool in the evaluation of ILD in patients with CVID. Differential cell counts from BAL effluent may hint at the presence of a lymphocytic alveolitis (eg, >25%), consistent with histopathologic lymphoid interstitial pneumonia, one of the key components in the GLILD lesion. Although BAL lymphocytosis can be an important piece in the diagnostic puzzle, it alone does not confirm GLILD. A lymphocyte-predominant BAL may be found in several ILDs, including hypersensitivity pneumonitis, drug-induced lung disease, and sarcoidosis. Flow cytometry and gene rearrangement studies on the effluent may identify the presence of a monoclonal population of lymphocytes, thus confirming lymphoma, which is always a concern in this patient population.[9,10]

Transbronchial biopsies (TBBx) are potentially useful in the diagnostic evaluation of peribronchovascular processes, such as lymphoma, and in airspace-filling diseases. However, small specimen size and sampling error are significant limitations to TBBx, and in general, a highly confident histopathologic diagnosis of GILID cannot be made from TBBx specimens. Video-assisted thoracoscopic surgery remains the surgical procedure of choice when a diagnosis cannot be obtained by less invasive methods and when the clinical, physiologic, radiographic, and laboratory features are not specific enough to provide diagnostic confirmation. However, histologic data need to be integrated with clinical and radiographic information to come to a final diagnosis.

Pathologic Patterns

The key histopathologic findings of GLILD (**Fig. 1**) are nonnecrotizing granulomas and a spectrum of lymphoproliferation, including LIP, follicular bronchiolitis, NLH, and low-grade B-cell lymphoma of mucosa-associated lymphoid tissue (MALT) or so-called MALToma (extranodal marginal zone B-cell lymphoma). Potentially confusing matters, any of these histopathologic components can be the sole finding, a feature that may be caused by sampling. For example, CVID patients can develop follicular bronchiolitis or LIP without granulomas. I prefer to reserve the term GLILD for those cases in which both granulomas and lymphoproliferative processes occur.

Granulomas

Microscopically, granulomas in GLILD are sarcoid-like, nonnecrotizing, and fairly well circumscribed in a perilymphatic distribution. The granulomas are generally described as morphologically dissimilar to those observed in infection, vasculitides, and hypersensitivity pneumonitis; however, whether this distinction actually can be made in practice has not been tested.

Because CVID predisposes to bacterial infections, special stains for acid-fast bacilli and fungi should be assessed in all cases. Randomly dispersed necrotizing granulomas may be seen (and hint at concomitant infection), but they are not the predominant feature. Localized or systemic nonnecrotizing granulomatous disease has been described in 8% to 20% of patients with CVID.[11–13] Of this subgroup, the lung is one of the most common involved sites, with granulomas reported to occur in 54% of affected patients.[12] I have found granulomatous inflammation in the livers, kidneys, gastrointestinal tract, and spleens of patients with GLILD.

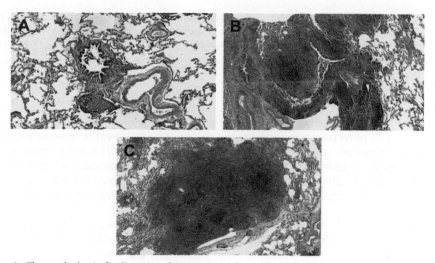

Fig. 1. The pathologic findings in a biopsy-proved patient with granulomatous lymphocytic interstitial lung disease. (A) Peribronchiolar, nonnecrotizing granuloma (hematoxylin and eosin, original magnification × 100). (B) Lymphoid hyperplasia with regions of nodular and conglomerate interstitial, peribronchiolar, and perivascular lymphocytic inflammation (hematoxylin and eosin, original magnification × 200). (C) Lymphoid hyperplasia with germinal centers (hematoxylin and eosin, original magnification × 200).

Lymphoproliferative features

The histologic appearance of LIP in GLILD is no different from LIP of other causes. LIP is characterized by cellular infiltrates composed of a mixture of lymphocytes, plasma cells, and histiocytes that diffusely expand the alveolar septae.[14,15] The interstitial lymphoid cells are mainly T cells, whereas polyclonal B cells are found in the lymphoid follicles. In LIP, germinal centers are common and sometimes prominent; however, in the setting of CVID they might be few and small.

Follicular bronchiolitis or follicular hyperplasia of bronchus-associated lymphoid tissue is present when the lymphoid infiltrate is limited to the bronchioles and adjacent peribronchiolar interstitium. The infiltrate can be so extensive as to cause bronchiolar obliteration.[16] In contrast to LIP, cellular and lymphoid extension into the distal parenchyma, or widespread alveolar septal infiltration, is not present in follicular bronchiolitis.[15]

NLH, sometimes referred as inflammatory pseudotumor, is histologically similar to LIP. However, NLH is a discrete mass lesion usually solitary, whereas LIP is a diffuse interstitial process.[14]

Because atypical lymphoid hyperplasia and malignant lymphoproliferative disorders enter the differential diagnosis of LIP, the histopathologic diagnosis of LIP cannot be made solely on morphologic grounds. Therefore, immunohistochemistry for monoclonality or molecular studies is advisable to support the diagnosis. Close clinical, physiologic, and radiographic follow-up with expert thoracic pathologic input is desirable when features of clonality are observed on surgical lung biopsy, because clonal lymphocyte populations can occur in patients with CVID without lymphoma (eg, infection-related atypical lymphoid hyperplasia) or may precede the development of lymphoma.[17] MALT is generally absent from the normal human lung.[18] However, it can be acquired during bronchial inflammatory processes and diseases involving chronic B-cell dysfunction. Acquired MALT tissue in patients with CVID can take the form of a benign lymphoid disorder or MALTomas.[18] MALTomas are the most frequent primary non-Hodgkin's lymphoma in the lungs and are far more prevalent than NLH. In contrast to LIP, the lymphoid infiltrate in MALTomas is monomorphic and denser, is often found in a lymphangitic distribution, may be associated with destruction of lung architecture, and extend into the parietal pleura and lymph nodes.[14] Unlike non-CVID immunodeficiencies, B-cell–derived lymphoma is rarely an Epstein-Barr virus–driven disease.[17]

Radiologic Evaluation

Chest CT findings in GLILD are dynamic. It is unclear if the chest CT pattern in GLILD correlates with other parameters of disease activity (eg, BAL or extrapulmonary manifestations). However, when integrated with clinical data chest CT plays an invaluable role in guiding the selection of invasive testing; helping discriminate the presence of lung fibrosis from other nonfibrotic patterns; in detecting and following specific complications (eg, superimposed cavitary lung lesion); and in assessing the response to therapy in GLILD.

Common chest CT findings in GLILD include multifocal airspace consolidation; smooth thickening of the interlobular septa and widespread centrilobular micronodules (both with lower zone predominance); mediastinal and hilar lymphadenopathy; bronchiectasis; patchy bilateral ground-glass opacities; and sometimes air trapping emanating from inflammatory small airways involvement, mucous plugging, or abnormal airway collapse (**Fig. 2**).[4,19,20] In more advanced cases, features of fibrosis characterized by fine and coarse reticulation and honeycombing have been observed.[19] Thin-walled cysts in a bronchovascular distribution, as seen often in LIP,[21] are not a frequent or dominant pattern in GLILD but can be helpful in distinguishing LIP from follicular bronchiolitis or diffuse lymphoma.[22] Conglomerate masses surrounding major airways and irregular or beaded bronchovascular bundles common in sarcoidosis are not a characteristic chest CT feature of GLILD.

A common and challenging problem is the waxing and waning of lung opacities in GLILD. Their differential diagnosis includes organizing pneumonia, eosinophilic lung disorders, infectious and noninfectious granulomatous disorders, and lymphoproliferative lesions. The frequently migratory nature of the nodules on serial CT often effectively excludes granuloma, infection, and lymphoma, and suggests organizing pneumonia. Evaluation of the specific morphologic characteristics (size, margins, contour, internal features), growth rate, and surrounding lung parenchyma of solitary or multifocal pulmonary nodules with CT can help differentiate benign from malignant nodules. How these nodules should be followed is unclear but requires striking a balance between diligence (so that malignant transformation to lymphoma is not missed) and exposing the patient to excessive radiation (with repeated CT scans) and multiple lung biopsies.

RISK FACTORS FOR THE DEVELOPMENT OF GLILD

The pathogenesis of GLILD is poorly understood. Although many questions remain, in the last one and half decades observations have uncovered important links between lymphoproliferation, granulomatous disease, and CVID, discussed next. (1) GLILD often occurs in patients with CVID with low switched memory B cells (CD27$^+$/IgM$^-$/IgD$^-$) and CD45RA$^+$CCR7$^+$CD4$^+$T cells. Such patients commonly have a severe clinical phenotype characterized by granulomatous disease, lymphadenopathy, hypersplenism, lymphoid hyperplasia, and chronic lung disease.[12,23–25] (2) Germinal center presence and dysfunction are prerequisites for the development of GLILD. The inducible costimulator (ICOS) that is found on activated T cells interacts with the ICOS-L receptor on B cells, allowing B cells to undergo class switch recombination

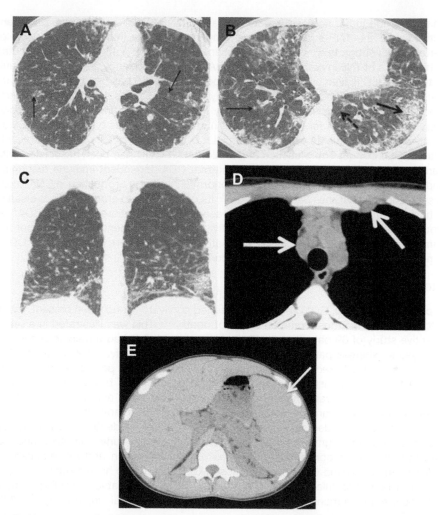

Fig. 2. Noncontrast chest CT in a 29-year-old man with typical findings of granulomatous lymphocytic interstitial lung disease in the setting of combined variable immunodeficiency syndrome. (*A, B*) Axial noncontrast CT images in lung windows show bronchovascular-predominant pulmonary nodules (*thick arrows*) of variable density. Patchy areas of consolidation (*thin arrows*) are present at the lung bases. Mild interlobular septal thickening (*dashed arrows*) is also noted. (*C*) Coronal reformation demonstrates the basilar preponderance of disease. (*D, E*) Axial images in soft tissue windows show paratracheal and left internal mammary lymphadenopathy (*arrows in D*) and splenomegaly (*arrow in E*).

and facilitating the development of follicular T helper cells.[26,27] ICOS deficiency represents a genetic human defect in which there is severe peripheral B-cell lymphopenia and germinal centers do not form. Therefore, in patients with ICOS deficiency[28] and subjects with X-linked agammaglobulinemia (a pure B-cell disorder), GLILD does not occur. Dysfunctional germinal centers provide a distorted cytokine environment for T-cell homeostasis contributing to defective T-cell proliferative responses, abnormal T-cell–dependent antibody responses, antigen sequestration, and granuloma formation.[11,17,27,29,30] (3) Granulomatous disease in CVID has been linked with an uncommon tumor necrosis factor (TNF) allele, TNF +488A.[31] Although, persistent activation of the TNF system has been implicated in the immunopathogenesis of certain CVID subgroups, whether the presence of the TNF +488A allele contributes to high levels of TNF in peripheral blood or BAL and subsequently granulomatous infiltration in GLILD is unknown. (4) Human herpes virus type 8 has been associated with lymphoproliferation and GLILD. In one study, genomic DNA isolated from peripheral blood mononuclear cells, and screened by nested and real-time quantitative polymerase chain reaction for the presence of human herpes virus type 8 genome, was positive in 6 of 9 patients with CVID with GLILD and only 1 of 21 patients with CVID without GLILD.[32] (5) The presence of granulomas in CVID has been associated with peripheral blood CD4$^+$ lymphopenia, abnormal CD4-dependent immune response, and CD8$^+$ lymphocytosis.[33,34] Although abnormal interferon production in CD8$^+$ cells in subjects with CVID has been described,[33] its contribution to granulomatous disease is unclear. Moreover, in sarcoidosis, increased CD4/CD8 ratio and excess CD4$^+$ T-lymphocyte activity at sites of disease activity is well documented.[35,36] Whether the same is observed in CVID-GLILD or alternatively whether there is "paradoxic" CD4$^+$ lymphopenia at sites of granuloma formation is unknown.

PROGNOSIS

In patients with CVID, GLILD predicts shortened survival,[3,37] and when present, respiratory failure is the most common cause of death.[3,12] This was illustrated in a retrospective study of 69 patients with CVID: subjects with ILD had a median survival of 13.7 years, whereas patients without ILD had a median survival of 28.8 years.[3] The prognosis is also linked to the severity of the disease, with severe restrictive lung dysfunction and extensive disease and fibrosis on chest CT being associated with worse outcome.[3] Extrapulmonary granulomatous disease is also relevant because when subjects with granulomatous-lymphocytic infiltration in any organ are analyzed, the median survival decreased to 10.9 years.[3] Causes of death in this subgroup included end-stage granulomatous liver disease, autoimmune hemolytic anemia, and systemic lymphoproliferative diseases. Early recognition and management of CVID when confronted with newly diagnosed GLILD may also have prognostic implications. Diagnostic delay of CVID is associated with considerable morbidity, particularly recurrent pneumonias, and probably secondary structural lung damage.[1,7,38,39]

MANAGEMENT

Immunoglobulin replacement therapy should be optimized to provide at near normal range immunoglobulin blood levels to help prevent and reduce the risk for sinopulmonary infections,[1,38,39] which can trigger GLILD deterioration. In one study of 12 patients with chronic lung disease and antibody deficiency, subjects were randomized to either 0.6 or 0.2 g/kg intravenous immunoglobulin and the frequency of acute infection was substantially reduced when serum IgG was 500 mg/dL or more. Pulmonary function worsened on the low-dose regimen and improved on the high-dose regimen.[40] Similarly, antimicrobial therapy plays an important role, because immunoglobulin replacement alone may not adequately prevent or treat superimposed lung infections aggravating GLILD.

Early diagnosis and treatment of GLILD might help prevent progressive and debilitating lung disease.[7] Pharmacologic treatment is generally reserved for those with persistent respiratory symptoms or evidence of radiographic or physiologic progressive lung disease. In this setting, a systemic corticosteroid trial is commonly first used. The dose and duration of corticosteroid therapy remain unknown. Furthermore, the quality of evidence informing the use of corticosteroids and other agents is very limited and based on observational uncontrolled data. In my practice, I continue corticosteroid therapy, in the absence of adverse side effects, for 3 to 6 months while reassessing the patient's symptoms, subjective exercise tolerance, pulmonary physiology, and chest imaging (**Fig. 3**). Therapy might be continued if there has been improvement (eg, improved dyspnea and pulmonary function, decreased oxygen requirements, and interstitial chest CT findings). To limit steroid-related toxicity and avoid intolerable side effects, steroid-sparing agents may be considered on a case-by-case basis. In refractory cases, the type of lymphocytic infiltration on surgical lung biopsy (eg, B-cell predominant vs T-cell process) and the presence of concomitant disorders, such as idiopathic thrombocytopenic purpura, may argue for the introduction of such agents as rituximab, although data to support its use are extremely limited.

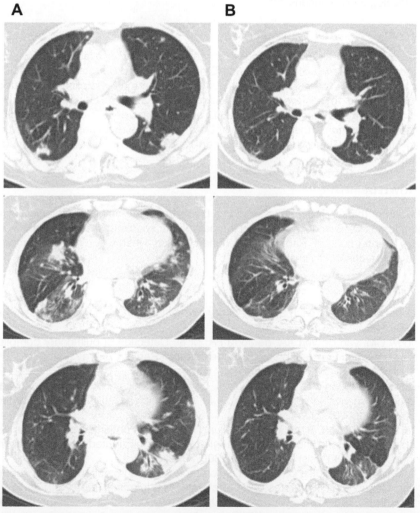

Fig. 3. Noncontrast chest CT in a 60-year-old woman with granulomatous lymphocytic interstitial lung disease before (*A*) and after 2 months of prednisone therapy (*B*).

The nonpharmacologic management of GLILD centers on close patient follow-up by a multidisciplinary team that includes pulmonary and allergy/immunology primarily and other subspecialties as indicated by the clinical scenario. Supportive measures include (1) supplemental oxygen when needed; (2) treatment and prevention of comorbid conditions, such as gastroesophageal reflux and bronchiectasis (eg, airway clearance techniques, mucolytic agents, bronchodilators, inhaled corticosteroids, antimicrobial agents); (3) smoking cessation; and (4) maintenance of nutrition and pulmonary rehabilitation therapy. Also, after the decision to initiate immunomodulatory therapy has been made management of potential side effects or complications is highly advisable. Therefore, if corticosteroids are used, screening (eg, periodic electrolytes and bone mineral density testing), prevention (eg, bone mineral–preserving therapies), treatment of glucocorticoid side effects (eg, diabetes, weight gain) and *Pneumocystis* prophylaxis are recommended. Lastly, lung transplantation may be an option for patients with severe and progressive GLILD that is not responsive to pharmacologic interventions.[3,41]

SUMMARY

As the use of high-dose intravenous gamma globulin and available antimicrobials expands, the incidence of noninfectious CVID-related disorders, such as GLILD, is likely to increase. A thorough clinical evaluation using a multidisciplinary care model is recommended to achieve accurate diagnosis of GLILD. Enough progress has been made in the understanding of GLILD over the last decade that clinicians are now poised to conduct therapeutic trials. Data from large registries and population-based studies of GLILD are needed to better understand the disease trends and burden.

ACKNOWLEDGMENTS

The author thanks Dr Steve D. Groshong, Department of Pathology, National Jewish Health, for his assistance in providing the pathologic specimens; and Dr Jonathan H. Chung, Department of Radiology, National Jewish Health, for his assistance in providing the chest CT films.

REFERENCES

1. Popa V, Colby TV, Reich SB. Pulmonary interstitial disease in Ig deficiency. Chest 2002;122(5):1594–603.
2. Touw CM, van de Ven AA, de Jong PA, et al. Detection of pulmonary complications in common variable immunodeficiency. Pediatr Allergy Immunol 2010; 21(5):793–805.
3. Bates CA, Ellison MC, Lynch DA, et al. Granulomatous-lymphocytic lung disease shortens survival in common variable immunodeficiency. J Allergy Clin Immunol 2004;114(2):415–21.
4. Tanaka N, Kim JS, Bates CA, et al. Lung diseases in patients with common variable immunodeficiency: chest radiographic, and computed tomographic findings. J Comput Assist Tomogr 2006;30(5):828–38.
5. Cunningham-Rundles C, Bodian C. Common variable immunodeficiency: clinical and immunological features of 248 patients. Clin Immunol 1999;92(1):34–48.
6. Chapel H, Cunningham-Rundles C. Update in understanding common variable immunodeficiency disorders (CVIDs) and the management of patients with these conditions. Br J Haematol 2009;145(6):709–27.

7. Arnold DF, Wiggins J, Cunningham-Rundles C, et al. Granulomatous disease: distinguishing primary antibody disease from sarcoidosis. Clin Immunol 2008; 128(1):18–22.

8. Ross RM. ATS/ACCP statement on cardiopulmonary exercise testing. Am J Respir Crit Care Med 2003;167(10):1451 [author reply: 1451].

9. Semenzato G, Poletti V. Bronchoalveolar lavage in lung cancer. Respiration 1992; 59(Suppl 1):44–6.

10. Poletti V, Romagna M, Gasponi A, et al. Bronchoalveolar lavage in the diagnosis of low-grade, MALT type, B-cell lymphoma in the lung. Monaldi Arch Chest Dis 1995;50(3):191–4.

11. Mechanic LJ, Dikman S, Cunningham-Rundles C. Granulomatous disease in common variable immunodeficiency. Ann Intern Med 1997;127(8 Pt 1):613–7.

12. Ardeniz O, Cunningham-Rundles C. Granulomatous disease in common variable immunodeficiency. Clin Immunol 2009;133(2):198–207.

13. Fasano MB, Sullivan KE, Sarpong SB, et al. Sarcoidosis and common variable immunodeficiency. Report of 8 cases and review of the literature. Medicine (Baltimore) 1996;75(5):251–61.

14. Travis WD, Galvin JR. Non-neoplastic pulmonary lymphoid lesions. Thorax 2001; 56(12):964–71.

15. Swigris JJ, Berry GJ, Raffin TA, et al. Lymphoid interstitial pneumonia: a narrative review. Chest 2002;122(6):2150–64.

16. Allen TC. Pathology of small airways disease. Arch Pathol Lab Med 2010;134(5): 702–18.

17. Gompels MM, Hodges E, Lock RJ, et al. Lymphoproliferative disease in antibody deficiency: a multi-centre study. Clin Exp Immunol 2003;134(2):314–20.

18. Wislez M, Cadranel J, Antoine M, et al. Lymphoma of pulmonary mucosa-associated lymphoid tissue: CT scan findings and pathological correlations. Eur Respir J 1999;14(2):423–9.

19. Park JE, Beal I, Dilworth JP, et al. The HRCT appearances of granulomatous pulmonary disease in common variable immune deficiency. Eur J Radiol 2005; 54(3):359–64.

20. Torigian DA, LaRosa DF, Levinson AI, et al. Granulomatous-lymphocytic interstitial lung disease associated with common variable immunodeficiency: CT findings. J Thorac Imaging 2008;23(3):162–9.

21. Cosgrove GP, Frankel SK, Brown KK. Challenges in pulmonary fibrosis. 3: cystic lung disease. Thorax 2007;62(9):820–9.

22. Honda O, Johkoh T, Ichikado K, et al. Differential diagnosis of lymphocytic interstitial pneumonia and malignant lymphoma on high-resolution CT. AJR Am J Roentgenol 1999;173(1):71–4.

23. Detkova D, de Gracia J, Lopes-da-Silva S, et al. Common variable immunodeficiency: association between memory B cells and lung diseases. Chest 2007;131(6):1883–9.

24. Wehr C, Kivioja T, Schmitt C, et al. The EUROclass trial: defining subgroups in common variable immunodeficiency. Blood 2008;111(1):77–85.

25. Warnatz K, Denz A, Drager R, et al. Severe deficiency of switched memory B cells (CD27(+)IgM(-)IgD(-)) in subgroups of patients with common variable immunodeficiency: a new approach to classify a heterogeneous disease. Blood 2002; 99(5):1544–51.

26. Vinuesa CG, Tangye SG, Moser B, et al. Follicular B helper T cells in antibody responses and autoimmunity. Nat Rev Immunol 2005;5(11):853–65.

27. King C, Tangye SG, Mackay CR. T follicular helper (TFH) cells in normal and dysregulated immune responses. Annu Rev Immunol 2008;26:741–66.

28. Grimbacher B, Hutloff A, Schlesier M, et al. Homozygous loss of ICOS is associated with adult-onset common variable immunodeficiency. Nat Immunol 2003; 4(3):261–8.

29. Park JH, Levinson AI. Granulomatous-lymphocytic interstitial lung disease (GLILD) in common variable immunodeficiency (CVID). Clin Immunol 2010; 134(2):97–103.

30. Giovannetti A, Pierdominici M, Mazzetta F, et al. Unravelling the complexity of T cell abnormalities in common variable immunodeficiency. J Immunol 2007; 178(6):3932–43.

31. Mullighan CG, Fanning GC, Chapel HM, et al. TNF and lymphotoxin-alpha polymorphisms associated with common variable immunodeficiency: role in the pathogenesis of granulomatous disease. J Immunol 1997;159(12):6236–41.

32. Wheat WH, Cool CD, Morimoto Y, et al. Possible role of human herpesvirus 8 in the lymphoproliferative disorders in common variable immunodeficiency. J Exp Med 2005;202(4):479–84.

33. North ME, Webster AD, Farrant J. Primary defect in CD8+ lymphocytes in the antibody deficiency disease (common variable immunodeficiency): abnormalities in intracellular production of interferon-gamma (IFN-gamma) in CD28+ ('cytotoxic') and CD28- ('suppressor') CD8+ subsets. Clin Exp Immunol 1998;111(1): 70–5.

34. Holm AM, Sivertsen EA, Tunheim SH, et al. Gene expression analysis of peripheral T cells in a subgroup of common variable immunodeficiency shows predominance of CCR7(-) effector-memory T cells. Clin Exp Immunol 2004;138(2): 278–89.

35. Greene CM, Meachery G, Taggart CC, et al. Role of IL-18 in CD4+ T lymphocyte activation in sarcoidosis. J Immunol 2000;165(8):4718–24.

36. Kolopp-Sarda MN, Kohler C, De March AK, et al. Discriminative immunophenotype of bronchoalveolar lavage CD4 lymphocytes in sarcoidosis. Lab Invest 2000;80(7): 1065–9.

37. Quinti I, Soresina A, Spadaro G, et al. Long-term follow-up and outcome of a large cohort of patients with common variable immunodeficiency. J Clin Immunol 2007; 27(3):308–16.

38. Eijkhout HW, van Der Meer JW, Kallenberg CG, et al. The effect of two different dosages of intravenous immunoglobulin on the incidence of recurrent infections in patients with primary hypogammaglobulinemia. A randomized, double-blind, multicenter crossover trial. Ann Intern Med 2001;135(3):165–74.

39. Busse PJ, Razvi S, Cunningham-Rundles C. Efficacy of intravenous immunoglobulin in the prevention of pneumonia in patients with common variable immunodeficiency. J Allergy Clin Immunol 2002;109(6):1001–4.

40. Roifman CM, Levison H, Gelfand EW. High-dose versus low-dose intravenous immunoglobulin in hypogammaglobulinaemia and chronic lung disease. Lancet 1987;1(8541):1075–7.

41. Burton CM, Milman N, Andersen CB, et al. Common variable immune deficiency and lung transplantation. Scand J Infect Dis 2007;39(4):362–7.

Immunosuppressive Therapy for Autoimmune Lung Diseases

Keith C. Meyer, MD, MS[a,b,c,d],*, Jennifer Bierach, MD[d]

KEYWORDS

- Autoimmunity • Interstitial lung disease • Connective tissue disorder
- Immunosuppressive drug • Lung disease

KEY POINTS

- Immunosuppressive drugs are typically administered when connective tissue disease (CTD)-interstitial lung disease (ILD) is diagnosed to try to prevent progressive loss of lung function by reducing inflammation and preventing pulmonary fibrosis or bronchiolitis obliterans.
- The lung is frequently involved and subject to inflammation and fibrosis in patients with CTD.
- Numerous drugs can be used for systemic autoimmune disorders, but none have US Food and Drug Administration labeling for treatment of CTD-ILD, and many have not been investigated for usefulness in treating autoimmune lung disease.
- Treatment with agents such as corticosteroids, azathioprine, cyclophosphamide, or mycophenolate may provide benefit to patients with CTD-ILD, and other therapies such as prevention of pathologic gastroesophageal reflux (GER) or treatment of bronchiolitis with macrolides may also prove beneficial.
- The therapeutic approach must be personalized to each individual patient and their specific disease process, clinical behavior of the disorder, and associated comorbidities.
- If lung disease relentlessly progresses despite medical therapy, lung transplantation is a therapeutic option, with acceptable outcomes if patients wish to pursue this option.

INTRODUCTION

Pulmonary disorders that patients with various types of connective tissue disease (CTD) are at risk to develop range from airway-centered disorders (eg, cellular or follicular bronchiolitis, or bronchiectasis) to parenchymal disorders (eg, nonspecific interstitial

[a] UW Lung Transplant & Advanced Pulmonary Disease Program, University of Wisconsin School of Medicine and Public Health, Madison, WI, USA; [b] Interstitial Lung Disease Program, Interstitial Lung Disease Clinic, University of Wisconsin School of Medicine and Public Health, Madison, WI, USA; [c] Adult Cystic Fibrosis Program, Adult Cystic Fibrosis Clinic, University of Wisconsin School of Medicine and Public Health, Madison, WI, USA; [d] Section of Allergy, Pulmonary and Critical Care Medicine, Department of Medicine, University of Wisconsin School of Medicine and Public Health, Madison, WI, USA
* Corresponding author. K4/910 Clinical Science Center, 600 Highland Avenue, Madison, WI 53792-9988.
E-mail address: kcm@medicine.wisc.edu

Immunol Allergy Clin N Am 32 (2012) 633–669
http://dx.doi.org/10.1016/j.iac.2012.07.001
0889-8561/12/$ – see front matter © 2012 Elsevier Inc. All rights reserved.

pneumonia [NSIP], usual interstitial pneumonia [UIP] or organizing pneumonia [OP]), pulmonary hypertension (PH) (with or without the presence of interstitial lung disease [ILD]) or pleural disease.[1–3] Because CTD-associated ILD or CTD-associated bronchiolitis may lead to progressive lung function impairment, respiratory insufficiency, and death, immunosuppressive drugs are typically administered when CTD-ILD is diagnosed to try to prevent progressive loss of lung function by reducing inflammation and preventing pulmonary fibrosis or bronchiolitis obliterans. Newer drugs that may benefit patients with CTD are being evaluated in clinical trials or reaching approval for clinical use, but virtually none of the immunosuppressive drugs currently used to treat inflammatory disorders has been properly assessed for efficacy in treating CTD-associated lung disease in adequately powered, randomized, placebo-controlled clinical trials, although many have been validated as capable of inducing partial or complete remission for systemic aspects of some forms of CTD, such as disease-modifying antirheumatic drugs (DMARDs) for the treatment of rheumatoid arthritis (RA).

Rheumatologic disorders have long been recognized as systemic autoimmune diseases, and diagnosis is made via a combination of clinical presentation and types/patterns of autoantibodies that are usually present in the peripheral circulation.[4] However, recent studies suggest that autoantibodies and T cells associated with reactivity to self-antigens can be found in disorders such as idiopathic pulmonary fibrosis (IPF),[5–8] which raises the question whether ILDs such as NSIP or UIP that do not seem to be associated with the presence of a CTD are also autoimmune disorders (ie, lung-dominant CTD) that lack extrapulmonary involvement and often lack typical CTD-associated autoantibodies (as would be perceived for CTD-ILD when diagnostic autoantibodies are detected in the peripheral circulation).[3] In addition, Feghali-Bostwick and colleagues[5] have reported abnormal proliferation of CD4+ T-cell clones and identified IgG autoantibodies directed against several cellular antigens in most of a cohort of 48 patients with IPF. Extracts of IPF lung were found to be capable of stimulating autologous CD4 T-cell proliferation (but not preparations from normal lung or non-IPF lung disease), suggesting that these responses were driven by autoantigens in the IPF lung. Other investigations have also suggested that autoimmunity may play a role in idiopathic UIP (IPF),[6,7,9,10] and some patients diagnosed with idiopathic NSIP or UIP who seem to have no evidence of CTD at the time of diagnosis may have occult CTD and may eventually develop systemic CTD syndromes with the appearance of associated autoantibodies.[11] ILD associated with undifferentiated CTD[12] is frequently seen in referral clinics, and CTD serologies should be obtained when patients are evaluated for new-onset ILD or possible IPF.[13]

The demarcation between lung diseases that are considered classic autoimmune lung disorders versus disorders that do not involve autoimmunity (**Box 1**) has become even more blurred because evidence for sensitization to self-antigens has also been reported for obstructive lung disease. Rinaldi and colleagues[14] examined plasma from 320 patients with chronic obstructive pulmonary disease (COPD) and found a significant increase in T-cell sensitization to collagen V in both smokers and patients with COPD versus never smokers. Similarly, Liu and colleagues[15] found that patients with asthma had higher concentrations of anticollagen V antibodies versus controls, and higher antibody levels correlated with more severe asthma and with use of corticosteroids. Antibodies to other self-antigens were also detected; these included epidermal growth factor receptor, activin A type 1 receptors, and α-catenin. In addition, Núñez and colleagues[16] detected circulating antitissue antibodies in 26% of 328 patients with COPD, suggesting a role of autoimmunity in its pathogenesis. Even sarcoidosis has been suggested to represent a form of autoimmune disease and is frequently associated with other autoimmune disorders,[17] but proof of this has been elusive.

> **Box 1**
> **Autoimmune disorders associated with lung disease**
>
> - Classic rheumatologic disorders
>   - RA
>   - Juvenile RA
>   - Systemic sclerosis
>   - Inflammatory myopathies
>   - Dermatopolymyositis
>   - Antisynthetase syndrome
>   - Systemic lupus erythematosus (SLE)
>   - Sjögren syndrome
>   - Mixed CTD
>   - Vasculitis
>   - Antineutrophil cytoplasmic antibody (ANCA)-associated
>   - Other
>   - Undifferentiated CTD
> - Goodpasture syndrome
> - IgG4-related disease
> - Lung disease associated with autoimmune phenomena
>   - IPF
>   - Asthma
>   - COPD
>   - Posttransplant bronchiolitis obliterans

In light of evolving evidence that autoimmunity may play a role in many lung disorders in addition to CTD-associated ILD, a discussion that covers treatment of autoimmune lung disorders could be expansive if a broad definition of autoimmune lung disease was used. This article focuses on issues of safety and monitoring when immunosuppressive pharmacologic therapies are prescribed for the treatment of CTD-associated interstitial pneumonias, vasculitides, and bronchiolitis. All such therapies are off-label, and prospective, randomized placebo-controlled clinical trials have yet to be performed to evaluate the efficacy and safety of various immunosuppressive agents used to treat patients with CTD-ILD or idiopathic interstitial pneumonias (IIP) other than IPF (idiopathic UIP) that are not associated with the presence of CTD. All of these agents, both nonbiologic and biologic, can cause serious adverse reactions that can be life-threatening.[18] Knowledge of their potential toxicities and interactions with other drugs combined with the adoption of a systematic approach to monitoring therapy can minimize the likelihood that life-threatening reactions occur.

CORTICOSTEROIDS

Corticosteroids were recognized to have potent antiinflammatory properties in the early twentieth century from their ability to decrease formation of granulation tissue.[19] These agents rapidly became the mainstay of treatment of a variety of diffuse lung disorders soon after the introduction of cortisone into clinical use in 1948, and steroids and other immunosuppressive therapies were also gradually introduced into treatment regimens for various rheumatic disorders. Consequently, clinicians who treated patients with various forms of ILD after the introduction of steroids into clinical medical practice perceived that treatment with corticosteroids could dampen the progression of ILD and prevent irreversible fibrosis, respiratory failure, and death.[20] Although nonsteroidal antiinflammatory drugs (NSAIDs) showed some benefit for systemic manifestations of RA, NSAIDs did not seem to have a significant impact on CTD-ILD.

Several reports in the 1970s and 1980s described beneficial clinical responses to methylprednisolone or prednisone for patients diagnosed with cryptogenic fibrosing alveolitis (CFA), which was considered to be essentially the same clinical entity as IPF as (IPF was perceived at that time).[21] Analysis of responders diagnosed as having CFA revealed that they were frequently younger, female, and had evidence of circulating autoantibodies or arthritis.[22] When bronchoalveolar lavage (BAL) was performed, the responders tended to have BAL lymphocytosis.[23] We now recognize that most of these responders likely had CTD-ILD, and the entities of CFA or IPF as recognized in the 1970s to the late 1990s encompassed and lumped together several entities that we now recognize as specific IIP entities, with IPF redefined as idiopathic UIP.[13,24] The entities of idiopathic cellular NSIP or OP can respond well to corticosteroid therapy,[25–27] and both of these forms of IIP are frequently present in patients with CTD-ILD. In addition, it is now recognized that NSIP or OP histopathologic patterns may be present in patients diagnosed with hypersensitivity pneumonitis.[28]

In pulmonary fibrosis associated with scleroderma, improvements in alveolitis and pulmonary function have been observed with steroid therapy.[29,30] Nearly half of patients with RA-associated ILD have been shown to have objective improvement with treatment, but complete remission is unlikely.[31,32] Patients with underlying SLE, mixed CTD, or undifferentiated CTD can have a good response to corticosteroids (which may be given with other pharmacologic immunosuppressive agents during acute inflammatory events), but a poorer response is observed for patients with established fibrosis.[33–35] For patients with Sjögren syndrome-associated ILD, corticosteroids are often recommended, but the effect on outcome remains unclear.[36,37] Despite the lack of clinical trial data, corticosteroids are usually used in conjunction with other immunosuppressive medications to treat CTD-ILD.

Although patients with autoimmune lung disease can show good (and sometimes dramatic) responses to corticosteroid therapy, systemic corticosteroid therapy, especially if high-dose and sustained, is associated with numerous, significant side effects (**Box 2**). If extensive fibrosis is present (eg, UIP or fibrotic NSIP associated with systemic sclerosis), corticosteroid therapy may not induce a significant response. As with treatment of systemic CTD, administration of nonsteroidal immunosuppressive agents can allow corticosteroid doses to be tapered to low levels that are better tolerated and less likely to induce unwanted side effects and complications such as diabetes, systemic hypertension, excessive weight gain, and osteoporosis.

CYTOTOXIC AGENTS

Cytotoxic (or antiproliferative) agents that have been used to treat various forms of CTD include azathioprine, cyclophosphamide, leflunomide, methotrexate, and mycophenolic acid derivatives (**Table 1**). These agents are used for a wide spectrum of inflammatory/autoimmune disorders and can allow corticosteroid dosage to be reduced, thereby decreasing the risk of adverse effects of corticosteroid therapy, especially if treatment is long-term and relatively high doses of steroid as a single

Box 2
Complications of chronic systemic corticosteroid therapy

- Weight gain
- Obesity
- Impaired glucose metabolism
- Diabetes mellitus
- Systemic hypertension
- Myopathy
- Infection
- Decreased bone mineral density
- Osteoporosis
- Avascular necrosis of bone
- Dyslipidemia
- Accelerated atherosclerosis
- Nervous system perturbation
  - Adverse psychological effects
  - Sleep disturbance
- Eye/vision changes
  - Cataract formation
  - Glaucoma
- Growth retardation
- Cushingoid changes
- Dyspepsia

immunosuppressive agent are needed to suppress disease activity and maintain clinical stability. In addition, many of these agents have been evaluated for safety and efficacy in the treatment of several other disorders such as various vasculitides, inflammatory bowel disease (IBD), posttransplant solid-organ rejection, and various forms of ILD.

Azathioprine

Azathioprine is a prodrug that inhibits the activity of T cells and, to a lesser extent, B cells, by interfering in the early phase of lymphoid cell proliferation.[38] It is metabolized to 6-mercaptopurine (6-MP), which inhibits purine metabolism, likely inhibiting DNA and RNA synthesis, and, therefore, protein synthesis. The mechanisms of action remain unclear, but it seems that 6-MP interacts with Rac1, blocking upregulation of Bcl-xL messenger RNA and protein,[39] which leads to suppression of delayed hypersensitivity reactions and cell-mediated cytotoxicity. Controlled clinical trials in RA, SLE, and other forms of CTD have supported the efficacy of azathioprine as a steroid-sparing agent, and it is labeled by the US Food and Drug Administration (FDA) for adjunct therapy for renal transplant rejection and RA. Azathioprine was shown to stabilize scleroderma-associated ILD (which is usually fibrotic NSIP but may also be UIP on lung histopathology) when initiated after 6 months of monthly

Table 1
Cytotoxic (antiproliferative) drugs

Specific Agent	Mechanism of Action	Major Side Effects	Precautions	Suggested Monitoring
Azathioprine	Purine metabolism antagonist May inhibit DNA, RNA, and protein synthesis Inhibits cellular mitosis	Leukopenia Pancreatitis Hepatitis Other bone marrow suppression	Check for thiopurine methyltransferase deficiency (avoid use if deficient) Avoid allopurinol Start with low dose (50 mg/d) and escalate gradually	Monthly CBC Monthly LFT
Cyclophosphamide	Alkylating agent Cross-links DNA and RNA (inhibits protein synthesis and cell function)	Bone marrow suppression Hemorrhagic cystitis Bladder cancer Pulmonary fibrosis	Maintain adequate fluid intake to avoid bladder toxicity	CBC with platelets every 2–4 wk Monthly urinalysis LFT
Methotrexate	Inhibits dihydrofolate reductase (reversible)	Pulmonary toxicity Hepatitis	Give prophylactic folic acid (1–2 mg/d)	Monthly CBC and LFT Periodic renal function laboratory tests
Mycophenolate	Blocks de novo guanosine nucleotide synthesis (inhibits nucleic acid synthesis, which impairs T-lymphocyte and B-lymphocyte proliferative responses)	Diarrhea Bone marrow suppression PML (black box warning)	Blood level can be assayed to assist assessment of GI toxicity (high value supports mycophenolate as cause)	Monthly CBC
Leflunomide	Dihydroorotate dehydrogenase inhibition May inhibit T-cell pyrimidine biosynthesis	GI (nausea, diarrhea) Systemic hypertension Hepatotoxicity Skin (alopecia, rash)	Obtain CBC, LFT, phosphate, and creatinine level tests before initiation of therapy	CBC, LFT, phosphate, creatinine level tests every 4–6 wk for first 6 mo; check every 6–12 wk beyond 6 mo

Abbreviations: CBC, complete blood count; GI, gastrointestinal; LFT, liver function testing; PML, progressive multifocal leukoencephalopapathy.

intravenous (IV) cyclophosphamide infusions.[40] However, a National Institutes of Health-sponsored IPF Network study recently showed a significant mortality and hospitalization risk for patients with IPF receiving azathioprine plus N-acetylcysteine (NAC) versus patient groups receiving placebo or monotherapy with NAC.[41] This outcome led to early termination of the azathioprine/NAC study arm and raised concern for treatment of IPF with azathioprine. It is unknown whether azathioprine therapy may pose a similar risk for patients with CTD-ILD.

Azathioprine and 6-MP are both oxidized or methylated in erythrocytes and liver. Thiopurine methyltransferase (TPMT) converts mercaptopurine, via thiol methylation, to thiopurine analogues. Approximately 1 in 300 individuals lack this enzyme and can develop severe myelosuppression with the initiation of azathioprine.[42] Low levels of this enzyme have been associated with severe gastrointestinal (GI) distress and bone marrow suppression when azathioprine is taken.[43] It is now considered cost-effective to evaluate TPMT levels before initiating treatment with azathioprine; the number of patients needed to test to avoid 1 adverse event is estimated at 20.[44,45]

Azathioprine side effects include acne, GI distress, cholestasis, increased liver function tests, arthralgias, bone marrow suppression, alopecia, dizziness, allergy, opportunistic infections, and pancreatitis.[46,47] Adverse reactions occur in up to 19% of patients treated with azathioprine,[47] and azathioprine administration has been linked to an increased risk of malignancy, particularly lymphomas.[18] Monitoring for bone marrow suppression and liver toxicity needs to be performed when initiating therapy with azathioprine. Complete blood count (CBC) and liver function testing has been recommended every 2 weeks for the first 4 weeks, then every 4 weeks for the duration of treatment.[48]

Cyclophosphamide

Cyclophosphamide is a synthetic alkylating agent that is related to the nitrogen mustards. It has been FDA-labeled for the treatment of hematologic and nonhematologic malignancies,[18] but it is not FDA-labeled for treatment of CTD. High doses suppress T-helper 1 (TH1) and enhance TH2 lymphocyte activity and also affect CD4+CD25+ regulatory T cells, leading to marked immunosuppression.[49] Cyclophosphamide has also been used to treat various forms of ILD[50] as well as CTD-related lung disease,[51] and it has become the drug of choice for the treatment of ANCA-associated vasculitis.[52] Controlled trials have shown efficacy for lupus nephritis, systemic vasculitis, and ILD associated with scleroderma. It has been reported to benefit patients with progressive scleroderma-ILD, with improved quality of life and stabilization of pulmonary function and radiographic progression of fibrosis,[40,51,53] but these gains can be lost after 12 months if maintenance immunosuppressive therapy is not continued.[53] In addition, a recent, follow-up analysis of the Scleroderma Lung Study data reported that only a subset of patients received benefit from cyclophosphamide.[54]

Cyclophosphamide is converted to active metabolites (aldophosphamide and phosphoramide mustard) by the liver, and the kidney excretes both cyclophosphamide and the active metabolites. The metabolites induce cell death by inhibiting DNA replication. Cyclophosphamide can be dosed orally or via intermittent IV pulse therapy. For both ANCA-related vasculitis[52] and scleroderma-related lung disease,[51] pulse therapy has been shown to be as effective and less toxic than daily dosing. IV pulse therapy allows for daily dosage adjustments based on the patient's white blood cell (WBC) count; however, that benefit must be weighed against the cost and support staff required for administration.

Both IV and oral dosing can cause hematuria, fibrosis of the urinary bladder, bladder cancer, and hemorrhagic cystitis, which can be a life-threatening complication. Both cyclophosphamide and its active metabolites have been implicated in the development of hemorrhagic cystitis; 1 step toward prevention of this complication is ensuring a daily intake of at least 3 L of fluid. Hematuria seems to be time-dependent and dose-dependent.[55] Up to 15% of patients treated with cyclophosphamide for a year develop hematuria.[55] Bladder cancer risk is increased in patients who smoke cigarettes and also in those who developed hemorrhagic cystitis during therapy with cyclophosphamide.[55] Like hemorrhagic cystitis, bladder cancer also seems to be time-dependent and dose-dependent. Every 10 g of cumulative exposure to cyclophosphamide leads to a 2-fold increased risk of bladder cancer.[56] Cancers may occur many years after cyclophosphamide has been stopped. Screening with urinalysis and appropriate evaluation of hematuria, if noted, seems to be sufficient.[55]

Cyclophosphamide can also cause bone marrow suppression. Leukopenia is a dose-related complication and leads to alteration in the dosing regimen in many patients.[57] Cyclophosphamide administration can also lead to lymphomas, leukemias, skin cancers, and likely solid-organ tumors.[58] Many of the disease states that cyclophosphamide is used to treat predispose patients to higher rates of various malignancies. One prospective 15-year study of 726 patients with lung cancer that had previously been treated with busulfan, cyclophosphamide, or placebo, found no difference in rate of malignancies between the placebo and the cyclophosphamide arms.[59]

Cyclophosphamide has been associated with congestive heart failure (CHF), hemorrhagic pericarditis, and hemopericardium after particularly high doses. These conditions typically reverse after cessation of the drug. Skin rashes and even toxic epidermal necrolysis have been reported. Alopecia is a common side effect, which often reverses with cessation of the drug. However, the new hair that returns may be a new texture or color. Bacterial, viral, fungal, and protozoan infections are increased with cyclophosphamide use, although no consensus on preventive prophylactic medications exists.

Lung pneumonitis/fibrosis has been described extensively in animals exposed to cyclophosphamide[60] and in patients exposed to the drug,[61] but this relationship has been difficult to clearly show in human studies because of confounding variables. If fibrosis is suspected, cessation of the drug is recommended; typically these manifestations resolve with or without the use of corticosteroids.

Patients who are receiving cyclophosphamide should have a CBC with platelet count performed every 2 weeks. Because of infection risk, WBC count should be maintained greater than 4000 and absolute neutrophil count greater than 2000 cells/mm^3, and dosing adjustments may be necessary to maintain this level. Urinalysis should be performed before the initiation of therapy and then at least every 3 months. If the patient has received greater than 10 g cumulative dose or developed hemorrhagic cystitis during treatment, urinalysis with cytology should be performed yearly after cessation of therapy.[18]

Leflunomide

Leflunomide inhibits de novo pyrimidine synthesis, thereby inhibiting T-lymphocyte and B-lymphocyte activation and proliferation.[62] It is metabolized in the bowel wall and liver to an active metabolite, which is then excreted primarily by the biliary system. Little renal excretion occurs,[63] and its half-life is approximately 2 weeks. Clinical trials have supported the use of leflunomide for polyangiitis with granulomatosis, ankylosing spondylitis, SLE, Sjögren syndrome, psoriatic arthritis, and psoriasis,[64–66] and it is FDA-labeled for the treatment of RA.[67]

There are multiple side effects, which seem to be dose-related and typically resolve with dose reduction of leflunomide. These side effects include rash, nausea, hypertension, increased liver enzymes, alopecia, and diarrhea. Reports of serious infection, angioedema, cytopenias, interstitial pneumonitis, Stevens-Johnson syndrome, toxic epidermal necrolysis, erythema multiforme, and fulminant hepatitis have been published; however, these data are difficult to interpret because of the presence of often severe, underlying disease and the simultaneous use of other immunosuppressive medications.

Hepatic toxicity was found in 2% to 4% of patients treated with leflunomide for RA[68] and typically occurred within 6 months of initiating therapy. Hepatic toxicity was more prevalent in patients also treated with methotrexate or who had preexisting liver dysfunction,[69] and decreased dosing or cessation of therapy typically resulted in laboratory value normalization. Folic acid supplementation can help to prevent hepatic toxicity in patients treated with both leflunomide and methotrexate. Hepatocellular necrosis has been reported, but is less common than increased transaminase levels.[70]

Perineural vasculitis associated with leflunomide administration seems to lead to peripheral neuropathy as early as 3 days after initiation of therapy.[71] The best outcomes have been reported when leflunomide is stopped as soon as symptoms of neuropathy arise. Up to 54% of patients with RA who are treated with leflunomide have neuropathic symptoms compared with 8% treated with other agents.[72] Oral cholestyramine administration may be a useful adjunct to leflunomide cessation in cases of severe neuropathy.[72] Fatal cases of interstitial pneumonitis associated with leflunomide administration have been reported.[73]

Before initiating treatment with leflunomide, baseline CBC, phosphate, creatinine, and liver function tests are recommended.[18] Once treatment has begun, these laboratory tests should be repeated every 4 to 6 weeks for the first 6 months, and if stable can then be checked every 6 to 12 weeks. If leflunomide is given with methotrexate, these tests should be repeated every 4 weeks until the treatment is stopped. Serious side effects require the cessation of leflunomide and the administration of cholestyramine. Leflunomide undergoes enterohepatic recirculation, resulting in a prolonged half-life. Cholestyramine binds and eliminates the active metabolite, and activated charcoal can also be used if cholestyramine is not tolerated.

Methotrexate

Methotrexate interrupts nucleic acid and protein metabolism by inhibiting dihydrofolate reductase, and it is metabolized in the liver, where it is converted to polyglutamates, which have an immunosuppressive effect via inhibition of extracellular adenosine metabolism.[74] Evidence of the immunosuppressive activity of methotrexate has been found in blood cells for up to 1 week, although the half-life is only 8 to 15 hours. Caffeine, theophylline, and other adenosine receptor antagonists have been shown to inhibit the antiinflammatory properties of methotrexate in animal models.[75] Methotrexate is FDA-labeled for juvenile RA (JRA), psoriasis, and RA.

Methotrexate is known to have multiple toxicities as well as many side effects. Major toxicities documented in association with methotrexate include cytopenias, liver damage, and pneumonitis. Common side effects include nausea, diarrhea, rash, fatigue, cognitive impairment, alopecia, and headaches. In trials for RA and psoriasis, side effects led to drug cessation in up to 30% of patients, most commonly for abnormal liver function tests, GI symptoms, and peripheral blood cytopenias.[76] Risk factors for toxicity from methotrexate include impaired renal function or advanced age.[77] Pulmonary toxicity most commonly presents as hypersensitivity pneumonitis.[78] It may also present as bronchitis with airway hyperreactivity, pneumonitis, OP, pulmonary fibrosis, or diffuse alveolar damage (DAD). Monitoring with pulmonary function testing or high-resolution computed tomography (HRCT) does not seem to be useful in this population.[79]

Up to 5% of patients must stop methotrexate because of hepatic toxicity. Most cases of hepatic toxicity present as increased transaminase levels, which typically reverse with cessation of the medication; however, as many as 1 in 1000 patients develop severe liver failure and cirrhosis.[76] Risk factors for severe hepatic toxicity include heavy alcohol use, large cumulative dose of methotrexate, and history of psoriasis. Based on data from a large meta-analysis, liver biopsy was suggested for patients with psoriasis after each 1-g to 1.5-g cumulative dose of methotrexate.[80] However, patients with RA are considered to be at lower risk for the development of severe liver toxicity associated with methotrexate, and liver function tests obtained on a regular basis are considered sufficient for monitoring.[81] Current American College of Rheumatology recommendations regarding monitoring for liver toxicity include checking transaminase levels every 4 to 12 weeks, and if the levels show sustained increases more than normal, then liver biopsy is recommended.

Folic acid supplementation (1–2 mg/d) may be used to prevent many side effects associated with methotrexate but does not seem to affect the efficacy of the drug.[82,83] Folic acid is able to bypass the blockade of nucleic acid synthesis by methotrexate. In 1 study, folic acid supplementation decreased the methotrexate cessation because of toxicity from 38% in the control group to 17% in the group that received folic acid.[83] Folic acid may be added or increased if patients report symptoms of stomatitis, diarrhea, and nausea.[82]

Monitoring for methotrexate toxicities requires routine measures of renal function and CBCs.[84] If leukopenia is noted, the dose of methotrexate should be adjusted. Up to 26% of patients studied showed hematologic abnormalities while taking methotrexate, resulting in cessation of the medication. Greater than 95% of these patients were found to have symptoms of viral infection, and the hematologic abnormality returned to normal after a 1-month holiday from methotrexate, and the abnormality did not return when methotrexate was resumed.[85]

Mycophenolic Acid

Mycophenolic acid inhibits the de novo purine pathway, causing potent inhibition of T lymphocytes and B lymphocytes.[86] It has FDA approval for use in solid-organ transplant (heart, kidney, and liver) for rejection prophylaxis. However, it has been used to treat a myriad of diseases, including SLE,[87] lupus nephritis,[88] RA,[89] polyangiitis with granulomatosis,[90] and CTD-ILD.[91] A retrospective review of patients with CTD-ILD showed that the drug was well tolerated, allowed a reduction in corticosteroid dose, and was associated with stabilization of lung function.[91] In addition, other small studies suggest benefit for patients with scleroderma-ILD or other CTD-ILD.[92–95]

Mycophenolate is available as mycophenolate mofetil, which is orally administered and rapidly hydrolyzed to mycophenolic acid, and mycophenolate sodium, which is an extended release enteric formulation. Mycophenolic acid is metabolized by binding to glucuronide, and this complex is then cleared via the kidneys; it may accumulate in renal failure, requiring dosage adjustments or dialysis. Mycophenolic acid has been linked to respiratory, cardiovascular, genitourinary, dermatologic, endocrinologic, ocular, neurologic, metabolic, musculoskeletal, infectious, GI, and hematologic adverse events but is generally well tolerated. Neutropenia may occur but typically responds to reduced mycophenolate dosing.[96]

Mycophenolate interacts with many drugs. Azathioprine and mycophenolate should not be coadministered because both inhibit purine metabolism. The absorption of mycophenolate can be inhibited by colesevalam, colestipol, activated charcoal, cholestyramine, iron, aluminum, or magnesium salts.[97] Plasma concentrations of acyclovir and ganciclovir may be increased when coadministered with mycophenolate, and renal failure can exacerbate this effect. Mycophenolate may diminish the immunologic response to vaccination,[98] and patients on mycophenolate should not receive live attenuated virus vaccines.

Monitoring for mycophenolate toxicities include weekly CBCs for the first month, then every 2 weeks for the next 2 months, then monthly. It has not been shown that monitoring mycophenolate blood levels detects toxicity reliably enough to decrease its incidence, and blood levels have not been shown to be useful for predicting rejection prophylaxis efficacy in solid-organ transplantation.[99] However, following blood levels may be useful in patients with renal dysfunction.[100]

BIOLOGIC AGENTS

An expanding number of anticytokine agents (antibodies that inhibit and/or bind cytokines or inhibit cytokine cell surface receptors) and anti-immune cell antibodies (eg, antilymphocyte agents that can mediate cytotoxicity or inhibit cytokine production) are being developed and coming into clinical use (**Tables 2** and **3**). Some of these agents have FDA approval for use as DMARDs for RA, and others have received approval for use in transplantation or hematologic malignancies. The clinical use of many of these agents is likely to expand in the coming years, but significant and potentially life-threatening adverse reactions can occur with these agents, and clinicians should be aware of these untoward reactions when these drugs are administered to patients. This section provides an overview of these drugs.

Tumor Necrosis Factor Antagonists

Tumor necrosis factor α (TNF-α) plays a central role in tissue inflammation including granuloma formation, and various anti-TNF agents have been developed and approved for treatment of RA, psoriasis, ankylosing spondylitis, and IBD (see **Table 2**). The first 2 anti-TNF agents approved for clinical use were etanercept, which acts by binding TNF and preventing its interaction with the p75 TNF receptor on cell membranes, and infliximab, a monoclonal antibody that binds both endogenous-soluble and membrane-bound TNF and renders it biologically inactive.[101] Three additional monoclonal antibody preparations (adalimumab, certolizumab, golimumab) are now available for clinical use. These biologic agents have allowed targeted therapy that has essentially revolutionized treatment of rheumatoid disorders,[102] but the effect of these agents on CTD-ILD remains unknown. A recently published meta-analysis systematically examined results of clinical trials for treatment of RA with each of the 5 anti-TNF agents, and there was no clear difference in efficacy among the agents.[103] The data suggested that etanercept might have the best safety profile, and efficacy could not be stated to be better with any TNF agent compared with methotrexate, which is a substantially less expensive treatment option.

Significant risks associated with anti-TNF agents are numerous and include infection, lymphomas and other malignancies, and nervous system disorders, including demyelination syndromes (data are extracted from Micromedex). The risk of tuberculosis has been suggested to be greater with infliximab versus other agents, and infliximab therapy has been associated with risk of worsened cardiac dysfunction. Rare or unusual adverse events associated with anti-TNF therapy include lupus-like syndromes, bone marrow suppression, hepatotoxicity, and reactivation of viral hepatitis. In addition to taking a detailed baseline history and obtaining routine blood chemistries, patients should be evaluated for latent or active tuberculosis infection with skin

Table 2
FDA-approved cytokine antagonists used in transplant prophylaxis or for treatment of autoimmune disorders[a]

Specific Agent	Mechanism of Action	FDA-Approved Indications	Common Adverse Effects (>5%)	Serious Adverse Effects Reported
Etanercept	Soluble fusion protein form of p75 TNF receptor (binds TNF-α and TNF-β, which inhibits binding of TNF-β and TNF-β to p75 receptors)	RA, psoriasis, AS, JRA	Injection site reaction; respiratory (rhinitis, URI)	CHF; dermatologic (erythema multiforme, fasciitis, Stevens-Johnson syndrome, toxic epidermal necrolysis, malignancy): anemia; leukopenia; neutropenia; pancytopenia; thrombocytopenia; malignancy (lymphoma, leukemia); autoimmune hepatitis; hypersensitivity reaction; neurologic (demyelinating CNS disease, Guillain-Barré syndrome, seizure, acute transverse myelitis, seizure); optic neuritis; infection (TB, *Legionella* pneumonia)
Infliximab	Monoclonal antibody (high-affinity binding to free and membrane TNF-α that neutralizes TNF-α activity)	RA, AS, psoriasis, IBD	Rash; abdominal pain; nausea; headache; pharyngitis or respiratory infection (children); fatigue	Cardiovascular (acute coronary syndrome, heart failure); dermatologic (erythema multiforme, Stevens-Johnson syndrome, toxic epidermal necrolysis); pancytopenia; leukopenia; neutropenia; thrombocytopenia; hepatotoxicity; hypersensitivity reaction; infusion reaction; drug-induced lupus erythematosus; malignancy (lymphoma); neurologic

				(demyelinating CNS disease, Guillain-Barré syndrome); infection (TB, *Legionella*, histoplasmosis, listeriosis)
Adalimumab	Monoclonal antibody (binds TNF-α, blocking interaction with p55 and p75 cell surface receptors)	RA, JRA, AS, psoriasis, IBD	Injection site reaction or pain; rash; headache; sinusitis; URI; antiadalimumab antibody development; positive ANA	CHF; dermatologic (erythema multiforme, Stevens-Johnson syndrome); agranulocytosis; aplastic anemia; erythrocytosis; leukopenia; pancytopenia; thrombocytopenia; acute hepatic failure; anaphylaxis; hypersensitivity reaction; malignancy (lymphoma); demyelinating CNS disease; infection (*Legionella* pneumonia, TB, listeriosis)
Certolizumab	Humanized Fab fragment conjugated to polyethylene glycol (binds TNF-α but not TNF-β)	RA, IBD	Arthralgia; UTI; URI	Cardiovascular (CHF; cardiac rhythm disturbance, MI, pericardial effusion, pericarditis); skin (erythema multiforma, erythema nodosum, Stevens-Johnson syndrome, toxic epidermal necrolysis, urticarial); bone marrow suppression; bowel obstruction; hypersensitivity reaction; lupus erythematosus; demyelinating CNS disease; seizure; suicide risk; nephrotic syndrome; renal failure; infection (TB, listeriosis); malignancy

(continued on next page)

Table 2
(continued)

Specific Agent	Mechanism of Action	FDA-Approved Indications	Common Adverse Effects (>5%)	Serious Adverse Effects Reported
Golimumab	Monoclonal antibody (binds soluble and cell surface membrane TNF-α)	RA, AS, psoriasis	Injection site reaction; URI	CHF; HBV reactivation; hypersensitivity reaction; lupus erythematosus and erythema multiformelike syndrome; neurologic (demyelinating CNS disease, Guillain-Barré syndrome, peripheral demyelinating neuropathy); optic neuritis; infection (TB, invasive mycosis, *Legionella* pneumonia; listeriosis); malignancy
Basiliximab	IL-2 receptor antagonist	Renal transplant prophylaxis	Vomiting; abdominal pain; asthenia; dizziness; insomnia	Infusion reaction (hypersensitivity); HTN; edema; anemia; dysuria; cough; dyspnea
Tocilizumab	IL-6 receptor antagonist	RA, JRA	HTN, rash, diarrhea, LFT increase, dizziness, headache, nasopharyngitis	Infection site reaction; GI perforation; thrombocytopenia, neutropenia; anaphylaxis or hypersensitivity reactions; URI; malignancy
Anakinra	IL-1 receptor antagonist	RA	Injection site reaction	Cardiorespiratory arrest; hypersensitivity reaction; malignancy

Abbreviations: ANA, antinuclear antibody; AS, ankylosing spondylitis; CNS, central nervous system; HBV, hepatitis B virus; HTN, systemic hypertension; LFT, liver function testing; MI, myocardial infarction; TB, tuberculosis; URI, upper respiratory infection; UTI, urinary tract infection.
[a] All agents are associated with increased risk of infection.

testing (or via peripheral blood testing for evidence of reactivity) and appropriate imaging to rule out active pulmonary infection before initiation of anti-TNF therapy.

Other Biologic Agents

Various antilymphocyte and nonanti-TNF anticytokine agents have been approved for clinical use for the treatment of malignancies, transplantation, and various forms of CTD. Some of these agents may prove useful for the treatment of autoimmune lung disorders, but none has been evaluated in clinical trials that specifically target CTD-ILD that could lead to FDA approval for such use. Currently available anticytokine agents include baxiliximab (interleukin 2 [IL-2] signaling inhibition, FDA-labeled for kidney transplantation), tocilizumab (IL-6 receptor antagonist, FDA-labeled for RA), and anakinra (IL-1 receptor antagonist, FDA-labeled for RA).

Antilymphocyte agents currently available for clinical use include rituximab, abatacept, belatacept, belimumab, bortezomib, alemtuzumab, anti-CD3, and antithymocyte globulin (see **Table 3**). Rituximab has received FDA approval for treatment of RA and vasculitis, and it is also under investigation as a treatment of other autoimmune disorders, acute exacerbations of IPF, refractory sarcoidosis, and pulmonary alveolar proteinosis. However, it has been associated with a considerable number of potential adverse events including fatal infusion reactions and pulmonary toxicity.[18,104] However, recent systematic analyses have found rituximab therapy for RA to be safe and relatively free of adverse events.[105–107] Frequent monitoring of vital signs during infusions is recommended, and clinicians must also be vigilant for the appearance of other complications such as infection including reactivation of latent viral infections, cardiac complications, and bowel perforation.

CHLOROQUINES

These synthetic 4-aminoquinolone antimalarial drugs (**Table 4**) have antiinflammatory properties via mechanisms that remain unclear. Chloroquine is rapidly absorbed from the GI tract and sequestered in many tissues, including the lung, kidney, liver, spleen, and nervous tissue, and its half-life is estimated to range from 30 to 60 days, with the drug remaining in tissues for years after therapy is discontinued. Prolonged therapy is associated with several adverse events, and some can be serious and life-threatening, but the drug is generally well tolerated. Hydroxychloroquine sulfate is FDA-labeled for SLE and RA and is commonly used in initial therapeutic regimens as an agent for mild CTD that is symptomatic; it may be useful in pediatric ILD[108] and may induce a clinical response in some patients with sarcoidosis.[109]

CALCINEURIN INHIBITORS

The calcineurin inhibitors, cyclosporine A and tacrolimus, are the key immunosuppressive agents in posttransplant immunosuppressive regimens and are usually administered along with an antiproliferative agent (mycophenolate or azathioprine) and prednisone, although mammalian target of rapamycin (mTOR) inhibitors (sirolimus, everolimus) may also be used to allow calcineurin dose reduction (or occasionally in place of a calcineurin inhibitor).[110] Calcineurin inhibitors have been administered to patients with refractory inflammatory myopathy or RA when other therapies have been ineffective,[111,112] but randomized, controlled clinical trials to evaluate such therapy have not been reported. Major concerns with these agents include opportunistic infections and nephrotoxicity, and many other adverse effects may occur. In addition, numerous drug-drug interactions can occur when other drugs that affect CYP 3A4 (cytochrome P450), the hepatic enzyme that degrades both the calcineurin inhibitors and mTOR inhibitors, are simultaneously

Table 3
Antilymphocyte antibodies available for clinical use[a]

Specific Agent	Mechanism of Action	FDA-Approved Indications	Common Adverse Effects (>5%)	Serious Adverse Effects
Rituximab	Anti-CD20 (monoclonal antibody [mediates B-cell cytotoxicity via binding of cell surface CD20])	RA, microscopic PAN, ANCA-associated vasculitis, CLL, lymphoma	Fever; cardiovascular (hypotension, edema); dermatologic (rash, night sweats, pruritus); GI (abdominal pain, nausea, diarrhea); anemia; arthralgia; myalgia; neurologic (headache, dizziness, asthenia, sensory neuropathy); cough	Cardiac (shock, CHF, dysrhythmia, MI); GI (obstruction, perforation, ileocolitis); PML; dermatitis/rash; angioedema; anemia (aplastic, hemolytic); neutropenia; lymphocytopenia; thrombocytopenia; HBV; infusion reaction; nephrotoxicity; respiratory (dyspnea, OB, pneumonitis/fibrosis)
Abatacept	CTLA-4 costimulation antagonist (suppresses T-cell proliferation, cytokine release)	RA, JRA	Nausea; UTI; headache; respiratory (acute exacerbation of COPD, nasopharyngitis, URI)	Sepsis; cellulitis; acute pyelonephritis; pneumonia; malignancy
Belatacept	Binds B7 ligand (CD80, CD86) (suppresses T-cell proliferation and cytokine release)	Renal transplant rejection or prophylaxis	Hypotension; peripheral edema; GI (nausea, vomiting, diarrhea, constipation); anemia; leukopenia; UTI; hyperkalemia or hypokalemia; cough; fever; headache	Severe infections; Guillain-Barré syndrome; PML; nephropathy (transplanted kidney)
Bortezomib	Anti-CD19 (inhibits plasma cells)	MM, lymphoma	Rash; hypotension; GI (nausea, vomiting, diarrhea, constipation, suppressed appetite; anemia; fever; musculoskeletal (arthralgia, myalgia, cramp, bone pain); neurologic (asthenia, dizziness, dysesthesia, headache, insomnia, paresthesia,	CHF; toxic epidermal necrolysis; neutropenia; thrombocytopenia; acute hepatic failure; angioedema; postherpetic neuralgia, TIA; respiratory (ARDS, interstitial pneumonitis)

Drug	Mechanism	Condition	Adverse Reactions	Serious Adverse Reactions
				peripheral neuropathy); psychiatric disorder; cough; dyspnea; pneumonia
Belimumab	Inhibits B cells (anti-B-lymphocyte stimulator-BlyS)	SLE	Diarrhea; nausea; fever; limb pain; insomnia; nasopharyngitis	Anaphylaxis; hypersensitivity reaction; infusion reaction; bronchitis; pneumonia
Ofatumumab	Anti-CD20 (B-cell lysis)	CLL	Respiratory (bronchitis, dyspnea, cough, pneumonia, URI); rash; nausea; diarrhea; anemia; fever; fatigue	Neutropenia; PML; HBV (fulminant, relapse); bowel obstruction; infusion reaction
Alemtuzumab	Binds CD52 (antibody-dependent cellular-mediated lysis of T and B lymphocytes, monocytes, macrophages, natural killer cells and some granulocytes)	CLL	Systemic hypotension; rash, urticarial; GI (nausea, vomiting, diarrhea); anemia; neutropenia; thrombocytopenia; musculoskeletal pain; insomnia; anxiety; bronchospasm; dyspnea; fever; fatigue; shivering; CMV infection	Cardiovascular (dysrhythmia, CHF, cardiomyopathy); anemia (aplastic or autoimmune hemolytic); thrombocytopenia (may be autoimmune); neutropenia; lymphocytopenia; PTLD; GVHD; neurologic (demyelinating CNS disease, Guillain-Barré syndrome); optic neuropathy; Goodpasture syndrome; severe infection; CMV or EBV infection
Muromonab	Murine monoclonal anti-CD3 antibody that inhibits T-cell proliferation and response to antigen challenge	Renal, liver, and heart transplant rejection	Fever; systemic hypotension; tachycardia; edema; rash; diarrhea; nausea; vomiting; headache; tremor; dyspnea; shivering	Cardiac dysrhythmia; hypertension; Stevens-Johnson syndrome; thrombosis; hepatitis; anaphylaxis; neurologic (cerebral edema, encephalopathy; seizure); pulmonary edema; respiratory failure and arrest

(continued on next page)

Table 3
(continued)

Specific Agent	Mechanism of Action	FDA-Approved Indications	Common Adverse Effects (>5%)	Serious Adverse Effects
ATG	Polyclonal immunoglobulin mixture (raised in rabbits or horses immunized with human thymus lymphocytes)	Aplastic anemia; renal transplant (rejection or prophylaxis)	Fever; shivering; chest or back pain; arthralgia; myalgia; hypertension; peripheral edema; tachycardia; rash; hyperkalemia; GI (nausea, vomiting, diarrhea, abdominal pain); leukopenia, thrombocytopenia; hemolysis; serum sickness; anti-ATG antibody development; asthenia; headache; nephrotoxicity; dyspnea	Anaphylaxis; ARDS; PTLD; hyperkalemia

Abbreviations: ARDS, acute respiratory distress syndrome; ATG, antithymocyte globulin; CLL, chronic lymphocytic leukemia; CMV, cytomegalovirus; CTLA-4, cytotoxic T-lymphocyte antigen 4; EBV, Epstein-Barr virus; GVHD, graft-versus-host disease; HBV, hepatitis B virus infection/reactivation; MI, myocardial infarction; MM, multiple myeloma; OB, obliterative bronchiolitis; PAN, polyarteritis nodosa; PML, progressive multifocal leukoencephalopathy; PTLD, posttransplant lymphoproliferative disease; TIA, transient ischemic attack; URI, upper respiratory infection; UTI, urinary tract infection.
[a] All agents are associated with increased risk of infection.

administered because of either enhanced degradation (CYP 3A4 stimulation) or competition (drug is metabolized by CYP 3A4). It is essential that treating physicians understand these interactions and carefully monitor drug blood levels, CBCs, and kidney function, with appropriate intervals between testing.

MISCELLANEOUS ADDITIONAL PHARMACOLOGIC THERAPIES

Several other agents (not necessarily immunosuppressive agents) may have a role in treating autoimmune lung disease, but relatively little clinical information is available to support their use. The mTOR inhibitors, sirolimus and everolimus, have potent immunosuppressive and antiproliferative effects.[18,110] Sirolimus binds to intracellular FK-binding protein, and this complex subsequently binds to the mTOR and suppresses the function of this serine/threonine kinase, which plays a key role in the cell cycle and T-cell proliferation. mTOR signaling has been shown to play a crucial role in joint destruction in animal models of experimental inflammatory arthritis,[113] and inhibition of mTOR by sirolimus has been shown to suppress activities of synovial fibroblasts in a rat model of RA.[114] In addition, everolimus coadministered with methotrexate produced a significantly greater response compared with patients receiving methotrexate alone in a 3-month prospective, double-blind, placebo-controlled proof of concept clinical trial.[115] However, one of the adverse events associated with sirolimus administration is pulmonary toxicity.[116]

Thalidomide has FDA approval for the treatment of multiple myeloma and has been studied in sarcoidosis, Langerhans cell histiocytosis, and RA. It has been shown to suppress TNF-α production and has antiangiogenic properties, although its mechanism of action remains unclear. It may benefit some patients with Langerhans cell histiocytosis,[117] but it did not clearly benefit patients with sarcoidosis,[118] although its maximal dosing was limited by side effects. Small studies have suggested potential benefit in JRA,[119–121] but thalidomide and its analogues, pomalidomide and lenalidomide, have been linked to acute pulmonary toxicity and interstitial pneumonitis as adverse events.[122,123]

Tetracyclines have antiinflammatory as well as antibacterial properties and have been used to treat several inflammatory disorders.[124] They can suppress matrix metalloproteinases, collagenase, and phospholipase A2 activity, suppress production of IL-1β and TNF-α, and may suppress neutrophil and T-cell function. Several placebo-controlled, randomized studies have been performed in RA with minocycline, and 1 large study showed significant improvement in joint disease and markers of inflammation over a 48-week treatment period.[125] Another trial reported superiority of minocycline over hydroxychloroquine for symptom control and prednisone-sparing over a 2-year study period.[126]

Macrolides (eg, erythromycin), neomacrolides (eg, clarithromycin), and azalides (eg, azithromycin) also have both antiinflammatory and antimicrobial properties,[127] and they have been shown to have clinical benefit or promise in treating bronchiolitis (eg, diffuse pan-bronchiolitis, bronchiolitis obliterans syndrome [BOS]) cystic fibrosis (CF) bronchiectasis, non-CF bronchiectasis, COPD, and asthma.[122–129] These agents can inhibit the respiratory burst of neutrophils, and they can also suppress cytokine production (eg, IL-8, IL-6, TNF-α). Azithromycin is highly concentrated in lung tissue and alveolar macrophages, and it can be safely used in patients with liver disease because it is not metabolized by the cytochrome P450 system. Several studies support their potential usefulness for the treatment of bronchial disorders (ie, bronchiolitis, bronchiectasis) associated with autoimmune disorders. Erythromycin has been shown to significantly improve symptoms of patients with RA-associated

Table 4
Miscellaneous drugs with potential benefit for autoimmune disorders

Drug Class	Specific Agent	Mechanism of Action	Potential Toxicities	Precautions and Monitoring
Chloroquines	Hydroxychloroquine sulfate	Antiinflammatory effects (FDA-labeled for SLE and RA)	Cardiac (cardiomyopathy, dysrhythmia); peripheral neuropathy; myopathy; CNS (headache, confusion, seizure, coma); GI upset; hepatic failure; visual disturbance; urticaria; pruritis; bone marrow suppression	Periodic ocular screening Avoid prolonged, high-dose therapy (associated with risk of irreversible retinopathy and ototoxicity)
Calcineurin inhibitor[a]	Cyclosporine A	Inhibits T-cell function by disrupting IL-2 signaling	Nephrotoxicity; hypertension; tremor; hyperkalemia; hypomagnesemia; hepatotoxicity; CNS (headache, tremor, seizure, coma, encephalopathy; leukoencephalopathy); hirsutism, gingival hyperplasia, burning sensation in eye	Frequent (as appropriate) monitoring of peripheral blood (drug level, renal function, serum K and Mg, and LFT)
	Tacrolimus	Inhibits T-cell function by disrupting IL-2 signaling via formation of FK 506-binding proteins	Cardiac (prolonged QT interval, hypertension, cardiomegaly); diabetes mellitus; nephrotoxicity; hypomagnesemia; hyperkalemia; neurologic (headache, tremor, insomnia, paresthesia, coma); leukoencephalopathy; skin (alopecia, pruritus, rash); GI upset; anemia; thrombocytopenia	Frequent (as appropriate) monitoring of peripheral blood (drug level, renal function, serum K and Mg, LFT, and glucose)

	Mechanism	Adverse effects	Monitoring
mTOR inhibitors[a]			
Sirolimus	Inhibits mTOR, which suppresses T cells, antibody production, and cytokine production	Fever; infection; pain; hypertension; edema; acne; rash; GI upset; anemia; thrombocytopenia; arthralgia; headache; PML; increased serum creatinine level; UTI; HUS; nephrotic syndrome; epistaxis; coronary artery stent thrombosis; dyslipidemia; DVT; PE; TTP; pancytopenia; hepatotoxicity; ILD; pulmonary hemorrhage; malignancy	Avoid use in early postoperative period Monitor CBC, renal function, serum cholesterol and triglycerides Monitor whole blood levels
Everolimus	Everolimus-FK506 binding protein complex binds and inhibits mTOR	Fever; infection; fatigue; asthenia; cough; dyspnea; URI; otitis; impaired wound healing; LFT increase; creatinine increase; HUS; anemia; leukopenia; thrombocytopenia; GI upset (stomatitis; nausea, vomiting, diarrhea, constipation); dyslipidemia; hyperlipidemia; thrombosis; thrombotic microangiopathy; TTP; PE; hyperglycemia; acne; rash	Avoid use in early postoperative period Monitor CBC, renal function, serum cholesterol, and triglycerides Monitor whole blood levels
Miscellaneous			
Macrolides and azalides	Various antiinflammatory and immunomodulatory effects	Prolonged QT interval; torsades de pointes or other ventricular dysrhythmia; GI upset; headache; allergic reaction; increased LFT; hepatitis; pancreatitis; rash; Stevens-Johnson syndrome; ototoxicity; seizure	Monitor LFTs with chronic therapy if P450-metabolized Consider pretherapy ECG and early on-therapy ECG to check QT interval

(continued on next page)

Table 4
(continued)

Drug Class	Specific Agent	Mechanism of Action	Potential Toxicities	Precautions and Monitoring
	Minocycline	Antiinflammatory effects	Dizziness; vertigo; tooth discoloration; anaphylaxis; drug hypersensitivity reaction; SLE; pseudotumor cerebri	
	NAC (oral)	Antioxidant effects (replenishes oxidized glutathione)	Rash; urticaria; angioedema; GI upset (nausea, vomiting, diarrhea) IV NAC has been associated with several additional (and potentially severe) adverse events	Bronchospasm has occurred in patients given IV drug
	Pirfenidone	Inhibits fibroblast growth and collagen production via TGF-β₁ and PDGF inhibition	GI (anorexia, nausea, abdominal discomfort/bloating, diarrhea, vomiting, constipation); skin (photosensitivity, rash); fatigue; weakness; increased LFT	Avoid sun exposure Take with food
	Thalidomide	Suppresses TNF-α production; antiangiogenic; modulates T-cell subsets	Edema; atrial fibrillation; other cardiac dysrhythmia; hypocalcemia; pneumonia; leukopenia; GI upset or perforation; rash; Stevens-Johnson syndrome; asthenia; confusion; drowsiness, somnolence; tremor; peripheral neuropathy; PE; teratogenesis	Watch for peripheral neuropathy Periodic CBC

Abbreviations: CNS, central nervous system; DVT, deep venous thrombosis; ECG, electrocardiogram; HUS, hemolytic uremic syndrome; LFT, liver function testing; Mg, magnesium; PDGF, platelet-derived growth factor; PE, pulmonary embolus; PML, progressive multifocal leukoencephalopathy; mTOR, mammalian target of rapamycin; TTP, thrombotic thrombocytopenic purpura; URI, upper respiratory infection; UTI, urinary tract infection.
ᵃ CYP 3A4 (P450)-metabolized drugs (monitor closely for drug-drug interactions if other drugs that affect P450 function or are metabolized by P450 are coadministered).

follicular bronchiolitis or bronchiolitis obliterans.[130,131] In addition, OP may be the cause of ILD in patients with CTD-ILD, and bronchiolar inflammation with variable alveolar involvement is typically present. Several studies have reported treatment responses to macrolide therapy for OP,[132–135] including OP refractory to corticosteroids.[134,135] Azithromycin can stabilize or improve BOS in lung transplant recipients, and 1 mechanism may be its ability to diminish acid reflux.[136–138]

GASTROESOPHAGEAL DYSMOTILITY AND REFLUX

An abnormal degree of GER has been increasingly recognized as playing a potential role in ILD.[139] Many patients with IPF or CTD-ILD have been shown to have significant (pathologic) GER, and patients with CTD-ILD frequently have esophageal dysmotility or GER.[140] Extent of pulmonary fibrosis has been correlated with the extent of GER in patients with scleroderma,[141] and extreme esophageal dysmotility (aperistalsis) is frequently detected in patients with scleroderma. Patients with IPF and abnormal GER can have disease stabilization when GER is adequately suppressed[142] or after antireflux surgery.[143] In addition, patients with IPF who receive proton pump inhibitor (PPI) therapy or undergo Nissen fundoplication have been shown to be associated with improved survival,[144] and GER may be linked to acute exacerbations of IPF.[145] Suppression of abnormal GER may benefit patients with CTD-ILD, but additional research is needed in this area, and chronic acid suppression may have significant adverse effects if sustained over long periods.

ANTIFIBROTIC AGENTS

Although predominantly inflammatory idiopathic pneumonia (eg, cellular NSIP) can remain stable over time, the appearance of progressive fibrosis is what usually leads to progressive loss of function and death in patients with CTD-ILD, and antiinflammatory/immunosuppressive therapies may be ineffectual in preventing lung function decline despite having an effect on systemic disease. Antifibrotic agents (eg, pirfenidone or BIBF-1120) have been shown to have a potential impact on disease progression in patients with IPF,[146,147] and antifibrotic therapies may hold benefit for patients with CTD associated with progressive pulmonary fibrosis. Another agent, NAC, which has putative antifibrotic activity via its antioxidant activity (replenishing glutathione) has been studied for treatment of IPF in a fairly well-powered study[148] that suggested possible benefit. However, this trial was flawed by lack of a true placebo group; a National Institutes of Health-sponsored trial of oral NAC versus placebo for IPF that is in progress showed that a third treatment arm with azathioprine plus NAC had significantly increased mortality risk versus NAC alone or placebo.[41] Clinical investigations with adequately powered clinical trials of antifibrotic therapies for treatment of CTD-ILD have yet to be performed.

LUNG TRANSPLANTATION

Lung transplantation is a well-accepted therapy for patients with advanced lung disease that is progressive and refractory to other therapies, and it can significantly prolong survival and improve quality of life for patients with IPF.[149] However, because patients with CTD-ILD may not only have debilitating systemic disease but also may have significant esophageal dysmotility and GER,[150] many centers may refuse to consider them for lung transplantation evaluation and wait-listing, although relatively good results have been reported in scleroderma.[151] A major consideration that can have a significant impact on posttransplant outcome is poorly controlled pathologic

GER, and posttransplant GER considerably increases the risk of allograft dysfunction, especially triggering of BOS, which can lead to graft loss.[152] Nonetheless, a substantial number of patients with CTD-ILD (scleroderma, inflammatory myositis, RA, SLE) have undergone successful lung transplantation and been reported to lung transplant databases, and we have had successful outcomes with many patients with CTD-ILD at our center. However, patients must be carefully evaluated for the presence of complications or comorbidities that predict a substantially increased risk of poor outcome.

A SUGGESTED APPROACH TO TREATMENT AND TO MONITORING RESPONSE TO THERAPY

A treatment plan must consider the specific type of lung disease, systemic manifestations (when present) of a specific systemic CTD or other autoimmune disorder, degree of respiratory impairment, and the temporal behavior of the disease. Aggressive immunosuppressive therapy is indicated with rapidly advancing or clearly progressive disease. However, some patients may be clinically stable without receiving immunosuppressive therapy for prolonged periods, and exposing them to the risk of significant (and occasionally severe) adverse events associated with immunosuppressive therapies is generally not warranted for stable patients. In addition, individual patients can have their lung disease complicated by the presence of secondary PH, venous thromboembolism, or several comorbidities (eg, cardiac disease, anemia, osteoporosis) that may have a significant impact on behavior of the disease or symptoms and quality of life. Patients may have a complex combination of disease processes such as pulmonary fibrosis combined with secondary PH, ILD accompanied by significant bronchiectasis, pathologic GER (which may be asymptomatic and not necessarily controlled by acid-suppressing therapies), or significant extrapulmonary end-organ dysfunction. Interventions must be tailored/personalized to match a given patient with their specific pulmonary disease manifestations and comorbidities. A multidisciplinary approach to disease management across specialties with pulmonologist, rheumatologist, and primary physicians communicating and comanaging patients (especially those with severe or aggressive disease) is desirable and in the best interest of the patient.

A suggested approach to management is summarized in **Box 3**. Patients should understand the nature of their disease as well as the risks and benefits associated with various therapies. If pharmacologic therapies are chosen, patients should be aware of the risks associated with the specific drugs to which they are to be exposed and be educated as to what symptoms or signs may indicate that an adverse, therapy-related event is occurring. Similarly, care providers should be aware of potential side effects of pharmacologic therapies and appropriate precautions to be taken before and during therapy, including appropriate laboratory monitoring with surveillance of bone marrow, liver, or kidney function. Drug levels need to be monitored if calcineurin or mTOR inhibitors are administered, and drug-drug interactions must be avoided. If an agent is metabolized by the P450 cytochrome system, care must be taken to carefully monitor and adjust therapy if other drugs that affect or are metabolized by P450 are administered. If medications such as rituximab are administered IV, patients must be carefully monitored for infusion reactions. In addition, some drugs (methotrexate, mTOR inhibitors) are more likely than others to cause pneumotoxic reactions, and worsened pulmonary function may be caused by drug-associated pneumotoxicity rather than disease progression. If intense immunosuppression is used, infection prophylaxis should be considered to prevent infectious complications such as *Pneumocystis jiroveci* pneumonia or reactivation of tuberculosis.

Box 3
Treating the patient with autoimmune lung disease: a suggested approach

- Establish patient-provider partnership for disease and symptom management
- Provide patient education
  - Information concerning disease characteristics and prognosis
  - Knowledge of potential side effects and toxicity of pharmacologic agents if prescribed
  - Smoking cessation
- Obtain adequate baseline testing
  - Imaging (HRCT or CXR as appropriate)
  - Pulmonary function testing (spirometry, DLCO, 6-MWT, dyspnea assessment)
- Thoughtful discussion of treatment options
  - Observation
  - Pharmacologic therapy (if appropriate) to induce remission or stabilize disease
    - Evidence-based (eg, DMARDs)
    - Off-label use (eg, cytotoxic drugs, corticosteroids, therapies for PH)
  - Therapies to relieve symptoms and improve quality of life (eg, cough, dyspnea, fatigue)
  - Enrollment in clinical trials if available and appropriate
  - Lung transplantation for advanced disease refractory to other therapies
  - Best supportive care
- Vaccinations
  - Pneumococcal and influenza
  - Other if appropriate and not contraindicated (hepatitis, *Herpes zoster*, papillomavirus)
- Pulmonary rehabilitation if appropriate
- Supplemental oxygen as indicated for:
  - Resting hypoxemia
  - Nocturnal desaturation during sleep
  - Significant exertional oxyhemoglobin desaturation ($\leq$88%)
- Screen for GER (may be asymptomatic) or esophageal dysmotility as appropriate
  - Associated with presence of hiatal hernia (can be seen on HRCT)
  - Consider other testing (impedance/pH esophageal probe, esophagram, endoscopy) to detect, quantitate, and characterize (eg, acid vs nonacid)
- Screen and treat comorbidities and disease complications:
  - PH
  - Coronary artery disease
  - Thromboembolism
  - Infectious complications
  - Obstructive sleep apnea
  - Airway obstruction (eg, bronchiectasis, ILD superimposed on emphysema)
  - Diabetes mellitus
  - Osteopenia, osteoporosis

○ Obesity (encourage weight-reduction)

○ Cachexia/malnutrition (nutritional supplements)

○ Anxiety and depression (refer for psychosocial support as needed)

○ Adverse drug reactions

• Monitor disease activity at appropriate intervals

○ Pulmonary function testing

○ Intermittent thoracic imaging

■ CXR (frequency as needed for the specific disease process)

■ HRCT of the thorax if routine CXR imaging not adequate

• Prompt evaluation and treatment of disease exacerbations

• Discuss advance care planning as appropriate

○ End-of-life issues (resuscitation, ventilator support)

○ Directives (living will, durable power of attorney)

• Palliative care for end-stage disease (relief of suffering)

Abbreviations: CXR, chest radiograph; DLCO, diffusion capacity of the lung for CO; 6-MWT, 6-minute walk test.

Treatment that adequately treats/stabilizes systemic CTD may control associated pulmonary disease, and we have occasionally had patients at our center whose ILD stabilizes or even improves when they have undergone kidney transplant and been placed on posttransplant immunosuppression with a calcineurin inhibitor plus an anti-proliferative agent and low-dose prednisone. Rapid-onset pneumonitis/fibrosis with rapid progression may require intense therapy (eg, high-dose pulse IV methylprednisolone or IV cyclophosphamide combined with high-dose steroid) to attempt to stabilize the disease and prevent progression. In addition, similarly to patients with IPF,[153] patients with CTD-ILD can have acute pulmonary exacerbations with rapid deterioration.[154,155] Infection must be sought and treated if present, but these exacerbations may be caused by acute worsening with superimposed OP, DAD, or pulmonary hemorrhage as the cause of acute deterioration. BAL may prove useful in evaluating an acute deterioration in lung function,[156] and the presence of significant BAL lymphocytosis suggests the presence of a hypersensitivity drug reaction or other complication that is likely to respond to augmented immunosuppression if other causes (eg, infection, alveolar hemorrhage) are not identified.

If airway disease (eg, bronchiolitis) is the primary manifestation of lung involvement, adequate control of a systemic disorder may control and stabilize the lung disease. In addition, treatment with a macrolide or azalide may provide benefit for treatment of bronchiolitis or OP, and we have had several individuals with progressive bronchiolitis associated with RA achieve remission with substantial improvement in lung function with macrolide therapy. Macrolides may also benefit patients with bronchiectasis (which is usually associated with the presence of ILD) if used as an adjunctive therapy. When CTD is complicated by PH, either primary or secondary to CTD-ILD, it is unclear whether therapies used for treating precapillary pulmonary arterial hypertension (PAH),[157] such as prostanoids, phosphodiesterase inhibitors, or endothelin antagonists, are beneficial, because existing evidence is only anecdotal. A recent retrospective study of 70 patients with scleroderma from 2 large referral centers could not find clear benefit associated with PAH pharmacologic therapies.[158]

When patients have pathologic GER, measures to prevent GER should be considered. Lifestyle changes and positional changes (eg, elevation of the head of bed when recumbent) may help prevent reflux. Although PPI therapy may suppress acid secretion and alleviate symptoms of acid reflux if patients have associated symptoms (many do not), reflux may still occur despite PPI therapy. Antireflux surgery can be considered, although the presence of esophageal dysmotility, especially aperistalsis, greatly increases the challenge of surgical approaches that are intended to prevent GER, and antireflux surgery should be performed only by surgeons who are skilled at the procedure and can modify their approach appropriately if foregut dysmotility is present.[140,159] We have observed several patients with undifferentiated CTD-ILD and associated pathologic reflux to have lung disease stabilization or improvement after successful antireflux surgery.

To monitor established lung disease behavior over time or evaluate response to therapies, dyspnea assessment and intermittent pulmonary function testing along with a 6-minute walk test can usually provide an adequate gauging of disease status. Change in forced vital capacity over time correlates well with stability versus significant decline (>10% decline) in IPF, and similar observations have been made for diffusion capacity of the lung for CO ($\geq$15% decline) and 6-minute walk test (distance and desaturation).[160] Although HRCT is useful for diagnosis and fibrosis score severity is predictive of disease severity and prognosis in IPF, obtaining serial HRCTs to gauge disease progression is generally not useful and substantially increases radiation exposure. However, HRCT imaging can be useful to evaluate disease exacerbations, and it may be useful to gauge response to therapies if routine chest radiography is likely to be insensitive to parenchymal changes that suggest therapeutic benefit. Useful biomarkers that can predict prognosis and correlate with disease activity are much needed; with acute onset of CTD-ILD, C-reactive protein (CRP) and erythrocyte sedimentation rate (ESR) may be considerably increased, and a significant decline or normalization of CRP and ESR generally correlates with response to therapy.

We need to know more about the natural history of autoimmune lung disorders, especially CTD-ILD. Autoimmune disorders occur because of loss of immune tolerance as the ability of regulatory mechanisms to maintain tolerance by suppressing autoreactive lymphocytes wanes,[161] which may correlate to some degree with advancing age.[162] A better understanding of regulatory mechanisms that depend on intact function of CD4+CD25+FoxP3+ regulatory T cells and the acquisition of knowledge that allows the manipulation or augmentation of this cell population such that immune tolerance can be reestablished may lead to a vastly improved ability to treat, control, or prevent various autoimmune disorders and avoid the many potential adverse side effects of currently used pharmacotherapeutic agents. Efforts to attain multidisciplinary consensus on criteria that can be used to measure disease activity and therapeutic response in CTD-ILD[163,164] are a step in the right direction and may lead to clinical trials that can establish therapies to improve our management of patients with autoimmune lung disease.

SUMMARY

The lung is frequently involved and subject to inflammation and fibrosis in patients with CTD. Other autoimmune disorders such as Goodpasture syndrome can also involve the lung, and evolving research has identified autoimmune phenomena associated with non-CTD lung disease such as IPF and COPD. There are numerous drugs that can be used for systemic autoimmune disorders, but none have FDA labeling for treatment of CTD-ILD, and many have not been investigated for usefulness in treating autoimmune lung disease. Nonetheless, treatment with agents such as corticosteroids, azathioprine, cyclophosphamide, or mycophenolate may provide benefit to patients with CTD-ILD, and other therapies such as prevention of pathologic GER or treatment of bronchiolitis with macrolides may also prove beneficial. The therapeutic approach must be personalized to each individual patient and their specific disease process, clinical behavior of the disorder, and associated comorbidities. Patients need to be educated concerning risks, benefits, and signs/symptoms of adverse reactions if immunosuppressive medications are prescribed, and treating medical personnel must be aware of potential adverse reactions and appropriate precautions and monitoring protocols for specific drugs when prescribed. If lung disease relentlessly progresses despite medical therapy, lung transplantation is a therapeutic option, with acceptable outcomes if patients wish to pursue this option. The natural history of CTD-ILD remains obscure, and clinical trials to evaluate efficacy of immunosuppressive therapies, especially promising new biologic or antifibrotic agents, are greatly needed.

ACKNOWLEDGMENT

Supported in part by the George and Julie Mosher Pulmonary Research Fund.

REFERENCES

1. Fischer A, West SG, Swigris JJ, et al. Connective tissue disease-associated interstitial lung disease: a call for clarification. Chest 2010;138(2):251–6.
2. Swigris JJ, Brown KK, Flaherty KR. The idiopathic interstitial pneumonias and connective tissue disease-associated interstitial lung disease. Curr Rheumatol Rev 2010;6:91–8.
3. Fischer A, du Bois RM. A practical approach to connective tissue disease-associated lung disease. In: Baughman RP, du Bois RM, editors. Diffuse lung disease. New York: Springer; 2011. p. 217–37.
4. Self SE. Autoantibody testing for autoimmune disease. Clin Chest Med 2010; 31(3):415–22.
5. Feghali-Bostwick CA, Tsai CG, Valentine VG, et al. Cellular and humoral autoreactivity in idiopathic pulmonary fibrosis. J Immunol 2007;179(4):2592–9.
6. Kurosu K, Takiguchi Y, Okada O, et al. Identification of annexin 1 as a novel autoantigen in acute exacerbation of idiopathic pulmonary fibrosis. J Immunol 2008;181(1):756–67.
7. Taillé C, Grootenboer-Mignot S, Boursier C, et al. Identification of periplakin as a new target for autoreactivity in idiopathic pulmonary fibrosis. Am J Respir Crit Care Med 2011;183(6):759–66.
8. Burlingham WJ, Love RB, Jankowska-Gan E, et al. IL-17-dependent cellular immunity to collagen type V predisposes to obliterative bronchiolitis in human lung transplants. J Clin Invest 2007;117(11):3498–506.
9. Gilani SR, Vuga LJ, Lindell KO, et al. CD28 down-regulation on circulating CD4 T-cells is associated with poor prognoses of patients with idiopathic pulmonary fibrosis. PLoS One 2010;5(1):e8959.
10. Kotsianidis I, Nakou E, Bouchliou I, et al. Global impairment of CD4+CD25+FOXP3+ regulatory T cells in idiopathic pulmonary fibrosis. Am J Respir Crit Care Med 2009;179(12):1121–30.
11. Tzelepis GE, Toya SP, Moutsopoulos HM. Occult connective tissue diseases mimicking idiopathic interstitial pneumonias. Eur Respir J 2008;31(1):11–20.

12. Kinder BW, Collard HR, Koth L, et al. Idiopathic nonspecific interstitial pneumonia: lung manifestation of undifferentiated connective tissue disease? Am J Respir Crit Care Med 2007;176(7):691–7.
13. Raghu G, Collard HR, Egan JJ, et al, ATS/ERS/JRS/ALAT Committee on Idiopathic Pulmonary Fibrosis. An official ATS/ERS/JRS/ALAT statement: idiopathic pulmonary fibrosis: evidence-based guidelines for diagnosis and management. Am J Respir Crit Care Med 2011;183(6):788–824.
14. Rinaldi M, Lehouck A, Heulens N, et al. Antielastin B-cell and T-cell immunity in patients with chronic obstructive pulmonary disease. Thorax 2012;67(8): 694–700.
15. Liu M, Subramanian V, Christie C, et al. Immune responses to self-antigens in asthma patients: clinical and immunopathological implications. Hum Immunol 2012;73(5):511–6.
16. Núñez B, Sauleda J, Antó JM, et al, PAC-COPD Investigators. Anti-tissue antibodies are related to lung function in chronic obstructive pulmonary disease. Am J Respir Crit Care Med 2011;183(8):1025–31.
17. Sharma OP. Sarcoidosis and other autoimmune disorders. Curr Opin Pulm Med 2002;8(5):452–6.
18. Meyer KC, Decker C, Baughman R. Toxicity and monitoring of immunosuppressive therapy used in systemic autoimmune diseases. Clin Chest Med 2010;31: 565–88.
19. Kim R, Meyer KC. Therapies of interstitial lung disease–past, present, and future. Ther Adv Respir Dis 2008;2:319–38.
20. Mapel DW, Samet JM, Coultas DB. Corticosteroids and treatment of idiopathic pulmonary fibrosis: past, present, and future. Chest 1996;110:1058–67.
21. Turner-Warwick M, Burrows B, Johnson A. Cryptogenic fibrosing alveolitis: response to corticosteroid treatment and its effect on survival. Thorax 1980; 35(8):593–9.
22. Turner-Warwick M, Burrows B, Johnson A. Cryptogenic fibrosing alveolitis: clinical features and their influence on survival. Thorax 1980;35(3):171–80.
23. Rudd RM, Haslam PL, Turner-Warwick M. Cryptogenic fibrosing alveolitis. Relationships of pulmonary physiology and bronchoalveolar lavage to response to treatment and prognosis. Am Rev Respir Dis 1981;124(1):1–8.
24. American Thoracic Society, European Respiratory Society. American Thoracic Society/European Respiratory Society International Multidisciplinary Consensus Classification of the Idiopathic Interstitial Pneumonias. This joint statement of the American Thoracic Society (ATS), and the European Respiratory Society (ERS) was adopted by the ATS board of directors, June 2001 and by the ERS Executive Committee, June 2001. Am J Respir Crit Care Med 2002;165(2):277–304.
25. King TE, Mortenson RL. Cryptogenic organizing pneumonitis. The North American experience. Chest 1992;102(Suppl 1):8S–13S.
26. Cordier JF. Cryptogenic organizing pneumonia. Eur Respir J 2006;28:422–46.
27. Flaherty KR, Martinez FJ. Nonspecific interstitial pneumonia. Semin Respir Crit Care Med 2006;27(6):652–8.
28. Gaxiola M, Buendía-Roldán I, Mejía M, et al. Morphologic diversity of chronic pigeon breeder's disease: clinical features and survival. Respir Med 2011; 105(4):608–14.
29. Rossi GA, Bitterman PB, Rennard SI, et al. Evidence for chronic inflammation as a component of the interstitial lung disease associated with progressive systemic sclerosis. Am Rev Respir Dis 1985;131:612–7.

30. Wallaert B, Hatron PY, Grosbois JM, et al. Subclinical alveolitis in immunological systemic disorders. Transition between health and disease? Eur Respir J 1990; 3:1206–16.

31. Turner-Warwick M, Evans RC. Pulmonary manifestations of rheumatoid disease. Clin Rheum Dis 1977;3:549–64.

32. Roschmann RA, Rothenberg RJ. Pulmonary fibrosis in rheumatoid arthritis: a review of clinical features and therapy. Semin Arthritis Rheum 1987;16: 174–85.

33. Sullivan WD, Hurst DM, Harmon CE. A prospective evaluation emphasizing pulmonary involvement in patients with mixed connective tissue disease. Medicine 1984;63:92–107.

34. Holgate ST, Glass DN, Haslam P, et al. Respiratory involvement in systemic lupus erythematosus: a clinical and immunological study. Clin Exp Immunol 1976;24:385–95.

35. Lamblin C, Bergoin C, Saelens T, et al. Interstitial lung disease in collagen vascular disease. Eur Respir J 2001;18(Suppl 32):69s–80s.

36. Papiris SA, Tsonis IA, Moutsopoulos HM. Sjogren's syndrome. Semin Respir Crit Care Med 2007;28:459–72.

37. Ito I, Nagl S, Kitalchi M, et al. Pulmonary manifestations of primary Sjogren's syndrome. Am J Respir Crit Care Med 2005;171:632–8.

38. Lennard L. The clinical pharmacology of 6-mercaptopurine. Eur J Clin Pharmacol 1992;43:329–39.

39. Tiede I, Fritz G, Strand S, et al. CD28-dependent Rac1 activation is the molecular target of azathioprine in primary human CD4+ T lymphocytes. J Clin Invest 2003;111:133–45.

40. Hoyles RK, Ellis RW, Wellsbury J, et al. A multicenter, prospective, randomized, double-blind, placebo-controlled trial of corticosteroids and intravenous cyclophosphamide followed by oral azathioprine for the treatment of pulmonary fibrosis in scleroderma. Arthritis Rheum 2006;54(12):3962–70.

41. Idiopathic Pulmonary Fibrosis Clinical Research Network, Raghu G, Anstrom KJ, King TE Jr, et al. Prednisone, azathioprine, and N-acetylcysteine for pulmonary fibrosis. N Engl J Med 2012;366(21):1968–77.

42. Carrico CK, Sartorelli AC. Effects of 6-thioguanine on macromolecular events in regenerating rat liver. Cancer Res 1977;37:1868–75.

43. Stolk JN, Boerbooms AM, de Abreu RA, et al. Reduced thiopurine methyltransferase activity and development of side effects of azathioprine treatment in patients with rheumatoid arthritis. Arthritis Rheum 1998;41(10): 1858–66.

44. Schedel J, Godde A, Schutz E, et al. Impact of thiopurine methyltransferase activity and 6-thioguanine nucleotide concentrations in patients with chronic inflammatory diseases. Ann N Y Acad Sci 2006;1069:477–91.

45. Marra CA, Esdaile JM, Anis AH. Practical pharmacogenetics: the cost effectiveness of screening for thiopurine S-methyltransferase polymorphisms in patients with rheumatological conditions treated with azathioprine. J Rheumatol 2002;29: 2507–12.

46. Mantia LL, Mascoli N, Milanese C. Azathioprine. Safety profile in multiple sclerosis patients. Neurol Sci 2007;28:299–303.

47. Kirschner BS. Safety of azathioprine and 6-mercaptopurine in pediatric patients with inflammatory bowel disease. Gastroenterology 1998;115:813–21.

48. Gaffney K, Scott DG. Azathioprine and cyclophosphamide in the treatment of rheumatoid arthritis. Br J Rheumatol 1998;37:824–36.

49. Baughman RP, Peddi R, Lower EE. Therapy: general issues. In: Baughman RP, du Bois RM, Lynch JP III, et al, editors. Diffuse lung disease: a practical approach. London: Arnold; 2004. p. 78–105.
50. Kondoh Y, Taniguchi H, Yokoi T, et al. Cyclophosphamide and low-dose prednisolone in idiopathic pulmonary fibrosis and fibrosing nonspecific interstitial pneumonia. Eur Respir J 2005;25:528–33.
51. Tashkin DP, Elashoff R, Clements PJ, et al. Cyclophosphamide versus placebo in scleroderma lung disease. N Engl J Med 2006;354:2655–66.
52. Haubitz M, Schellong S, Gobel U, et al. Intravenous pulse administration of cyclophosphamide versus daily oral treatment in patients with antineutrophil cytoplasmic antibody-associated vasculitis and renal involvement: a prospective, randomized study. Arthritis Rheum 1998;41:1835–44.
53. Tashkin DP, Elashoff R, Clements PJ, et al, Scleroderma Lung Study Research Group. Effects of 1-year treatment with cyclophosphamide on outcomes at 2 years in scleroderma lung disease. Am J Respir Crit Care Med 2007;176(10):1026–34.
54. Roth MD, Tseng CH, Clements PJ, et al, Scleroderma Lung Study Research Group. Predicting treatment outcomes and responder subsets in scleroderma-related interstitial lung disease. Arthritis Rheum 2011;63(9):2797–808.
55. Talar-Williams C, Hijazi YM, Walther MM, et al. Cyclophosphamide-induced cystitis and bladder cancer in patients with Wegener granulomatosis. Ann Intern Med 1996;124:477–84.
56. Radis CD, Kahl LE, Baker GL, et al. Effects of cyclophosphamide on the development of malignancy and on long-term survival of patients with rheumatoid arthritis. A 20-year followup study. Arthritis Rheum 1995;38:1120–7.
57. Martin-Suarez I, D'Cruz D, Mansoor M, et al. Immunosuppressive treatment in severe connective tissue diseases: effects of low dose intravenous cyclophosphamide. Ann Rheum Dis 1997;56:481–7.
58. Dorr FA, Coltman CA Jr. Second cancers following antineoplastic therapy. Curr Probl Cancer 1985;9:1–43.
59. Girling DJ, Stott H, Stephens RJ, et al. Fifteen-year follow-up of all patients in a study of post-operative chemotherapy for bronchial carcinoma. Br J Cancer 1985;52:867–73.
60. Siemann DW, Macler L, Penney DP. Cyclophosphamide-induced pulmonary toxicity. Br J Cancer Suppl 1986;7:343–6.
61. Malik SW, Myers JL, DeRemee RA, et al. Lung toxicity associated with cyclophosphamide use. Two distinct patterns. Am J Respir Crit Care Med 1996; 154(6 Pt 1):1851–6.
62. Cherwinski HM, Cohn RG, Cheung P, et al. The immunosuppressant leflunomide inhibits lymphocyte proliferation by inhibiting pyrimidine biosynthesis. J Pharmacol Exp Ther 1995;275:1043–9.
63. Li EK, Tam LS, Tomlinson B. Leflunomide in the treatment of rheumatoid arthritis. Clin Ther 2004;26:447–59.
64. Nash P, Thaci D, Behrens F, et al. Leflunomide improves psoriasis in patients with psoriatic arthritis: an in-depth analysis of data from the TO-PAS study. Dermatology 2006;212:238–49.
65. van Woerkom J, Kruize AA, Geenen R, et al. Safety and efficacy of leflunomide in primary Sjögren's syndrome: a phase II pilot study. Ann Rheum Dis 2007;66: 1026–32.
66. Tam LS, Li EK, Wong CK, et al. Double-blind, randomized, placebo-controlled pilot study of leflunomide in systemic lupus erythematosus. Lupus 2004;13: 601–4.

67. Cohen S, Cannon GW, Schiff M, et al. Two-year, blinded, randomized, controlled trial of treatment of active rheumatoid arthritis with leflunomide compared with methotrexate. Utilization of Leflunomide in the Treatment of Rheumatoid Arthritis Trial Investigator Group. Arthritis Rheum 2001;44: 1984–92.

68. Emery P, Breedveld FC, Lemmel EM, et al. A comparison of the efficacy and safety of leflunomide and methotrexate for the treatment of rheumatoid arthritis. Rheumatology (Oxford) 2000;39:655–65.

69. Prakash A, Jarvis B. Leflunomide: a review of its use in active rheumatoid arthritis. Drugs 1999;58:1137–64.

70. Olsen NJ, Stein CM. New drugs for rheumatoid arthritis. N Engl J Med 2004;350: 2167–79.

71. Bharadwaj A, Haroon N. Peripheral neuropathy in patients on leflunomide. Rheumatology (Oxford) 2004;43:934.

72. Richards BL, Spies J, McGill N, et al. Effect of leflunomide on the peripheral nerves in rheumatoid arthritis. Intern Med J 2007;37(2):101–7.

73. Suissa S, Hudson M, Ernst P. Leflunomide use and the risk of interstitial lung disease in rheumatoid arthritis. Arthritis Rheum 2006;54:1435–9.

74. Chan ES, Cronstein BN. Molecular action of methotrexate in inflammatory diseases. Arthritis Res 2002;4(4):266–73.

75. Montesinos MC, Yap JS, Desai A, et al. Reversal of the antiinflammatory effects of methotrexate by the nonselective adenosine receptor antagonists theophylline and caffeine: evidence that the antiinflammatory effects of methotrexate are mediated via multiple adenosine receptors in rat adjuvant arthritis. Arthritis Rheum 2000;43:656–63.

76. Kinder AJ, Hassell AB, Brand J, et al. The treatment of inflammatory arthritis with methotrexate in clinical practice: treatment duration and incidence of adverse drug reactions. Rheumatology (Oxford) 2005;44:61–6.

77. McKendry RJ, Dale P. Adverse effects of low dose methotrexate therapy in rheumatoid arthritis. J Rheumatol 1993;20:1850–6.

78. Zisman DA, McCune WJ, Tino G, et al. Drug-induced pneumonitis: the role of methotrexate. Sarcoidosis Vasc Diffuse Lung Dis 2001;18:243–52.

79. Dawson JK, Graham DR, Desmond J, et al. Investigation of the chronic pulmonary effects of low-dose oral methotrexate in patients with rheumatoid arthritis: a prospective study incorporating HRCT scanning and pulmonary function tests. Rheumatology (Oxford) 2002;41:262–7.

80. Roenigk HH, Auerbach R, Mailbach HI, et al. Methotrexate guidelines revised. J Am Acad Dermatol 1982;6:145–55.

81. Walker AM, Funch D, Dreyer NA, et al. Determinants of serious liver disease among patients receiving low-dose methotrexate for rheumatoid arthritis. Arthritis Rheum 1993;36(3):329–35.

82. Morgan SL, Baggott JE, Vaughn WH, et al. Supplementation with folic acid during methotrexate therapy for rheumatoid arthritis. Ann Intern Med 1994; 121:833–41.

83. van Ede AE, Laan RF, Rood MJ, et al. Effect of folic or folinic acid supplementation on the toxicity and efficacy of methotrexate in rheumatoid arthritis: a forty-eight week, multicenter, randomized, double-blind, placebo-controlled study. Arthritis Rheum 2001;44:1515–24.

84. Pavy S, Constantin A, Pham T, et al. Methotrexate therapy for rheumatoid arthritis: clinical practice guidelines based on published evidence and expert opinion. Joint Bone Spine 2006;73:388–95.

85. Ortiz-Alvarez O, Morishita K, Avery G, et al. Guidelines for blood test monitoring of methotrexate toxicity in juvenile idiopathic arthritis. J Rheumatol 2004;31: 2501–6.
86. Allison AC, Eugui EM. The design and development of an immunosuppressive drug, mycophenolate mofetil. Springer Semin Immunopathol 1993;14:353–80.
87. Samad AS, Lindsley CB. Treatment of pulmonary hemorrhage in childhood systemic lupus erythematosus with mycophenolate mofetil. South Med J 2003; 96:705–7.
88. Contreras G, Pardo V, Leclercq B, et al. Sequential therapies for proliferative lupus nephritis. N Engl J Med 2004;350:971–80.
89. Goldblum R. Therapy of rheumatoid arthritis with mycophenolate mofetil. Clin Exp Rheumatol 1993;11(Suppl 8):S117–9.
90. Langford CA, Talar-Williams C, Sneller MC. Mycophenolate mofetil for remission maintenance in the treatment of Wegener's granulomatosis. Arthritis Rheum 2004;15:278–83.
91. Swigris JJ, Olson AL, Fischer A, et al. Mycophenolate mofetil is safe, well tolerated, and preserves lung function in patients with connective tissue disease-related interstitial lung disease. Chest 2006;130:30–6.
92. Liossis SN, Bounas A, Andonopoulos AP. Mycophenolate mofetil as first-line treatment improves clinically evident early scleroderma lung disease. Rheumatology (Oxford) 2006;45(8):1005–8.
93. Zamora AC, Wolters PJ, Collard HR, et al. Use of mycophenolate mofetil to treat scleroderma-associated interstitial lung disease. Respir Med 2008;102(1): 150–5.
94. Gerbino AJ, Goss CH, Molitor JA. Effect of mycophenolate mofetil on pulmonary function in scleroderma-associated interstitial lung disease. Chest 2008;133(2): 455–60.
95. Saketkoo LA, Espinoza LR. Experience of mycophenolate mofetil in 10 patients with autoimmune-related interstitial lung disease demonstrates promising effects. Am J Med Sci 2009;337(5):329–35.
96. Nogueras F, Espinosa MD, Mansilla A, et al. Mycophenolate mofetil-induced neutropenia in liver transplantation. Transplant Proc 2005;37(3):1509–11.
97. Morii M, Ueno K, Ogawa A, et al. Impairment of mycophenolate mofetil absorption by iron ion. Clin Pharmacol Ther 2000;68:613–6.
98. Smith KG, Isbel NM, Catton MG, et al. Suppression of the humoral immune response by mycophenolate mofetil. Nephrol Dial Transplant 1998;13:160–4.
99. van Gelder T, Silva HT, de Fijter JW, et al. Comparing mycophenolate mofetil regimens for de novo renal transplant recipients: the fixed-dose concentration-controlled trial. Transplantation 2008;86(8):1043–51.
100. van Gelder T, le Meur Y, Shaw LM, et al. Therapeutic drug monitoring of mycophenolate mofetil in transplantation. Ther Drug Monit 2006;28:145–54.
101. Thalayasingam N, Isaacs JD. Anti-TNF therapy. Best Pract Res Clin Rheumatol 2011;25(4):549–67.
102. Furst DE, Keystone EC, Braun J, et al. Updated consensus statement on biological agents for the treatment of rheumatic diseases, 2010. Ann Rheum Dis 2011; 70(Suppl 1):i2–36.
103. Aaltonen KJ, Virkki LM, Malmivaara A, et al. Systematic review and meta-analysis of the efficacy and safety of existing TNF blocking agents in treatment of rheumatoid arthritis. PLoS One 2012;7(1):e30275.
104. Hadjinicolaou AV, Nisar MK, Parfrey H, et al. Non-infectious pulmonary toxicity of rituximab: a systematic review. Rheumatology (Oxford) 2012;51(4):653–62.

105. Buch MH, Smolen JS, Betteridge N, et al, Rituximab Consensus Expert Committee. Updated consensus statement on the use of rituximab in patients with rheumatoid arthritis. Ann Rheum Dis 2011;70(6):909–20.
106. Covelli M, Sarzi-Puttini P, Atzeni F, et al. Safety of rituximab in rheumatoid arthritis. Reumatismo 2010;62(2):101–6.
107. Lee YH, Bae SC, Song GG. The efficacy and safety of rituximab for the treatment of active rheumatoid arthritis: a systematic review and meta-analysis of randomized controlled trials. Rheumatol Int 2011;31(11):1493–9.
108. Fan LL. Evaluation and therapy of chronic interstitial pneumonitis in children. Curr Opin Pediatr 1994;6(3):248–54.
109. Baughman RP, Nunes H. Therapy for sarcoidosis: evidence-based recommendations. Expert Rev Clin Immunol 2012;8(1):95–103.
110. Bhorade SM, Stern E. Immunosuppression for lung transplantation. Proc Am Thorac Soc 2009;6(1):47–53.
111. Labirua A, Lundberg IE. Interstitial lung disease and idiopathic inflammatory myopathies: progress and pitfalls. Curr Opin Rheumatol 2010;22(6):633–8.
112. Kawai S, Takeuchi T, Yamamoto K, et al. Efficacy and safety of additional use of tacrolimus in patients with early rheumatoid arthritis with inadequate response to DMARDs–a multicenter, double-blind, parallel-group trial. Mod Rheumatol 2011; 21(5):458–68.
113. Cejka D, Hayer S, Niederreiter B, et al. Mammalian target of rapamycin signaling is crucial for joint destruction in experimental arthritis and is activated in osteoclasts from patients with rheumatoid arthritis. Arthritis Rheum 2010;62(8): 2294–302.
114. Laragione T, Gulko PS. mTOR regulates the invasive properties of synovial fibroblasts in rheumatoid arthritis. Mol Med 2010;16(9–10):352–8.
115. Bruyn GA, Tate G, Caeiro F, et al, RADD Study Group. Everolimus in patients with rheumatoid arthritis receiving concomitant methotrexate: a 3-month, double-blind, randomised, placebo-controlled, parallel-group, proof-of-concept study. Ann Rheum Dis 2008;67(8):1090–5.
116. Pham PT, Pham PC, Danovitch GM, et al. Sirolimus-associated pulmonary toxicity. Transplantation 2004;77(8):1215–20.
117. McClain KL, Kozinetz CA. A phase II trial using thalidomide for Langerhans cell histiocytosis. Pediatr Blood Cancer 2007;48(1):44–9.
118. Judson MA, Silvestri J, Hartung C, et al. The effect of thalidomide on corticosteroid-dependent pulmonary sarcoidosis. Sarcoidosis Vasc Diffuse Lung Dis 2006;23(1):51–7.
119. Scoville CD, Reading JC. Open trial of thalidomide in the treatment of rheumatoid arthritis. J Clin Rheumatol 1999;5(5):261–7.
120. Lehman TJ, Schechter SJ, Sundel RP, et al. Thalidomide for severe systemic onset juvenile rheumatoid arthritis: a multicenter study. J Pediatr 2004;145(6): 856–7.
121. García-Carrasco M, Fuentes-Alexandro S, Escárcega RO, et al. Efficacy of thalidomide in systemic onset juvenile rheumatoid arthritis. Joint Bone Spine 2007;74(5):500–3.
122. Chen Y, Kiatsimkul P, Nugent K, et al. Lenalidomide-induced interstitial lung disease. Pharmacotherapy 2010;30(3):325.
123. Geyer HL, Viggiano RW, Lacy MQ, et al. Acute lung toxicity related to pomalidomide. Chest 2011;140(2):529–33.
124. Voils SA, Evans ME, Lane MT, et al. Use of macrolides and tetracyclines for chronic inflammatory diseases. Ann Pharmacother 2005;39:86–94.

125. Tilley BC, Alarcón GS, Heyse SP, et al. Minocycline in rheumatoid arthritis. A 48-week, double-blind, placebo-controlled trial. MIRA Trial Group. Ann Intern Med 1995;122(2):81–9.
126. O'Dell JR, Blakely KW, Mallek JA, et al. Treatment of early seropositive rheumatoid arthritis: a two-year, double-blind comparison of minocycline and hydroxychloroquine. Arthritis Rheum 2001;44(10):2235–41.
127. Kanoh S, Rubin BK. Mechanisms of action and clinical application of macrolides as immunomodulatory medications. Clin Microbiol Rev 2010;23:590–615.
128. Friedlander AL, Albert RK. Chronic macrolide therapy in inflammatory airways diseases. Chest 2010;138(5):1202–12.
129. Crosbie PA, Woodhead MA. Long-term macrolide therapy in chronic inflammatory airway diseases. Eur Respir J 2009;33(1):171–81.
130. Hayakawa H, Sato A, Imokawa S, et al. Bronchiolar disease in rheumatoid arthritis. Am J Respir Crit Care Med 1996;154:1531–6.
131. Matsui S, Yamashita N, Narukawa M, et al. Rheumatoid arthritis-associated bronchiolitis successfully treated with erythromycin. Nihon Kokyuki Gakkai Zasshi 2000;38(3):195–200 [in Japanese].
132. Hotta M. Neutrophil chemotactic activity in cryptogenic organizing pneumonia and the response to erythromycin. Kurume Med J 1996;43(3):207–17.
133. Stover DE, Mangino D. Macrolides: a treatment alternative for bronchiolitis obliterans organizing pneumonia? Chest 2005;128(5):3611–7.
134. Chang WJ, Lee EJ, Lee SY, et al. Successful salvage treatment of steroid-refractory bronchiolar COP with low-dose macrolides. Pathol Int 2012;62(2):144–8.
135. Lee J, Cha SI, Park TI, et al. Adjunctive effects of cyclosporine and macrolide in rapidly progressive cryptogenic organizing pneumonia with no prompt response to steroid. Intern Med 2011;50(5):475–9.
136. Vos R, Vanaudenaerde BM, Verleden SE, et al. Antiinflammatory and immunomodulatory properties of azithromycin involved in treatment and prevention of chronic lung allograft rejection. Transplantation 2012;94(2):101–9.
137. Mertens V, Blondeau K, Pauwels A, et al. Azithromycin reduces gastroesophageal reflux and aspiration in lung transplant recipients. Dig Dis Sci 2009;54(5):972–9.
138. Rohof WO, Bennink RJ, de Ruigh AA, et al. Effect of azithromycin on acid reflux, hiatus hernia and proximal acid pocket in the postprandial period. Gut 2012. [Epub ahead of print].
139. Raghu G, Meyer KC. Silent gastro-oesophageal reflux and microaspiration in IPF: mounting evidence for anti-reflux therapy? Eur Respir J 2012;39(2):242–5.
140. Patti MG, Gasper WJ, Fisichella PM, et al. Gastroesophageal reflux disease and connective tissue disorders: pathophysiology and implications for treatment. J Gastrointest Surg 2008;12:1900–6.
141. Savarino E, Bazzica M, Zentilin P, et al. Gastroesophageal reflux and pulmonary fibrosis in scleroderma: a study using pH-impedance monitoring. Am J Respir Crit Care Med 2009;179(5):408–13.
142. Raghu G, Yang ST, Spada C, et al. Sole treatment of acid gastroesophageal reflux in idiopathic pulmonary fibrosis: a case series. Chest 2006;129:794–800.
143. Linden PA, Gilbert RJ, Yeap BY, et al. Laparoscopic fundoplication in patients with end-stage lung disease awaiting transplantation. J Thorac Cardiovasc Surg 2006;131:438–46.

144. Lee JS, Ryu JH, Elicker BM, et al. Gastroesophageal reflux therapy is associated with longer survival in patients with idiopathic pulmonary fibrosis. Am J Respir Crit Care Med 2011;184(12):1390–4.

145. Lee JS, Song JW, Wolters PJ, et al. Bronchoalveolar lavage pepsin in acute exacerbation of idiopathic pulmonary fibrosis. Eur Respir J 2012; 39:352–8.

146. Richeldi L, Costabel U, Selman M, et al. Efficacy of a tyrosine kinase inhibitor in idiopathic pulmonary fibrosis. N Engl J Med 2011;365(12):1079–87.

147. Noble PW, Albera C, Bradford WZ, et al, CAPACITY Study Group. Pirfenidone in patients with idiopathic pulmonary fibrosis (CAPACITY): two randomised trials. Lancet 2011;377(9779):1760–9.

148. Demedts M, Behr J, Buhl R, et al. High-dose acetylcysteine in idiopathic pulmonary fibrosis. N Engl J Med 2005;353(21):2229–42.

149. George TJ, Arnaoutakis GJ, Shah AS. Lung transplant in idiopathic pulmonary fibrosis. Arch Surg 2011;146(10):1204–9.

150. Gasper WJ, Sweet MP, Golden JA, et al. Lung transplantation in patients with connective tissue disorders and esophageal dysmotility. Dis Esophagus 2008; 21(7):650–5.

151. Shitrit D, Amital A, Peled N, et al. Lung transplantation in patients with scleroderma: case series, review of the literature, and criteria for transplantation. Clin Transplant 2009;23(2):178–83.

152. Mertens V, Dupont L, Sifrim D. Relevance of GERD in lung transplant patients. Curr Gastroenterol Rep 2010;12(3):160–6.

153. Kim DS. Acute exacerbation of idiopathic pulmonary fibrosis. Clin Chest Med 2012;33(1):59–68. http://dx.doi.org/10.1016/j.ccm.2012.01.001.

154. Silva CI, Müller NL, Fujimoto K, et al. Acute exacerbation of chronic interstitial pneumonia: high-resolution computed tomography and pathologic findings. J Thorac Imaging 2007;22:221–9.

155. Park IN, Kim DS, Shim TS, et al. Acute exacerbation of interstitial pneumonia other than idiopathic pulmonary fibrosis. Chest 2007;132:214–20.

156. Meyer KC, Raghu G, Baughman RP, et al, American Thoracic Society Committee on BAL in Interstitial Lung Disease. An official American Thoracic Society clinical practice guideline: the clinical utility of bronchoalveolar lavage cellular analysis in interstitial lung disease. Am J Respir Crit Care Med 2012; 185(9):1004–14.

157. Polomis D, Runo JR, Meyer KC. Pulmonary hypertension in interstitial lung disease. Curr Opin Pulm Med 2008;14(5):462–9.

158. Le Pavec J, Girgis RE, Lechtzin N, et al. Systemic sclerosis-related pulmonary hypertension associated with interstitial lung disease: impact of pulmonary arterial hypertension therapies. Arthritis Rheum 2011;63(8):2456–64. http://dx.doi.org/10.1002/art.30423.

159. Watson DI, Jamieson GG, Bessell JR, et al. Laparoscopic fundoplication in patients with an aperistaltic esophagus and gastroesophageal reflux. Dis Esophagus 2006;19(2):94–8.

160. Meyer KC. Management of interstitial lung disease in elderly patients. Curr Opin Pulm Med 2012;18(5):483–92.

161. Valencia X, Lipsky PE. CD4+CD25+FoxP3+ regulatory T cells in autoimmune diseases. Nat Clin Pract Rheumatol 2007;3(11):619–26.

162. Selman M, Rojas M, Mora AL, et al. Aging and interstitial lung diseases: unraveling an old forgotten player in the pathogenesis of lung fibrosis. Semin Respir Crit Care Med 2010;31(5):607–17.

163. Saketkoo LA, Matteson EL, Brown KK, et al, Connective Tissue Disease-related Interstitial Lung Disease Special Interest Group. Developing disease activity and response criteria in connective tissue disease-related interstitial lung disease. J Rheumatol 2011;38(7):1514–8.

164. Huscher D, Saketkoo LA, Pittrow D, et al. Development of clinical trial assessments for the study of interstitial lung disease in patients who have connective tissue diseases-methodological considerations. Curr Rheumatol Rev 2010;6(2): 145–50.

Printed and bound by CPI Group (UK) Ltd, Croydon, CR0 4YY

03/10/2024

01040448-0018

Index

Note: Page numbers of article titles are in **boldface** type.

A

Abatacept, 647–648

ACE-IPF (Anticoagulant Effectiveness in Idiopathic Pulmonary Fibrosis) trial, 479

N-Acetylcysteine, 477–478, 654–655

Acute reversible hypoxemia, syndrome of, 525

Adalimumab, 504–505, 643, 645

"Air-trapping," in bronchiolitis, 604

Airways disease, in connective tissue disease, 518, 520–523

Alemtuzumab, 647, 649

Allergic bronchopulmonary aspergillosis, 571–574

Allergy, eosinophilia in. *See* Eosinophilic lung disease.

Alveolar epithelial cells, in pulmonary fibrosis, 474–475

Alveolar hemorrhage, diffuse. *See* Diffuse alveolar hemorrhage.

Alveolitis, extrinsic allergic. *See* Hypersensitivity pneumonitis.

American College of Rheumatology criteria, for Churg-Strauss syndrome, 570

American College Pathology criteria, for Churg-Strauss syndrome, 569–570

American Thoracic Society consensus guideline, 464–465

Aminocaproic acid, for diffuse alveolar hemorrhage, 592

Amiodarone, pulmonary toxicity of, 457

Anakinra, 646–647

Angiotensin-converting enzyme, in sarcoidosis, 498

Animal proteins, exposure to, hypersensitivity pneumonitis in. *See* Hypersensitivity pneumonitis.

Anticoagulant Effectiveness in Idiopathic Pulmonary Fibrosis (ACE-IPF) trial, 479

Antifibrotic agents, 655

Antineutrophil cytoplasmic antibodies

    in Churg-Strauss syndrome, 568

    in diffuse alveolar hemorrhage, 590, 593

Antiphospholipid syndrome, diffuse alveolar hemorrhage with, 595–596

Antisynthetase syndrome, in connective tissue disease, 520

Antithymocyte globulin, 647, 650

Asbestosis, 458

Aspergillosis, allergic bronchopulmonary, 571–574

Aspiration, in connective tissue disease, 519, 521

Asthma

    in allergic bronchopulmonary aspergillosis, 571–574

    in Churg-Strauss syndrome, 567, 570

Autoimmune disorders

    history of, 456

    immunosuppressive therapy for, **633–669**

    versus disorders not involving autoimmunity, 634–635

Immunol Allergy Clin N Am 32 (2012) 671–684

http://dx.doi.org/10.1016/S0889-8561(12)00125-7

0889-8561/12/$ – see front matter © 2012 Elsevier Inc. All rights reserved.

immunology.theclinics.com

United States Postal Service

Statement of Ownership, Management, and Circulation
(All Periodicals Publications Except Requestor Publications)

1. Publication Title
Immunology and Allergy Clinics of North America

2. Publication Number
0 0 6 1 - 3 6 1 1

3. Filing Date
9/14/12

4. Issue Frequency
Feb, May, Aug, Nov

5. Number of Issues Published Annually
4

6. Annual Subscription Price
$294.00

7. Complete Mailing Address of Known Office of Publication (Not printer) (Street, city, county, state, and ZIP+4®)
Elsevier Inc.
360 Park Avenue South
New York, NY 10010-1710

Contact Person
Stephen Bushing

Telephone (Include area code)
215-239-3688

8. Complete Mailing Address of Headquarters or General Business Office of Publisher (Not printer)
Elsevier Inc., 360 Park Avenue South, New York, NY 10010-1710

9. Full Names and Complete Mailing Addresses of Publisher, Editor, and Managing Editor (Do not leave blank)

Publisher (Name and complete mailing address)
Kim Murphy, Elsevier, Inc., 1600 John F. Kennedy Blvd. Suite 1800, Philadelphia, PA 19103-2899

Editor (Name and complete mailing address)
Pamela Hetherington, Elsevier, Inc., 1600 John F. Kennedy Blvd. Suite 1800, Philadelphia, PA 19103-2899

Managing Editor (Name and complete mailing address)
Sarah Barth, Elsevier, Inc., 1600 John F. Kennedy Blvd. Suite 1800, Philadelphia, PA 19103-2899

10. Owner (Do not leave blank. If the publication is owned by a corporation, give the name and address of the corporation immediately followed by the names and addresses of all stockholders owning or holding 1 percent or more of the total amount of stock. If not owned by a corporation, give the names and addresses of the individual owners. If owned by a partnership or other unincorporated firm, give its name and address as well as those of each individual owner. If the publication is published by a nonprofit organization, give its name and address.)

Full Name	Complete Mailing Address
Wholly owned subsidiary of	1600 John F. Kennedy Blvd., Ste. 1800
Reed/Elsevier, US holdings	Philadelphia, PA 19103-2899

11. Known Bondholders, Mortgagees, and Other Security Holders Owning or Holding 1 Percent or More of Total Amount of Bonds, Mortgages, or Other Securities. If none, check box ☐ None

Full Name	Complete Mailing Address
N/A	

12. Tax Status (For completion by nonprofit organizations authorized to mail at nonprofit rates) (Check one)
The purpose, function, and nonprofit status of this organization and the exempt status for federal income tax purposes:
☐ Has Not Changed During Preceding 12 Months
☐ Has Changed During Preceding 12 Months (Publisher must submit explanation of change with this statement)

PS Form 3526, September 2007 (Page 1 of 3 (Instructions Page 3)) PSN 7530-01-000-9931 PRIVACY NOTICE: See our Privacy policy in www.usps.com

---

13. Publication Title
Immunology and Allergy Clinics of North America

14. Issue Date for Circulation Data Below
August 2012

15. Extent and Nature of Circulation

		Average No. Copies Each Issue During Preceding 12 Months	No. Copies of Single Issue Published Nearest to Filing Date
a. Total Number of Copies (Net press run)		580	468
b. Paid Circulation (By Mail and Outside the Mail)	(1) Mailed Outside-County Paid Subscriptions Stated on PS Form 3541 (Include paid distribution above nominal rate, advertiser's proof copies, and exchange copies)	229	255
	(2) Mailed In-County Paid Subscriptions Stated on PS Form 3541 (Include paid distribution above nominal rate, advertiser's proof copies, and exchange copies)		
	(3) Paid Distribution Outside the Mails Including Sales Through Dealers and Carriers, Street Vendors, Counter Sales, and Other Paid Distribution Outside USPS®	63	71
	(4) Paid Distribution by Other Classes Mailed Through the USPS (e.g. First-Class Mail®)		
c. Total Paid Distribution (Sum of 15b (1), (2), (3), and (4))		362	326
d. Free or Nominal Rate Distribution (By Mail and Outside the Mail)	(1) Free or Nominal Rate Outside-County Copies Included on PS Form 3541	59	49
	(2) Free or Nominal Rate In-County Copies Included on PS Form 3541		
	(3) Free or Nominal Rate Copies Mailed at Other Classes Through the USPS (e.g. First-Class Mail)		
	(4) Free or Nominal Rate Distribution Outside the Mail (Carriers or other means)		
e. Total Free or Nominal Rate Distribution (Sum of 15d (1), (2), (3) and (4))		59	49
f. Total Distribution (Sum of 15c and 15e)		421	375
g. Copies not Distributed (See instructions to publishers #4 (page #3))		159	93
h. Total (Sum of 15f and g)		580	468
i. Percent Paid (15c divided by 15f times 100)		85.99%	86.93%

16. Publication of Statement of Ownership

If the publication is a general publication, publication of this statement is required. Will be printed in the **November 2012** issue of this publication.

Publication not required

17. Signature and Title of Editor, Publisher, Business Manager, or Owner

Stephen R. Bushing –Inventory/Distribution Coordinator

Date September 14, 2012

I certify that all information furnished on this form is true and complete. I understand that anyone who furnishes false or misleading information on this form or who omits material or information requested on the form may be subject to criminal sanctions (including fines and imprisonment) and/or civil sanctions (including civil penalties).

PS Form 3526, September 2007 (Page 2 of 3)